PERSIAN MEDICAL MANUSCRIPTS
AT THE UNIVERSITY OF CALIFORNIA, LOS ANGELES

Humana Civilitas

Sources and Studies
Relating to the Middle Ages and the Renaissance

Volume 4

Editorial Board:

Michael J. B. Allen
Robert L. Benson
Fredi Chiappelli

Editorial Coordinator:

Carol D. Lanham

Published under the auspices of

THE CENTER FOR MEDIEVAL AND RENAISSANCE STUDIES

University of California, Los Angeles

Persian Medical Manuscripts

at the

University of California, Los Angeles

A Descriptive Catalogue

Lutz Richter-Bernburg

UNDENA PUBLICATIONS

Malibu, 1978

The emblem of
the Center for Medieval and Renaissance Studies
reproduces the imperial eagle of the gold *augustalis*
struck after 1231 by Emperor Frederick II;
Elvira and Vladimir Clain-Stefanelli,
The Beauty and Lore of Coins, Currency and Medals
(Croton-on-Hudson, 1974), fig. 130 and p. 106.

Library of Congress Card Number: 77-094986
ISBN: 0-89003-026-X (hard cover only)

Undena Publications, P.O. Box 97, Malibu, Ca. 90265

© 1978 by The Regents of the University of California

All rights reserved. No part of this publication may be reproduced or transmitted in any form or by any means, electronic or mechanical, including photo-copy, recording, or any information storage and retrieval system, without permission in writing from the author or the publisher.

Contents

Illustrations

(following page 78)

Note on the Transcription of Arabic Script

Consonants

ا	ʾ	ص	ṣ
ب	b	ض	ḍ/ż
پ	p	ط	ṭ
ت	t	ظ	ẓ
ث	th/s̱	ع	ʿ
ج	j	غ	gh
چ	č	ف	f
ح	ḥ	ق	q
خ	kh	ك	k
د	d	گ	g
ذ	dh/ẕ	ل	l
ر	r	م	m
ز	z	ن	n
ژ	zh	و	w/v
س	s	ه	h
ش	sh	ى	y

Vowels

Arabic	*Persian*	*Turkish*
a, i, u	a, e, ä, o, wo	a, e, i, o, u, ı
ā, ī, ū	ā, wā, ī, ow, ū	ö, ü (macron used only
au, ai	ai	to indicate spelling)

The Library of Congress system of transcription has not been adopted here, because it does not take account of Persian or Turkish deviations from the Arabic sound system, especially as regards vowels.

Preface

The manuscript collections of the University of California, Los Angeles (UCLA) include a large section of manuscripts in Near Eastern languages. Within the scope of Islamic literatures, medicine has been one area of special collecting activity. Thus, UCLA's medical manuscripts in Islamic languages, mainly in Arabic and Persian, match its considerable holdings in the fields of Western as well as Chinese medical history. The present catalogue contains descriptions of Persian medical manuscripts in the collections at UCLA; Persian texts in predominantly Arabic collectaneous MSS are included, but the description of these volumes, as well as a discussion of Persian works of non-medical contents, is reserved for catalogues of those works.

The bulk of UCLA's holdings in the field of Persian medicine is formed by a collection brought together by a Western-educated physician in contemporary Iran who was interested in the medical literature of his country and tried to obtain as much material as possible, including a relatively large number of duplicate copies. Most of the manuscripts clearly were used as textbooks and reference works in day-to-day medical practice, as is shown by numerous marginal entries of prescriptions, excerpts from other medical texts, etc. This provenance of most manuscripts may also account for the damage apparent in many, such as missing leaves, especially at the beginning and end, stains, spots, loss of original binding, etc. Sometimes this renders impossible the identification of title and author.

Numerically, UCLA's collection of Persian medical manuscripts ranks among the first in Western countries. In this catalogue, 135 Persian and two Arabic titles are discussed; they are contained in 134, including 41 collectaneous (*majmūᶜā*), manuscripts. Nearly the whole period during which the Persian language has been used for writing on medical subjects is covered by the collection. Of the 137 titles mentioned, 68 can be dated with reasonable certainty, either because the authors included a date in the texts, or because they are dedicated to known rulers or other prominent personages, or on the basis of some other textual evidence. The earliest author represented is the oculist "Zarrīndast" of the late fifth/eleventh century, approximately one hundred years after the first appearance of medical writing in Neo-Persian. Many of the better-known later medieval authors are also represented, e.g., Esmāᶜīl Jorjānī, Najmoddīn Maḥmūd Shīrāzī, "Ḥājjī Zaino l-ᶜAṭṭār," and Manṣūr b. Moḥammad . . . b. Elyās. But the majority of manuscripts and works catalogued dates from Ṣafavid and post-Ṣafavid, or Mughal, times; some of the more prominent authors are Bahāᵓo d-dowlä Nūrbakhshī, Yūsofī, Moẓaffar Shefāᵓī, ᶜEmādoddīn Maḥmūd Shīrāzī, Nūroddīn ᶜAbdollāh, Moḥammad Moᵓmen Tonakābonī, Moḥammad Arzānī, Moḥammad Ḥosain b. Moḥammad Hādī, and Moḥammad ᶜAlī al-Fānī. Among the latest writers, active not long after modern European medicine had first been introduced into Iran towards the middle of the nineteenth century, is Moṣṭafā b. ᶜAqīl, who collaborated with Joseph Désiré Tholozan, French doctor to Nāṣeroddīn Shāh.

Considering the present state of knowledge in the field of Persian medical literature, it is admittedly of only relative value to call a given author better known. No judgment as to the interest his works deserve is to be implied; to the contrary, some of the less well known, or hitherto unknown, authors whose works this collection contains may warrant even more detailed study. The following datable works and authors may be mentioned here: Ḥosain, son of "Ḥājjī Zaino l-ᶜAṭṭār" (**No. 31 : MS 45**); abū Zain Kaḥḥāl's book on surgery, *Sharāyeṭ-e jarrāḥī* (**No. 41 : MS 61 I**); Qoṭb Moḥammad's version of ibn an-Nafīs's *Mūjiz* (**No. 45 : MS 98**); *Favāyed-e Saᶜdīyä* by Esmāᶜīl, a brother of Yūsofī (**No. 86 : MS 57 III**); Kamāloddīn Ḥosain Shīrāzī's tract on *teryāq-e kabīr* (**No. 105 : MS 88**); Amānollāh Fīrūz-Jang's (?) treatise on Indian medicine, *Dastūro l-Honūd* (**No. 109 : MS**

105 III); *Roʾūso l-masāʾel* by Moḥammad Ḥakīm b. Moḥammad Rashīd, who composed it during the reign of Shāh Solaimān Ṣafavī, in 1082/1671, taking Manṣūr b. Moḥammad's *Kefāyä-ye Mojāhedīyä* as his model (**No. 125 : MS 50**); a late, early nineteenth-century version of Avicenna's *Qānūn* in its author's, Moḥammad Mahdī b. Moḥammad Qāsem's, own hand (**No. 141 : MS 104**); an even later, autograph copy of *Majmaʿo t-tajāreb*, on syphilis, by Moḥammad Bāqer b. Moḥammad Ḥosain Monajjem (**No. 148 : MS 61 III**).

The group of non-datable texts includes some versions of Arabic works done at an unknown time, such as a relatively early rendering of ʿAlī b. ʿĪsā's *Tadhkirat al-kaḥḥālīn* (**No. 154 : MS 74 II**), and some works of evident importance for the history of Persian medical writing that unfortunately cannot yet be assigned to a definite period: ʿAbdo r-Razzāq's *Kholāṣato t-tashrīḥ* (**No. 157 : MS Ar. 60 II**); *Mūjez-e Kommī* (**Nos. 161–162 : MSS 18–19**); Ebrāhīmo l-Ḥosainī's *Menhājo l-mobtadeʾīn* (**No. 174 : MS 53**); two anonymous medical textbooks, in **Nos. 163** and **171 : MSS 95** and **99**; *Merṣādo l-aṭebbāʾ* by Sharafoddīn b. Shāh Ḥosain Bairamī Lārī (**No. 175 : MS 52**); a big *qarābāzīn* in **No. 176 : MS 92**; an anonymous, untitled treatise on ophthalmology in **No. 181 : MS 75**; *Kanzo l-kaḥḥālīn*, by an anonymous author who quotes from a wealth of (partly unknown) sources, in **No. 182 : MS 76**; a treatise on pharmaceutical weights and measures (**No. 204 : MS 120 II**); a *resālä* on alchemy, magic, and medicine (**No. 220 : MS 96**); and, outside the field of medicine proper and related sciences, the allegory *Qeṣṣä-ye rūḥ* (**No. 222 : MS 69**).

A group of some thirty of the non-datable texts consists of lists of simple medicines, prescription books, Persian-Arabic glossaries of drug names, etc., most of which cover only a few pages and lack a title or author's name; some are no longer than a paragraph and might rather be called notes than formal writings. With reasonable certainty, they can be said to have been written within the last 200–250 years.

This catalogue's main objective is to present material to the student of the history of Persian medicine. The basic unit of description is therefore not the individual manuscript, but an individual text. A collectaneous manuscript is discussed as such along with the first text from that manuscript; cross references to other works represented in it are added in order to facilitate reconstruction of the volume as a unit. Datable works have been grouped together according to their authors and are listed in chronological order, as far as the available evidence allows. The context of literary tradition common to most medical writings in Persian appears to be too strong to warrant a distinction between specialized fields of medicine in the catalogue section of datable texts.

Conversely, in the section of non-datable works, an arrangement according to subject matter has been adopted: texts on anatomy, the days of crisis (*boḥrān*), and other parts of *ṭebb-e ʿelmī* are followed by medical handbooks, general works on therapy, treatises on ophthalmology, sexual medicine, *materia medica*, synonyms of drug names, pharmacy, weights and measures, and at the end by miscellaneous texts not strictly belonging to medicine or related sciences. Arabic texts in Persian versions that cannot themselves be dated are listed after the section of datable works.

References to other extant manuscripts of a given text follow the description of the (first) manuscript of that text in this catalogue. Exceptions have been made in the case of unidentifiable works. Usually, these references are to the bibliographies of Storey (cited as PL) and Monzavī; only those catalogues not included in their works are listed separately. Within an individual entry, description of the MS precedes discussion of the text. The orthography of Incipits and Explicits follows the peculiarities of a given copy, but *majhūl* consonants are written as such. Specific references to a manuscript are by folio and line number, e.g., "fol. 24b, 5 and -8" indicates, respectively, line 5 from the top and line 8 from the bottom of fol. 24b. Indices of proper names, other than those of cataloguers of manuscripts, and of titles of sources, with the exception of modern secondary materials, have been included in this catalogue along with a list of Incipits, chronological lists of datable works and MSS, an index of uncatalogued MSS or MS parts, and two concordances of catalogue and MS numbers.

In the preparation of this catalogue I have enjoyed the help and support of a number of colleagues and friends on the faculty and library staff at UCLA. Professors Gustave Edmund von Grunebaum, late director of the Center for Near Eastern Studies which now bears his name, and Andreas Tietze, past professor of Persian and Turkish, first suggested that I undertake this work, and they followed it with continuing interest and comment for which I am deeply grateful. Professors Speros Vryonis, former director of the Von Grunebaum Center, and Albert Dietrich, professor of Arabic at the University of Göttingen, watched the slow growth of this work with great patience. At UCLA's Research Library, I found all the help I needed, in Dr. Miriam Lichtheim, past Near Eastern bibliographer, and my hosts in the Department of Special Collections, especially Saundra B. Taylor, Brooke Whiting, and Wilbur J. Smith. My fellow cataloguer, Dr. Albert Zaki Iskandar, also made helpful suggestions based on his own rich experience.

Work on this catalogue, which was substantially finished by the end of 1974, was generously supported by the Von Grunebaum Near Eastern Center for two years. Its publication has been assured by the liberal financial aid of the Center for Medieval and Renaissance Studies, a generous contribution from the Pahlavi Library of Medicine, Imperial Medical Center of Iran, and by further financial assistance from the Von Grunebaum Center, the Friends of the UCLA Library, the UCLA School of Medicine, and the Sidney Stern Memorial Trust, Los Angeles. I am deeply indebted to Professor Fredi Chiappelli, Director of the Center for Medieval and Renaissance Studies, whose interest in this work was instrumental in providing the necessary funds. Dr. Carol D. Lanham of the Center for Medieval and Renaissance Studies has edited a difficult manuscript with all the interest and care an author could wish for.

Those passages of this catalogue that make smooth reading, as far as that can be expected from a work of this kind, are owed to the expert and patient help of my wife, Dr. Melanie Richter-Bernburg; without denying my own sole responsibility, I should like to thank her for her contribution and her constant encouragement.

Göttingen
January 1978

Bibliography

All reference works quoted in this catalogue are included in the following list; for a bibliography of catalogues of Persian MSS other than those listed here, see Huisman, Monzavī, and PL. Abbreviations used in this catalogue are alphabetized as they stand. In the section of Arabic, Persian, and Urdu works, the order is that of the Arabic alphabet; differences of pronunciation between these languages have not been taken into account. Words like *ibn*, *abū*, or the Arabic article have not been considered in determining alphabetical order. No *eżāfä* has been used in Persian names.

I. Works in Arabic, Persian, and Urdu

Āghā Buzurg aṭ-Ṭihrānī, Muḥammad Muḥsin *nazīl* Sāmarrā᾽ *ash-shahīr bi*-sh-Shaikh. *adh-Dharī*ʿ*a ilā taṣānīf ash-Shī*ʿ*a*. 22 vols. to date. an-Najaf and Ṭihrān 1355- .

Ibn al-Athīr, ʿIzz ad-Dīn a. l-Ḥasan ʿAlī. *Chronicon quod perfectissimum inscribitur* [*al-Kāmil fī-t-ta*᾽*rīkh*]. Edited by Carolus Johannes Torberg. 13 vols. Leiden 1867–74.

Aḥmad b. Ḥosain b. Yaḥyā Kāteb. *Tārīkh-e jadīd-e Yazd*. Edited by Īraj Afshār. Tehrān 1345 (*Enteshārāt-e Farhang-e Īrān-Zamīn, Selselä-ye motūn va-taḥqīqāt, sh.* 10).

Aḥmad Rāzī, Amīn. *Haft-Iqlîm . . . Encyclopaedia*, vol. 1. Edited by E. Denison Ross, ʿAbdul Muqtadir, A. H. Harley, and M. Mahfuz-ul Haq. Calcutta 1939 (*Bibliotheca Indica*, Work No. 215).

Ebn Esfandyār: *see* Part II, Browne, Edward G., *An abridged translation . . .*

Eskandar Bēg Torkmān. *Tārīkh-e* ʿ*ālamārā-ye* ʿ*Abbāsī*. 2 vols. *az rū-ye čāp-e sangī* (Tehrān 1314 *q.*) *čāp shodä, fehresthā be-kūshesh-e* Īraj Afshār. Tehrān 1334–35.

Eskandar Bēg Torkmān *va*-Moḥammad Yūsof Movarrekh. *Zail-e Tārīkh-e* ʿ*ālamārā-ye* ʿ*Abbāsī*. Edited by Sohailī Khwānsārī. Tehrān 1317.

Esmāʿīl b. al-Ḥosain b. Moḥammad . . . al-Jorjānī, Zainoddīn a. Ebrāhīm. *K. Aghrāżo ṭ-ṭebbīyä va-l-mabāḥeṣo l-*ʿ*Alā*᾽*īyä* (offset reproduction of a MS in Teheran University Library, copied in A.H. 789). Tehrān 1344 (*Enteshārāt-e Bonyād-e Farhang-e Īrān* 10. ʿ*Elm dar Īrān* 3).

———. *Zakhīrä-ye Khwārezmshāhī, ketāb* 1–2. Edited by M. H. Eʿtemādī, M. Shahrād, and J. Moṣṭafavī. 2 vols. Tehrān 1344–49 (*Selselä-ye Enteshārāt-e Anjoman-e Āṣār-e Mellī* 51, 76).

———. *Zakhīrä-ye Khwārezmshāhī*, vol. 1. Edited by M. T. Dāneshpazhūh and Ī. Afshār. Tehrān 1344 (*Enteshārāt-e Dāneshgāh-e Tehrān* 1002).

Ibn a. Uṣaibiʿa, Muwaffaq ad-Dīn a. l-ʿAbbās Aḥmad b. al-Qāsim as-Saʿdī al-Khazrajī *al-ma*ʿ*rūf bi-*. ʿ*Uyūn al-anbā*᾽ *fī ṭabaqāt al-aṭibbā*᾽. Edited by August Müller. Königsberg i. Pr. and Cairo 1884.

———. ʿ*Uyūn al-anbā*᾽. . . . Edited by Nizār Riḍā. Beirut 1965.

Afshār, Īraj. "Maḥmūd b. Elyās-e Ṭabīb." *Majallä-ye Mehr* VIII 3-4 (Tehrān 1331/1952-53), pp. 158-60, 234-36.

———. *Yādgārhā-ye Yazd*, vol. I: *Khāk-e Yazd*. Tehrān 1348 (*Selselä-ye Enteshārāt-e Anjoman-e Āṣār-e Mellī* 68).

Eqbāl, ʿAbbās. "Ghīāṣoddīn Yasodar [Yesüder] b. Jarghūṭai." *Majallä-ye Yādgār* III 3 (Tehrān 1325), pp. 65-67.

Ūktā᾽ī: *see* Mashhad.

Bozorg Tehrānī, Āqā: *see* Āghā Buzurg aṭ-Ṭihrānī.

al-Baihaqī, Ẓahīr ad-Dīn a. l-Ḥasan ʿAlī b. Zaid "Ibn Funduq." *Tatimmat Ṣiwān al-ḥikma.* Edited by Moḥammad Shafīʿ. Vol. I: Arabic text. Lahore 1351.

———. *Tatimmat Ṣiwān al-ḥikma.* Persian translation: *Dorrato l-akhbār va-lomʿato l-anvār,* by Nāṣeroddīn b. ʿOmdato l-molk Montakhaboddīn Monshī Yazdī. Reprint of the Indian edition. Tehrān 1318 (*Majallä-ye Mehr* V, Supplement).

Panjāb P. L.: *see* ʿAbbāsī, Manẓūr Aḥsan.

Tārīkh-e jadīd-e Yazd: *see* Aḥmad b. Ḥosain b. Yaḥyā Kāteb.

Tārīkh-e Qoṭbī: *see* Khworshāh b. Qobād.

Tārīkh-e Gozīdä: *see* Ḥamdollāh Mostowfī Qazvīnī.

Tārīkh-e Yazd: *see* Jaʿfar b. Moḥammad b. Ḥasan Jaʿfarī.

Tabrīz. *Fehrest-e Ketābkhānä-ye Mellī-ye Tabrīz. Jeld-e avval*: *kotob-e khaṭṭī-ye ehdāʾī-ye marḥūm-e Ḥājj Moḥammad Nakhjovānī, shāmel-e "405 jeld" az alef-kh.* By Mīrvadūd Yūnosi. Tabrīz 1348 (*Az Enteshārāt-e Ketābkhānä-ye Mellī-ye Tabrīz*).

Tehrān, Dāneshgāh. *Fehrest-e noskhähā-ye khaṭṭī-ye ketābkhānä-ye markazī-ye Dāneshgāh-e Tehrān.* By ʿAlī Naqī Monzavī (vols. 1–2) and M. T. Dāneshpazhūh (vols. 3–15). 15 vols. Tehrān 1330–45 (*Enteshārāt-e Dāneshgāh-e Tehrān*).

Tehrānī, Āqā Bozorg: *see* Āghā Buzurg aṭ-Ṭihrānī.

Jāmeʿ-e Mofīdī: *see* Moḥammad Mofīd.

Jaʿfar b. Moḥammad b. Ḥasan Jaʿfarī. *Tārīkh-e Yazd.* Edited by Ī. Afshār. Tehrān 1338 (*Enteshārāt-e Bongāh-e Tarjamä va-Nashr-e Ketāb* 94. *Majmūʿä-ye Motūn-e Fārsī* 2).

Junaid ash-Shīrāzī, Muʿīn ad-Dīn a. l-Qāsim. *Shadd al-izār fī ḥaṭṭ al-auzār ʿan zawār al-mazār.* Edited by M. Qazvīnī and ʿAbbās Eqbāl. Tehrān 1329.

al-Čalabī al-Mauṣilī, Dāwūd: *see* Mauṣil.

Čahār Maqālä: *see* Neẓāmī ʿArūżī.

Ḥājjī Khalīfa, Muṣṭafā b. ʿAbdallāh "Kātib Čelebī." *Kashf aẓ-ẓunūn ʿan asāmī l-kutub wa-l-funūn.* Edited by G. Fluegel. 7 vols. London 1835–58.

Ḥabībo s-sīar: *see* Khwāndmīr.

Ḥasan Shīrāzī Fasāʾī: *see* Fasāʾī.

Ḥusain, Muḥammad Bashīr. *Fihrist-i Makhṭūṭāt-i Shīrānī,* jild 2. Lāhūr 1969 (Idāra-yi Taḥqīqāt-i Pākistān. Dānishgāh-i Panjāb, Lāhūr).

Ḥamārina, Sāmī Khalaf. *Fihris Dār al-kutub aẓ-Ẓāhirīya, aṭ-ṭibb wa-ṣ-ṣaidala.* Dimashq 1389/1969 (*Maṭbūʿāt Majmaʿ al-Lugha al-ʿArabīya bi-Dimashq*).

Ḥamdollah Mostowfī Qazvīnī, *Tārīkh-e Gozīdä.* Edited by Edward G. Browne. London 1910 (*"E. J. W. Gibb Memorial" Series* XIV 1).

al-Khāliṣī: *see* Hadw, Ḥamīd Majīd.

Khworshāh b. Qobād al-Ḥosainī. *Tārīkh-e Qoṭbī* (or *Tārīkh-e ēlčī-ye Neẓāmshāhī*), *maqālä* 5. Edited by Mojāhed Ḥosain Zaidī. New Delhi 1965.

Khwāndmīr, Ghīāṣoddīn b. Homāmoddīn al-Ḥosainī *al-madʿūv be-. Tārīkh-e ḥabībo s-sīar fī akhbār-e afrād-e bashar.* 4 vols. Tehrān 1333 (*Enteshārāt-e Ketābkhānä-ye Khayyām* 2).

Dāneshpazhūh, Moḥammad Taqī: *see* Sepahsālār and Meshkāt III (2).
Dāneshgāh-e Tehrān: *see* Tehrān, Dāneshgāh.
Dībājī: *see* Nūrbakhsh.

adh-Dharīʿa: *see* Āghā Buzurg aṭ-Ṭihrānī.
Ẕail-e Tārīkh-e ʿālamārā-ye ʿAbbāsī: *see* Eskandar Bēg.

Rāzī, Amīn Aḥmad: *see* Aḥmad Rāzī, Amīn.
Rashīdoddīn Fażlollāh. *Taʾrīḫ-i-Mubārak-i-Ġāzānī. Des Rašīd . . . Geschichte der Ilḫāne Abāġā bis Gaiḫātū (1265–1295).* Edited by Karl Jahn. Prague 1941 (Abhandlungen der deutschen Gesellschaft der Wissenschaften und Künste in Prag. Philos.-histor. Abtlg., Heft I); reprint, The Hague 1957 (*Central Asiatic Studies* II).
———. *Geschichte Ġāzān-Ḫān's aus dem Taʾrīḫ-i-Mubārak-i-Ġāzānī.* Edited by Karl Jahn. London 1940 (*"E. J. W. Gibb Memorial" Series*, n.s. XIV).
———. *Ketāb-e Mokātabāt-e Rashīdī*, from Moḥammad Abarqūhī's collection. Edited by Moḥammad Shafīʿ. Lahore 1364/1945.
Rashīd ad-Dīn al-Waṭwāṭ: *see* al-Waṭwāṭ.
Rahāvard, Ḥasan. *Fehrest-e kotob-e khaṭṭī-ye ketābkhānä-ye Dāneshkadä-ye Pezeshkī.* Tehrān 1333 (*Enteshārāt-e Dāneshkadä-ye Pezeshkī*).

Sepahsālār. *Fehrest-e [noskhähā-ye khaṭṭī-ye] ketābkhānä-ye Sepahsālār*, vol. III (*ā* to *thāʾ*). By M. T. Dāneshpazhūh and ʿAlī Naqī Monzavī. Tehrān 1341.
Ibn Sīnā, a. ʿAlī al-Ḥosain. *al-Qānūn fī ṭ-ṭibb*, vols. I (*kitāb* 1–2), II (*k.* 3), III (*k.* 4–5). Būlāq 1294.

Shākerī, Ramażānʿalī. *Fehrest-e kotob-e khaṭṭī-ye Ketābkhānä-ye ʿOmūmī-ye Farhang va-Honar-e Mashhad.* Mashhad 1348 (*Az Enteshārāt-e Edārä-ye Koll-e Farhang va-Honar-e Khorāsān*).
Shabbūḥ, Ibrāhīm. *Fihris al-makhṭūṭāt al-muṣawwara* III 2: *aṭ-Ṭibb.* al-Qāhira 1959 (*Jāmiʿat ad-Duwal al-ʿArabīya. Maʿhad al-Makhṭūṭāt al-ʿArabīya*).
Shehāboddīn ʿAbdollāh b. ʿEzzoddīn Fażlollāh Shīrāzī "Vaṣṣāf-e Ḥażrat": *see* "Vaṣṣāf."
Shīrānī: *see* Ḥusain, Muḥammad Bashīr.

Ṭāher Vaḥīd Qazvīnī, Moḥammad: *see* Vaḥīd.
aṭ-Ṭihrānī, Āghā Buzurg: *see* Āghā Buzurg aṭ-Ṭihrānī.

aẓ-Ẓāhirīya: *see* Ḥamārina.

ʿAbbāsī, Manẓūr Aḥsan. *Tafṣīlī fihrist-i makhṭūṭāt-i fārsīya-yi Panjāb Pablik Lāʾibrīrī Lāhūr.* [Lāhūr] 1963.
ʿAbdo l-Ḥosain Khān Zonūzī Tabrīzī, Failasūfo d-dowlä. *Maṭraḥo l-anẓār fī tarājem-e aṭebbāʾo l-aʿṣār*, vol. I. Tabrīz 1334/1915–16.

Fārsnāmä-ye Nāṣerī: *see* Fasāʾī.
Farhang-e joghrāfyāʾī-ye Īrān. Edited by Dāyerä-ye Setād-e Artesh. 9 vols. [Tehrān?] 1328–32.
Fasāʾī, Ḥasan Shīrāzī *mashhūr be-*. *Fārsnāmä-ye Nāṣerī.* 2 vols. in 1, lithograph. Tehrān 1313.
Ebn Fondoq: *see* al-Baihaqī, Ẓahīr ad-Dīn . . . ʿAlī b. Zaid.
Failasūfo d-dowlä: *see* ʿAbdo l-Ḥosain Khān. . . .

al-Kāshānī: *see* Hadw, Ḥamīd Majīd.

Maʾāṣer-e ʿĀlamgīrī: *see* Mostaʿedd Khān, Moḥammad Sāqī.

Majles. *Fehrest-e ketābkhānä-ye Majles-e Shūrā-ye Mellī.* By Y. Eʿteṣāmī (vols. 1–2), Ebn-e Y. Shīrāzī (vol. 3), and ʿAbdo l-Ḥ. Ḥāʾerī (vols. 4–). 19 [?] vols. to date. Tehrān 1305/1927– .

Maḥfūẓ, Ḥusain ʿAlī. "Nafāʾis al-makhṭūṭāt al-ʿarabīya fī Īrān." *MMMA/RIMA* [*Majallat Maʿhad al-Makhṭūṭāt al-ʿArabīya*] III 1 (al-Qāhira 1376/1957), pp. 3–78.

———. "al-Makhṭūṭāt al-ʿarabīya fī l-ʿIrāq." *MMMA/RIMA* IV 2 (al-Qāhira 1378/1958), pp. 195–258.

Moḥammad Ṭāher Vaḥīd Qazvīnī: *see* Vaḥīd.

Moḥammad Mofīd Mostowfī Bāfeqī. *Jāmeʿ-e Mofīdī*, vol. III. Edited by Ī. Afshār. Tehrān 1340 (*Enteshārāt-e Ketābforūshī-ye Asadī*, sh. 2).

Moḥammad Yūsof Movarrekh: *see* Eskandar Bēg.

Maḥmūd b. Moḥammad ʿAbdollāh b. ʿObaidollāh. *Toḥfä-ye Khānī.* Edited by Alhaj Meer Tufail Ahmed Sahib. Madras 1959 (*Madras Government Oriental Series* No. CLII).

Mostaʿedd Khān, Moḥammad Sāqī. *Maāsir-i ʿĀlamgírí. A History of . . . Aurangzib. . . .* Translated into English . . . by Sir Jadu-Nath Sarkar. Calcutta 1947 (*Bibliotheca Indica*, Work No. 269, Issue No. 1556).

Meshkāt III (2). *Fehrest-e ketābkhānä-ye ehdāʾī-ye Āqā-ye Sayyed Moḥammad Meshkāt be ketābkhānä-ye Dāneshgāh-e Tehrān*, vol. III (2). By M. T. Dāneshpazhūh. Tehrān 1332 (*Enteshārāt-e Dāneshgāh-e Tehrān* 181).

Mashhad. *Fehrest-e kotob-e ketābkhānä-ye Āstān-e Qods-e Reżavī.* By Ūktāʾī. 4 vols. Mashhad 1305–29.

Mashhad, Honar: *see* Shākerī.

Muʿīn ad-Dīn a. l-Qāsim Junaid ash-Shīrāzī: *see* Junaid.

Mokātabāt-e Rashīdī: *see* Rashīdoddīn Fażlollāh.

[al-Munajjid, Ṣalāḥ ad-Dīn.] "Baʿthat Maʿhad al-Makhṭūṭāt ilā Īran," *MMMA/RIMA* VI (al-Qāhira 1379/1960), pp. 325–32.

———. "Maṣādir jadīda ʿan taʾrīkh aṭ-ṭibb ʿind al-ʿArab." *MMMA/RIMA* V 2 (al-Qāhira 1379/1959), pp. 229–337.

———. "Nawādir al-makhṭūṭāt fī maktabat Malik bi-Ṭihrān." *MMMA/RIMA* VI 1 (al-Qāhira 1379/1960), pp. 67–76.

Monzavī, Aḥmad. *Fehrest-e noskhähā-ye fārsī*, vol. I. Tehrān 1348 (*Moʾassasä-ye Farhangī-ye Menṭaqäʾī. Nashrīyä* 14).

al-Mauṣil. *Kitāb makhṭūṭāt al-Mauṣil.* By Dāwūd al-Čalabī al-Mauṣilī. Baghdād 1346/1927.

Nāṣeroddīn b. ʿOmdato l-molk Montakhaboddīn Monshī Yazdī: *see* al-Baihaqī.

Nashrīyä. *Nashrīyä-ye Ketābkhānä-ye Markazī-ye Dāneshgāh-e Tehrān "Dar bārä-ye noskhähā-ye khaṭṭī."* Edited by M. T. Dāneshpazhūh and Ī. Afshār. Tehrān 1340– (many MS catalogues of libraries in and outside Iran in this periodical).

Neẓāmī ʿArūżī Samarqandī, Aḥmad b. ʿOmar b. ʿAlī. *Čahār Maqālä.* Edited by M. Qazvīnī; revised edition by Moḥammad Moʿīn. Tehrān 1333–35/1955–57.

Nūrbakhsh. *Fehrest-e noskhähā-ye khaṭṭī-ye Ketābkhānä-ye Nūrbakhsh-e Khānqāh-e Neʿmatollāhī*, vol. I. By Sayyed Ebrāhīm Dībājī. Tehrān 1352 (*Enteshārāt-e Khānqāh-e Neʿmatollāhī* 51).

Vaḥīd Qazvīnī, Moḥammad Ṭāher. *ʿAbbāsnāmä.* Edited by Ebrāhīm Dehgān. [Tehrān?] 1329.

"Vaṣṣāf"[-e Ḥażrat], Shehāboddīn ʿAbdollāh b. ʿEzzoddīn Fażlollāh Shīrāzī. *Tajzīato l-amṣār va-tazjīato l-aʿṣār.* Lithograph. Bombay 1269/1853.

al-Waṭwāṭ, Rashīd ad-Dīn Muḥammad al-ʿUmarī. *Majmūʿat rasāʾil.* Edited by Muḥammad Afandī Fahmī. 2 vols. Miṣr 1358/1939, 1315, resp.

Hadw, Ḥamīd Majīd. *Makhṭūṭāt khizānat jāmiʿat Madīnat al-ʿIlm li-l-imām al-Khāliṣī al-kabīr fī l-Kāẓimīya.* Baghdād 1972.

———. *Maktabat al-ʿallāma al-ḥujja as-sayyid ʿAbbās al-Ḥusainī al-Kāshānī fī Karbalāʾ.* Karbalāʾ 1358/1966.

Yāqūt b. ʿAbdallāh ar-Rūmī. [*Muʿjam al-buldān*] *Geographisches Wörterbuch*. . . . Edited by Ferdinand Wüstenfeld. 7 vols. Leipzig 1866–73 (reprint: *Manshūrāt Maktabat al-Asadī*, raqm 7, Ṭihrān 1965).
Yūnosī: *see* Tabrīz.

II. Works in Other Languages

Ahlwardt, Wilhelm. *Verzeichnis der Arabischen Handschriften der Königlichen Bibliothek zu Berlin*, vol. VII. Berlin 1895 (*Die Handschriftenverzeichnisse der Königlichen Bibliothek zu Berlin*. Neunzehnter Band).
Akad. Nauk: *see* Miklukho-Maklaĭ.
Amritsar. *"Akal Sahāi." A Catalogue of Persian and Sanskrit Manuscripts in the Sikh History Research Department uptil* [sic] *March 31, 1962*. By Kirpal Singh. . . . Sikh History Research Department, Amritsar 1962.
Aretaeus. Edited by Carolus Hude. 2d ed. Berlin 1958 (*Corpus Medicorum Graecorum* II).
Aubin, Jean. "Le mécénat timouride à Chîrâz." *Studia Islamica* VIII (1957), pp. 71–88.
———. *Matériaux pour la biographie de Shâh Niʿmatullâh Walî Kermânî. Textes persans publiés avec une introduction*. Teheran and Paris 1956 (*Bibliothèque Iranienne*, vol. 7).
Aziz Pasha. "Treatises of Historical Interest in the Osmania University Library." *Bulletin of the Department of History of Medicine, Osmania Medical College*, I (Hyderabad, India 1963), pp. 54–56.

Bankipore. *Catalogue of the Arabic and Persian Manuscripts in the Oriental Public Library at Bankipore*, vols. IV (*Arabic Medical Works*), IX and XI (*Persian MSS. Philology, Sciences, and Arts*), and XVII (*Persian MSS. of Mixed Contents*). By Maulavî ʿAzîmuʾd-Dîn Ahmad (vol. IV), Maulaví Abdul Muqtadir *Khan Bahadur* (vols. IX, XI, and XVII). Calcutta and Patna 1910, 1925, 1927, 1930, resp.
Beale, Thomas William. *The Oriental Biographical Dictionary*. . . . Calcutta 1881.
Bibliothèque impériale [nationale]. Manuscrits orientaux. *Catalogue des manuscrits hébreux et samaritains de la Bibliothèque impériale*. Paris 1866.
Bibliothèque nationale. Département des manuscrits. *Catalogue des manuscrits arabes*. By M. le baron [W. MacGuckin] de Slane. Paris 1883–95 (issued in 3 parts).
———. *Index général des manuscrits arabes musulmans*. . . . By Georges Vajda. Paris 1953 (Centre national de la recherche scientifique. *Publications de l'Institut de recherche et d'histoire des textes* IV).
Bibliothèque nationale, manuscrits persans: *see* Blochet.
Blochet, Edgar. *Catalogue des manuscrits persans de la Bibliothèque nationale*. 4 vols. Paris 1905–34.
Blochmann, Heinrich Ferdinand. "Contributions to Persian Lexicography." *Journal of the Asiatic Society of Bengal* 37 (1868), pp. 1–72.
Bodleian. *Catalogue of the Persian, Hindûstânî, and Pushtû Manuscripts in the Bodleian Library*. By Ed[uard] Sachau (began part I), Hermann Ethé (parts I–II), and A. F. L. Beeston (part III). 3 vols. Oxford 1889, 1930, 1954, resp. (*Catalogi Codd. Mss. Bibliothecae Bodleianae Pars XIII*).
Bosworth, Clifford Edmund. *The Islamic Dynasties*. Edinburgh 1967 (*Islamic Surveys* 5).
British Museum: *see* Meredith-Owens and Rieu.
Brockelmann, Carl. *Geschichte der Arabischen Litteratur*. 2 vols. 2d ed. Leiden 1943 and 1949, resp. *Supplement*. 3 vols. Leiden 1937–42.
Browne, Catalogue. *A Descriptive Catalogue of the Oriental Mss. belonging to the late E. G. Browne*. By Edward G. Browne; completed and edited by Reynold A. Nicholson. Cambridge 1932.
Browne, Edward G. *A Literary History of Persia*, vol. IV: *Modern Times (1500–1924)*. Cambridge 1928.
———, trans. *An abridged translation of the* History of Ṭabaristán, . . . *by Muḥammad b. al-Ḥasan b. Isfandiyár*. Leiden and London 1905 (*"E. J. W. Gibb Memorial" Series* II).
Bursa. *Une liste des manuscrits choisis parmis les bibliothèques de Bursa, publiée à l'occasion du XXII. Congrès International des Orientalistes*. Istanbul 1951.

Calcutta Madrasah. *Catalogue of the Arabic and Persian Manuscripts in the Library of the Calcutta Madrasah.* By Kamálu ᵓd-Dîn Ahmad and ᶜAbdu ᵓl-Muqtadir. . . . Calcutta 1905.

Cambridge, *Supp. A Supplementary Handlist of the Muhammadan Manuscripts . . . preserved in the Libraries of the University and Colleges of Cambridge.* By Edward G. Browne. Cambridge 1922.

Charminar. "Persian Medical Manuscripts in Government Unani Medical College, Charminar, Hyderabad." *Bulletin of the Department of History of Medicine, Osmania Medical College,* I (Hyderabad, India 1963), pp. 237-42.

Chester Beatty. The Chester Beatty Library. *A Catalogue of the Turkish Manuscripts and Miniatures.* By V[ladimir] Minorsky. Dublin 1958.

Dietrich, Albert. *Medicinalia Arabica. Studien über arabische medizinische Handschriften in türkischen und syrischen Bibliotheken.* Göttingen 1966 (*Abhandlungen der Akademie der Wissenschaften in Göttingen, Philologisch-Historische Klasse.* Dritte Folge, Nr. 66).

Diocles Carystius: *see* Jaeger and Wellmann.

EI[1]: see *Enzyklopaedie des Islam. . . .*

EI[2]: see *Encyclopaedia of Islam. . . .*

Eilers-Heinz. *Persische Handschriften,* Teil I. Edited by Wilhelm Eilers and described by Wilhelm Heinz. Wiesbaden 1968 (*Verzeichnis der orientalischen Handschriften in Deutschland.* Band XIV, 1).

Elgood, Cyril. *A Medical History of Persia and the Eastern Caliphate, from the Earliest Times until the Year A.D. 1932.* Cambridge 1951.

———. "Translation of a Persian Monograph on Syphilis, entitled Risála-i-Átis͟hak by Imád-ul-Dín Maḥmúd Bin Masᶜúd bin Maḥmúd-ul-Ṭabíb." *Annals of Medical History,* n.s. 3 (1931), pp. 465-86.

———. "A treatise on the bezoar stone by the late Mahmud ibn Masud the Imad-ul-Din the physician of Ispahan. Translated from the original Persian." *Annals of Medical History,* n.s. 7 (1935), pp. 73-80.

Encyclopaedia of Islam, The, New Edition. . . . Edited by H. A. R. Gibb et al. Vols. I- . Leiden and London 1960- .

Enzyklopaedie des Islam. Geographisches . . . Wörterbuch der Muhammedanischen Völker. . . . Edited by M. Th. Houtsma et al. 4 vols. Leiden and Leipzig 1913-34.

Escorial. *Les manuscrits arabes de l'Escurial,* vol. I. By Hartwig Derenbourg. Paris 1884.

Ethé. *Catalogue of Persian Manuscripts in the Library of the India Office,* vols. I-II. By Hermann Ethé and Edward Edwards (revised vol. II). Oxford 1903 and 1937, resp.

Fleischer: *see* Leipzig.

Fonahn, Adolf. *Zur Quellenkunde der Persischen Medizin.* Leipzig 1910 (reprint Leipzig 1968).

GAL: *see* Brockelmann.

Galen. *Claudii Galeni opera omnia.* Edited by Carolus Gottlieb Kühn. 20 vols. Leipzig 1821-33 (reprint Hildesheim 1965).

GAS: *see* Sezgin.

Gujarat. *Descriptive Catalogue of Arabic and Persian Manuscripts* [*Gujarat Vidya Sabha Collection*]. 2 vols. Edited by Chhotubhai Ranchhodji Naik. Published by Gujarat Vidya Sabha. Ahmedabad 1964.

Haas, E[rnst]. "Über die Ursprünge der Indischen Medizin, mit besonderem Bezug auf Susruta." *ZDMG* 30 (1876), pp. 617-70.

Heinz: *see* Eilers-Heinz.

Hirschberg, Julius (assisted by J. Lippert and E. Mittwoch). *Die arabischen Lehrbücher der Augenheilkunde. . . .* Berlin 1905 (*Aus dem Anhang zu den Abhandlungen der Königl. Preuss. Akademie der Wissenschaften vom Jahre 1905*).

Hoghoughi, Ascar [ʿAskar Ḥoqūqī]. *Catalogue critique des manuscrits persans de la Bibliothèque nationale et universitaire de Strasbourg.* Strasbourg 1964 (*Publications de la Bibliothèque nationale et universitaire de Strasbourg* II). (No more medical MSS catalogued in this volume than by Landauer; see PL II.)

Horn, Paul. "Persische Handschriften in Constantinopel." *ZDMG* 54 (1900), pp. 275-332, 475-509.

———. "Der Schatz des Khvarezmšāh." *WZKM* 4 (1890), pp. 131-43.

Huisman, A. J. W. *Les manuscrits arabes dans le monde. Une bibliographie des catalogues.* Leiden 1967.

IAU: *see* Part I, Ibn a. Uṣaibiʿa.

India Office: *see* Ethé.

Inst. Hist. Med., New Delhi. *A Catalogue of Arabic and Persian Medical Manuscripts in the Library of Institute of History of Medicine and Medical Research,* vol. I. By Shabbir Ahmad Khan Ghori, Tazeemuddin Síddíqí, and S. A. Ali. New Delhi, n.d. [ca. 1968].

Ivanow, Wladimir. *Concise descriptive catalogue of the Persian manuscripts in the collection of the Asiatic Society of Bengal.* Calcutta 1924 (*Bibliotheca Indica.* Work No. 240).

———. *Concise descriptive catalogue of the Persian manuscripts in the Curzon collection, Asiatic Society of Bengal.* Calcutta 1926 (*Bibliotheca Indica.* Work No. 241).

———. *Concise descriptive catalogue of the Persian manuscripts in the collections of the Asiatic Society of Bengal. First* and *Second Supplement.* Calcutta 1927, 1928 (*Bibliotheca Indica.* Works No. 244, 248, resp.).

Jaeger, Werner. *Diokles von Karystos. Die griechische Medizin und die Schule des Aristoteles.* Berlin 1938.

Jolly, Julius. *Indian Medicine.* Translated from German [see next item] by C. G. Kashikar. Poona 1951.

———. "Medizin." *Grundriss der Indo-Arischen Philologie und Altertumskunde,* vol. III, no. 10. Strasbourg 1901.

———. "Zur Quellenkunde der indischen Medizin." *ZDMG* 54 (1900), pp. 260-74.

de Jong: *see* Leiden.

Justi, Ferdinand. *Iranisches Namenbuch.* Marburg 1895.

Katrak, Jamshed Cawasji. *Oriental Treasures. Being Condensed Tabular Statements of over a thousand Manuscripts . . . in Iranian and Indian Languages . . . in private Libraries of Parsis in . . . Gujarat.* [Bombay?] 1311 A.Y./1941 A.D.

Kayseri. *Une liste des manuscrits choisis parmis les bibliothèques de Kayseri, Akşehir, Bor, Gülşehir, Nevşehir, Niğde, Ürgüp, publiée à l'occasion du XXII. Congrès International des Orientalistes.* Istanbul 1951.

Kekelidze. Akademiīa Nauk Gruzinskoĭ SSR. Institut Rukopiseĭ im. K. S. Kekelidze. *Katalog arabskikh, tiurskikh i persidskikh rukopiseĭ instituta rukopiseĭ im. K. S. Kekelidze (kollektsiīa K).* Sostavili: Ts[isana] A[lexandrowna] Abuladze, R. V. Gvaramiīa, M. G. Mamatsashvili. . . . Tbilisi 1969 (catalogue in Georgian).

Konya. *Une liste des manuscrits choisis parmis les bibliothèques de Konya, publiée à l'occasion du XXII. Congrès International des Orientalistes.* Istanbul 1951.

Kudlien, Fridolf. *Untersuchungen zu Aretaios von Kappadokien.* Mainz and Wiesbaden 1964 (*Akademie der Wissenschaften und der Literatur [Mainz]. Abhandlungen der geistes- und sozialwissenschaftlichen Klasse.* 1963, 11).

Lane-Poole, Stanley. *The Mohammedan Dynasties.* Westminster [London] 1894 (reprint Beirut 1966).

Lazard, Gilbert. "Un amateur de sciences au Vème siècle de l'hégire: Shahmardân de Rai." *Mélanges Massé* (Teheran 1963), pp. 219-28.

Leeds. The University of Leeds, Department of Semitic Languages and Literatures. *Catalogue of Oriental Manuscripts.* By A. H. M. Muhiuddin and John Macdonald. Vol. IX: *Persian MSS 1-50.* Leeds 1960.

Leiden. *Catalogus codd. orientalium Bibliothecae academiae Lugduno Batavae*, vol. III. By Pieter de Jong and M. J. de Goeje. Leiden 1865.

Leipzig. *Catalogus librorum manuscriptorum qui in Bibliotheca senatoria civitatis Lipsiensis asservantur. . . . Codices orientalium linguarum*. By Henr. Orthob. [Heinrich Leberecht] Fleischer and Franc. Delitzsch. Grimma 1838.

Liddell, Henry George, Robert Scott, and Sir Henry Stuart Jones. *A Greek-English Lexicon*. 9th ed. Oxford 1940. *A Supplement*. . . . Edited by E. A. Barber et al. Oxford 1968.

Lindesiana. Bibliotheca Lindesiana. Hand-List of Oriental Manuscripts. Arabic, Persian, Turkish. Privately Printed. [Aberdeen] 1898.

LSJ: *see* Liddell.

Luzac. *Bibliotheca Orientalis XII. Being a Catalogue of Oriental Manuscripts (Arabic, Hindustani, Persian, and Turkish) . . . on sale by Luzac and Co.* London 1913.

MacKinney, Loren (assisted by Thomas Herndon). *Medical Illustrations in Medieval Manuscripts*, part I: *Early Medicine in Illustrated Manuscripts*; part II: *Medical Miniatures in Extant Manuscripts*. Berkeley and Los Angeles 1965.

Madras. *A Descriptive Catalogue of the Islamic Manuscripts in the Government Oriental Manuscripts Library, Madras*, vols. I, III, and IV. By Vidyasagara Vidyavacaspati et al. (vol. I) and T. Chandrasekharan et al. (vols. III and IV). Madras 1939, 1954, and 1961, resp.

Manisa. *Une liste des manuscrits choisis parmis les bibliothèques de Manisa, Akhisar, publiée à l'occasion du XXII. Congrès International des Orientalistes*. Istanbul 1951.

Meredith-Owens, G. M. *Handlist of Persian Manuscripts 1895–1966*. Published by the Trustees of the British Museum. [London 1968].

Miklukho-Maklaĭ, N. D., O. F. Akimushkin, V. V. Kushev, and M. A. Salakhetdinova. *Persidskīe i Tadzhikskīe Rukopisi Instituta Narodov Azii Akademii Nauk SSSR (Kratkiĭ Alfavitnyĭ Katalog)*, pod redaktsiīeĭ N. D. M.-M. Časti I–II. Moscow 1964.

Moattar [Moʿaṭṭar], Fariborz. *Ismāʿīl Ǧorǧānī und seine Bedeutung für die iranische Heilkunde, insbesondere Pharmazie. Unter Berücksichtigung seiner Verdienste für die Gestaltung der neupersischen Schriftsprache*. Diss. Marburg Nat. Fak. 1971.

Mossul: *see* Part I, Mauṣil.

Müller, August. "Arabische Quellen zur Geschichte der indischen Medizin." *ZDMG* 34 (1880), pp. 465–556.

Naficy, Abbas [Nafīsī, ʿAbbās]. *Les fondements théoriques de la médecine persane, d'après l'encyclopédie médicale de Gorgani, avec un aperçu sommaire sur l'histoire de la médecine en Perse*. Diss. Paris 1933.

Naniana. *Catalogo de' codici manoscritti orientali della Bibliotheca Naniana*. Compiled by Simone Assemani. . . . 2 vols. Padua 1787–92.

Oribasius. *Oribasii collectionum medicarum reliquiae*, vol. III. Edited by Ioannes Raeder. Leipzig and Berlin 1931 (*Corpus Medicorum Graecorum* VI 2, 1).

Osmania Med. Coll. "List of Arabic, Persian . . . Medical Manuscripts in the Department of History of Medicine." *Bulletin of the Department of History of Medicine, Osmania Medical College*, I (Hyderabad, India 1963), pp. 110–12.

Osmania Univ. "List of Arabic and Persian Medical Manuscripts in Osmania University." *Bulletin of the Department of History of Medicine, Osmania Medical College*, I (Hyderabad, India 1963), pp. 50–53.

Oudh. *Catalogue of the Reference Library of the Provincial Museum, N*[orth]-*W*[est] *P*[rovinces] *and Oudh* [Lucknow] *corrected to 1st December . . . by. . . .* Appendix II, *Classified Lists of Arabic, Persian, and Urdu Manuscripts in the Reference Library. . . .* By Munshi Chhote Lal. Allahabad 1892.

Pertsch. Berlin: *see* Pertsch, Wilhelm, *Verzeichnis. . . .*

Pertsch. Gotha: *see* Pertsch, Wilhelm, *Die Persischen. . . .*

Pertsch, Wilhelm. *Die Arabischen Handschriften der Herzoglichen Bibliothek zu Gotha . . .*, vol. 3. Gotha 1881 (*Die Orientalischen Handschriften der Herzoglichen Bibliothek zu Gotha. . . .* Dritter Theil . . .).

———. *Die Persischen Handschriften der Herzoglichen Bibliothek zu Gotha. . . .* Vienna 1859 (*Die Orientalischen Handschriften der Herzoglichen Bibliothek zu Gotha. . . .* Erster Theil . . .).

———. *Verzeichnis der Persischen Handschriften der Königlichen Bibliothek zu Berlin.* Berlin 1888 (*Die Handschriften-Verzeichnisse der Königlichen Bibliothek zu Berlin.* Vierter Band).

Pizzi, Italo. *Cataloghi dei Codici orientali di alcune Biblioteche d'Italia. . . .* fasc. 3: *Biblioteca Medicea Laurenziana: Codici persiani.* Florence 1886.

PL: *see* Storey.

Rampur. *Catalogue of Persian and Arabic Manuscripts of Saulat Public Library.* Compiled by Abid Raza Bedar. . . . Rampur, U.P. 1966.

Rehatsek, Edward. *Catalogue Raisonné of the Arabic, Hindostani, Persian, and Turkish MSS. in the Mulla Firuz Library. . . .* Bombay 1873.

Richter-Bernburg, Lutz. *Eine arabische Version der pseudogalenischen Schrift De Theriaca ad Pisonem.* Diss. Göttingen 1969.

Rieu, Charles. *Catalogue of the Persian Manuscripts in the British Museum.* 3 vols. London 1879-83. *Supplement to the Catalogue. . . .* London 1895.

Romaskewicz, A. *Indices alphabetici codicum manu scriptorum Persicorum Turcicorum Arabicorum qui in Bibliotheca Literarum Universitatis Petropolitanae adservantur. Supplementum.* Leningrad 1925.

Rosen, Baron Victor. *Collections scientifiques de l'Institut des langues orientales du Ministère des affaires étrangères,* vol. III: *Les manuscrits persans de l'Institut des langues orientales.* Saint Petersburg 1886.

Royal College of Physicians. "Catalogue of Oriental Manuscripts in the Royal College of Physicians." By A. S. Tritton. *Journal of the Royal Asiatic Society* (1951), pp. 182-92.

Rypka, Jan. *History of Iranian Literature. . . .* Edited by Karl Jahn. Dordrecht 1968.

Sellheim, Rudolf. *Materialien zur arabischen Literaturgeschichte,* I. Wiesbaden 1976 (*Verzeichnis der orientalischen Handschriften in Deutschland,* Band XVII, Reihe A: Arabische Handschriften).

Semenov, Aleksandr Aleksandrovič: *see* Tashkent.

Sezgin, Fuat. *Geschichte des arabischen Schrifttums,* vol. III: *Medizin, Pharmazie, Zoologie, Tierheilkunde bis ca. 430 A.H.* Leiden 1970.

Sprenger, A[loys]. *A Catalogue of the Arabic, Persian and Hindústány Manuscripts of the Libraries of the King of Oudh. . . .* vol. I: *Containing Persian and Hindústány Poetry.* Calcutta 1854.

Stewart, Charles. *A Descriptive Catalogue of the Oriental Library of the late Tippoo Sultan of Mysore. . . .* Cambridge 1809.

Storey, Charles Ambrose. *Persian Literature, a Bio-Bibliographical Survey,* vol. I: *Qur'anic Literature, History, Biography*; vol. II, part 1: A. *Mathematics . . .* ; part 2, E. *Medicine.* London 1927-71.

Tashkent. *Sobraniïe Vostočnykh rukopiseĭ Akademii Nauk Uzbekskoĭ SSR.* By A[leksandr] A[leksandrovič] Semenov and D. G. Voronovskiĭ. 10 vols. Tashkent 1952-75.

Tauer, Felix. "Persian Learned Literature from Its Beginnings to the End of the 18th Century." In Jan Rypka, *History of Iranian Literature. . . .* edited by Karl Jahn (Dordrecht 1968), pp. 419-82.

Teheran, University of: *see* Part I, Tehrān, Dāneshgāh.

Tritton, A. S.: *see* Royal College of Physicians.

Ullmann, Manfred. *Die Medizin im Islam.* Leiden and Cologne 1970 (*Handbuch der Orientalistik,* Erste Abteilung, Ergänzungsband VI, 1).

Versailles. Ministère de l'instruction publique. . . . *Catalogue général des manuscrits . . . .* vol. IX: *Départements Salins, Lure, Pontarlier, . . . Versailles, Lagny, . . .* Paris 1888.

Vogel, Claus. *Vāgbhaṭa's Aṣṭāṅgahṛdayasaṃhitā, The First Five Chapters of Its Tibetan Version.* Wiesbaden 1965 (*Abhandlungen für die Kunde des Morgenlandes* 37 II).

Wellmann, M[ax]. *Fragmentsammlung der griechischen Ärzte*, vol. I: *Die Fragmente der sikelischen Ärzte Akron, Philistion und des Diokles von Karystos.* Berlin 1901.

Winternitz, Moritz. *Geschichte der indischen Literatur*, vol. III. Leipzig 1920.

Wulff, Hans E. *The Traditional Crafts of Persia.* Cambridge, Mass. and London 1966.

Yale, Persian: a card catalogue of Yale University's Persian manuscript collection, at Beinecke Library, Yale University.

Yunusov, A[bdullodzhan]. *Fehrasti dastnavishoi Todzhikī-Forsii Kitobkhonai Davlatii RSS Todzhikiston ba nomi Abulqosim Firdavsī.* Dzhild I. Dushanbe 1971 (Vazorati Madaniĭati RSS Todzhikiston. Kitobkhonai Davlatii Respublikavii ba nomi Firdavsī. Shuʿbai dastnavishoi sharqī.).

PERSIAN MEDICAL MANUSCRIPTS AT THE UNIVERSITY OF CALIFORNIA, LOS ANGELES

No. 1 : MS 74 I

abū Rowḥ Moḥammad b. Manṣūr b. a. ʿAbdollāh al-Jorjānī "Zarrīndast"

Nūro l-ʿoyūn نور العيون

MS 74 (ex Coll. Min.), 284 fols., 175 x 133 mm; scribe's collection of two works. (See also **No. 154 : MS 74 II**.) *Nūro l-ʿoyūn* on fols. 1–222.

Bound in grey-patterned paper over thick, stiff cardboard, corners and spine brown leather; simple blind tooling on spine; inner covers pasted with light pink paper. Binding not original. Written on Eastern paper, medium thick, burnished, cream-colored. Some margins torn, mended; some fols. mouse-eaten; stains; some fols. loose, one fol. torn out between fols. 222 and 223; MS trimmed down from original size.

I. Fols. 1–222: 18–19 lines, 127 x 97 mm; II. fols. 223–284: 21 lines, 140 x 105 mm. Both on blind-ruled frame and lines; black with red rubrics and overlinings; medium-sized even, but undistinguished, *naskh*. Catchwords. Fols. 222b and 223a blank.

Collations by scribe.

Anonymous, undated copy; tenth/sixteenth century.

Recipes by readers on inner covers, fols. 1a, 284a, and in margins.

Several owner's stamps on fols. 1a and 284b, most of them effaced; one, on fol. 1a, reads, ibn Sayyid ʿAlī . . . (illegible) Muḥammad Ismāʿīl [؟] العريضى and is dated 1154/1741.

Incipit, fol. 1b

بسمله. الحمد لله رب العالمين والعاقبة للمتقين ولا عدوان الا
على الظالمين وصلى الله على خير خلقه محمد واله الطاهرين اجمعين
وسلم تسليما كثيرا چنين گويد ابو روح محمد بن منصور بن ابى
عبد الله الجرجانى المعروف بزرين دست كه...

Explicit, fol. 222a

وچشم بينائى نقصان گرفته ان ازخشكى باشد

The MS contains the well-known treatise *Nūro l-ʿoyūn* (fol. 3b, 6) by abū Rowḥ Moḥammad b. Manṣūr b. a. ʿAbdollāh al-Jorjānī "Zarrīndast" (fol. 1b, 3).[1] He composed it at the command of the Seljūq sultan abū l-Fatḥ Malekshāh b. Moḥammad b. Dāvūd in the year 480/1087 (fol. 3a, -6). It comprises ten *maqālā* in question and answer form.

1. Ullmann, p. 211; Hirschberg, pp. 9, 50–59.

PL II 205, no. 359; Monzavī I 607b, nos. 5667–74.

No. 2 : MS 1

Zainoddīn Esmāʿīl b. al-Ḥosain al-Jorjānī

Ẕakhīrä-ye Khwārezmshāhī ذخيرهٔ خوارزمشاهی

MS 1 (ex Coll. Min.), 381 fols., 340 x 206 mm

Bound in plain moss-green leather over thick, stiff cardboard; inner covers pasted with pink paper; bound in European fashion, spine slightly rounded, covers larger than fols. of MS. Binding partly faded, worn. Written on Russian paper of four provenances (four different blind stamps), medium thin to medium thick, partly glazed, white; some waterstains, few spots; few wormholes. On lacunae see below.

21 lines, 250 x 135 mm, on blind-ruled frame and lines; black with crimson overlinings and rubrics; medium-sized even *shekastä-āmīz*. Catchwords. Fols. 1b, 2b, 3a, 378a, 379, 380a, and 381a blank.

Occasional collations by scribe.

Anonymous copy, dated (fol. 70b) Saturday, 1 Moḥarram 1282/27 May 1865, after fourteen months of daily, but slow, work.

Medical notes on fols. 1a and 378b in the same hand; poetical quotations on fols. 2a and 381b, among them a *ghazal* by Saʿdī; on fol. 280b an Arabic anecdote about al-Aṣmaʿī.

Incipit, fol. 3b

بسمله. وبه نستعين. الحمد لله رب العالمين حمد
الشاكرين والصلوة على نبيه المصطفى واله اجمعين
چون بتقدير ايزد منان چنان بود كه جمع كننده
اين كتاب بنده دعاگوى خداوند خوارزمشاه ...
قطب الدين ... أبو الفتح محمد بن يمين الدين امير
المومنين [كذا] ...

Explicit, fol. 377b

وبسيار باشد كه تن از ماده بيمارى پاك]

The MS contains *ketāb* 1-5 of *Ẕakhīrä-ye Khwārezmshāhī* (fol. 3b, -9) by Esmāʿīl b. al-Ḥosain b. Moḥammad b. Aḥmad al-Ḥosainī al-Jorjānī (fol. 4a, 5). The text was not completely transcribed here; it breaks off on fol. 377b, -1 within *bāb* 3, *goftār* 6, *ketāb* 5, so that most of this *bāb* and *bāb* 4-5 of this *goftār* are missing.

A short table of contents, listing only the nine *ketāb* originally planned,[1] is on fols. 4b-5a. *Ketāb* 1, 2, 4, and 5 are each preceded by a very detailed list of contents, giving all the subdivisions—*goftār, jozv, bāb* (see fols. 5a-7a, 71a-75b, 280a-b, 311a-312a, resp.). *Ketāb* 3 lacks such a list (see fol. 138b); it is divided into two *bakhsh*, each further divided into numerous *goftār, jozv*, and *bāb*.[2]

So far, *Ẕakhīrä-ye Khwārezmshāhī* has mainly been viewed as just a Persian adaptation of Avicenna's *Qānūn*. In long passages, the author indeed translated almost verbatim from his predecessor's great work that was also his model for the disposition of his own book. Esmāᶜīl's reading in medicine covered a much more extended field, however, than Avicenna's works. Ar-Rāzī[3] and [Pseudo-]Thābit b. Qurra[4] are frequently quoted, less often ᶜAlī b. al-ᶜAbbās's *Kāmil*,[5] aṭ-Ṭabarī at-Turunjī's *Muᶜālajāt Buqrāṭīya*,[6] ibn al-Khammār,[7] and ibn a. Ṣādiq's commentary on Galen's anatomy.[8] In the section on ophthalmology, ᶜAlī b. ᶜĪsā's *Tadhkira*[9] and Aḥmad-e Farrokh[10] are important sources. In addition to these authors whose books, it may reasonably be assumed, Esmāᶜīl quoted directly, there are numerous earlier Islamic authorities adduced,[11] most of them probably quoted indirectly by way of such sources as already mentioned.[12]

Among Greek medical writers, the most frequently named are naturally Hippocrates and Galen, the former often first quoted in Arabic and then translated into Persian.[13] Other names of Greek authors appearing in *Ẕakhīrä* are Empedocles,[14] Plato,[15] Aristotle,[16] Asclepiades Bithynus,[17] Rufus Ephesius,[18] Dioscorides,[19] Archigenes,[20] Oribasius,[21] Alexander Trallianus,[22] Paulus Aegineta,[23] and Ahrun.[24] Two of these quotations, which were most certainly taken from intermediary sources, warrant special mention: one from Diocles Carystius,[25] on cotyledones in the uterus, and the other from Aretaeus Cappadox,[26] on the effect of blood on the innate heat.

The author of *Ẕakhīrä-ye Khwārezmshāhī*, Sharafo s-Sādāt[27] Zainoddīn a. Ebrāhīm[28] Esmāᶜīl b. al-Ḥosain[29] b. Moḥammad b. Aḥmad[30] al-Mūsavī[31] al-Ḥosainī al-ᶜAlavī al-Eṣfahānī[32] al-Jorjānī,[33] came to Khwārezm in the year 504/1110.[34] Little is known of his life up to that point, except that he studied medicine with ibn a. Ṣādiq[35] and Aḥmad-e Farrokh[36] and *ḥadīth* with abū l-Qāsim al-Qushairī,[37] on whose authority he transmitted *Arbaᶜūn ḥadīthā*, according to Yāqūt's testimony;[38] and Esmāᶜīl himself mentions that he saw the works of the astronomer Kīā Kūshyār in the hands of his descendants at Qom.[39]

At Khwārezm, Esmāᶜīl presented himself to the court of the Khwārezm-Shāh Qoṭboddīn Moḥammad b. Yamīnoddīn Anūshtegīn[40] and was appointed by him to the dispensary of Bahāʾo d-dowlä, a position that left him little leisure to pursue his writing.[41] According to ibn a. Uṣaibiᶜa, he earned 1,000 *dīnār* a month from the shāh's treasury.[42] Esmāᶜīl's importance for Khwārezmian health services can also be gathered from two nearly identical letters Rashīdoddīn Vaṭvāṭ wrote in the Khwārezm-Shāh's name to the two foremost physicians of Baghdād after Esmāᶜīl's departure or death: abū l-Barakāt al-Baghdādī[43] and ibn at-Tilmīdh[44] are both asked to recommend a physician from among their students who could take Esmāᶜīl's position at the *dār al-adwiya* and as physician-in-ordinary to the shāh.[45]

Esmāᶜīl stayed, highly honored, at the court of Qoṭboddīn and, after his death in 521/1127, at that of his son and successor ᶜAlāʾo d-dowlä Atsız,[46] until at some unspecified time he went to Marv.[47] At the court of Solṭān Sanjar, he was accorded an equally honorable treatment and, still active in the teaching of medicine,[48] died there, very old, in 530/1135, 531/1136, or 535/1140.[49] His age was nearly one hundred lunar years.[50] "Ebn-e Fondoq" Baihaqī writes that he met him at Sarakhs in 531, nearly consumed by age.[51] It cannot be determined whether Samᶜānī's study of *ḥadīth* under Esmāᶜīl took place while the latter was still at Khwārezm, or in Marv.[52]

Aside from Esmāᶜīl's work on *Arbaᶜūn ḥadīthā*, his *K. fī ḥifẓ aṣ-ṣiḥḥa*,[53] and his *at-Tuḥfa as-saᶜdīya*,[54] all his other books are said to have been composed in Khwārezm,[55] i.e., after 504/1110, when Esmāᶜīl was already seventy lunar years old.[56] The first, most voluminous and greatest, work was *Ẕakhīrä-ye Khwārezmshāhī*, dedicated to Qoṭboddīn Moḥammad and written between 504 and 506/1112, a time considered long for the compilation of a book of that size.[57] But Esmāᶜīl's position at the *dārūkhānä* did not leave him much time, and since he wanted to give his best, he set to work only when he felt productive.[58] If a MS described by Stewart[59] can be trusted, *Khoffī-ye ᶜAlāʾī* was written in 506.

As its title intimates, it was dedicated to Qoṭboddīn's son ᶜAlāᵓo d-dowlä Atsız, who was only sixteen years old at the time[60] and already charged with difficult military assignments if his title *eṣfahsālār* can be taken seriously.[61] Esmāᶜīl wrote it in two small oblong volumes so that Atsız could take it along on his campaigns in the shafts of his riding boots.[62]

Al-aghrāżo ṭ-ṭebbīyä va-l-mabāḥeṣo l-ᶜalāᵓīyä, Esmāᶜīl's third partly datable work on medicine, was written at the suggestion of the vizier Majdoddīn a. Moḥammad Ṣāḥeb b. Moḥammad al-Bokhārī,[63] after ᶜAlāᵓo d-dowlä Atsız had succeeded his father as Khwārezm-Shāh, i.e., after 522/1128.[64] It cannot at present be determined when Esmāᶜīl wrote his *Yādgār*[65] or *aṭ-Ṭibb al-mulūkī,*[66] except that he is reported to have composed them in Khwārezm.[67] In the preface to his Arabic translation of *Ẕakhīrä,* Esmāᶜīl states that he will be devoting the rest of his life to this task, but that is too little evidence to consider it his last work.[68] When his Arabic work *Zubdat aṭ-ṭibb* was composed also remains unknown. Possibly it belongs in the time when he worked at the Arabic version of *Ẕakhīrä.*[69]

In addition to the just listed works on medicine, Esmāᶜīl composed a number of philosophical tracts the dates of which are not known either: *K. ar-radd ᶜalā l-falāsifa,*[70] *K. al-yaum wa-l-laila* for the Qāḍī abū Saᶜīd ash-Shāriᶜī,[71] *Vaṣīyatnāmä,*[72] *Risāla munabbiha,*[73] and two short commentaries on Aristotle's *Organum, Fī l-qiyās* and *Fī t-taḥlīl.*[74]

The fame of Esmāᶜīl's medical writings spread fast. Neẓāmī ᶜArūżī recommends them as textbooks: among works of intermediate length he mentions Esmāᶜīl's *Aghrāż,* and among voluminous compendia for the advanced student *Ẕakhīrä*; as short reference works he names his *Yādgār* and *Khoffī.*[75] Esmāᶜīl's own translation of his *Ẕakhīrä* into Arabic has already been mentioned. His *Khoffī* was translated into Arabic under the title *at-Tadhkira al-ashrafīya fī ṣ-ṣināᶜa aṭ-ṭibbīya,* possibly for Saladin's nephew al-Malik al-Ashraf Mūsā.[76] *Al-ajwiba aṭ-ṭibbīya wa-l-mabāḥith al-ᶜalāᵓīya,* listed by Brockelmann from the Āṣafīya catalogue, could be an Arabic rendering of *Aghrāż.*[77]

Ẕakhīrä was moreover translated into Turkish, by ebū l-Fażl Meḥemmed b. Idrīs ed-Defterī el-Bidlīsī,[78] and into Hebrew: parts of *ketāb* 5 and *ketāb* 6–9.[79] An Urdu translation of *Ẕakhīrä* was published at Lucknow in 1878.[80]

The recognition Esmāᶜīl won even outside the circles of men professionally concerned with medicine is attested to by the historian Rāvandī, who quotes him at length on the subject of wine and whose testimony should, as just an example, not go unmentioned here.[81]

Biographical notes on Esmāᶜīl are found in all pertinent works of biography and history, but as can be seen from this account, they do not provide many details and moreover do not agree with each other on those they do report.[82]

1. The tenth *ketāb,* on simple and compound drugs, was added later; see Meshkāt III (2) 760, 2. According to Dāneshpazhūh (ibid., 761, 15), this tenth *ketāb,* the *qarābādīn,* was written later than the Arabic translation of *Ẕakhīrä.*
2. For an abridged table of contents see Fonahn, p. 7, no. 15; Bankipore XI 3–6, nos. 962–63.
3. One quotation from works of his is explicitly stated to be from *K. at-tajārib* (**MS 4**, fol. 19a, 1). For more quotations from ar-Rāzī see **MS 4** (*ketāb* 6), passim.
4. Passim in **MS 4** (*ketāb* 6).
5. **MS 4**, fol. 276b, 4; etc.
6. **MS 4**, fol. 253b, 11; etc.
7. He is quoted on *mālīkhūlīā* and the etymology of its name: a compound of *mālī,* "black," and *khūlī,* "humor" (**MS 4**, fol. 11a, 1).
8. In *ketāb* 1: **MS 1**, fols. 36b, -5; 38b, 2.
9. In *ketāb* 6, *goftār* 2: **MS 4**, fol. 77a, 6; etc.
10. Esmāᶜīl's *Ẕakhīrä* is the earliest source mentioning this physician, of whose life nothing is known but whose work *Kefāyä* enjoyed a good reputation at Esmāᶜīl's time and later (see **MSS 18–19:** *Mūjez-e Kommī,* and *Čahār Maqālä,* p. 110, 4, where it is recommended as one of the best intermediate textbooks of medicine). It may be surmised that Esmāᶜīl was a student of Aḥmad's, since he calls him *ostād* and adds the eulogy *raḥimahū llāh* to his name (**MS 4**, fol. 103b, 9, -7; without eulogy, **MS 4**, fol. 180a, 8).
11. Horn, WZKM 4 (1890), 142f., lists the following Islamic sources, besides those already mentioned here: ibn Juraij, ibn Māsawaih, Masīḥ, Sāhir; to be added are Jurjīs, ᶜAlī b. Rabban aṭ-Ṭabarī, Māsarjawaih, al-Fārisī, Qusṭā b. Lūqā, Ḥunain b. Isḥāq, al-Kindī, abū Māhir, ibn Sarābiyūn.

12. It cannot be determined whether the quotation from abū Muʿādh al-Jawādkānī (**MS 4**, fol. 227b, 6) was taken directly from his works or not. Al-Bīrūnī quotes him in his *K. aṣ-ṣaidana* (cf. GAS III 312).
13. E.g., **MS 1**, fol. 113a, 7.
14. **MS 1**, fol. 421b, 4; a quotation from Galen via Avicenna's *Qānūm*.
15. **MS 1**, fol. 186a, 8: children shall not drink wine.
16. E.g., **MS 1**, fol. 64a, 11, on the origin of the *quwwa nafsānīya*.
17. **MS 1**, fol. 185a, 10; called *ostād-e ṭabībān*; cf. Pseudo-Galen, Kühn XIV 683, 5 (*Introductio sive Medicus*), where he is mentioned as one of the heads of the logical, i.e., dogmatic, school.
18. **MS 1**, fols. 109b, -8; 184b, 9; **MS 4**, fols. 12b–13a.
19. **MS 1**, fol. 184b, -5.
20. See note 14 above.
21. See Horn, WZKM 4 (note 11 above), 142f.; Moattar, p. 83, no. 6.
22. **MS 4**, fol. 360a, 7: on "stones" in the sputum.
23. See Horn (note 21 above); Moattar, p. 82, no. 5.
24. **MS 4**, fols. 275a, 7; 308b, 8.
25. **MS 1**, fol. 63b, 2. The wording of the quotation appears to go back to a paraphrase combining the transmission of the fragment (fr. 27 Wellmann), as Galen gives it on one side (Kühn II 905, 15), and Oribasius on the other (Raeder III 44, 16).
26. **MS 4**, fol. 272b, -4, corresponds to Aretaeus, p. 142, 6 Hude. This passage was not quoted in Dioscorides, Pseudo-Alexander of Aphrodisias's *De febribus*, Aetius Amidenus, or in Paulus Aegineta; see Kudlien, *Untersuchungen zu Aretaios von Kappadokien*, pp. 11, 42.
27. This honorific title is given Esmāʿīl in Rashīdoddīn Vaṭvāṭ's letters (I 64, 66; see also note 45 below); it appears likely that ibn a. Uṣaibiʿa, in calling him Sharaf ad-Dīn instead of Zain ad-Dīn, confused this title with his *laqab* (II 31, -2 [Beirut 1965], p. 472).
28. This *kunya* in Yāqūt (II 54, 2) and in MSS of his works; ebn-e Esfandyār has "abū l-Fażl" (p. 86 bottom, no. 2), a MS in the British Museum has "abū l-Fażāyel" (Rieu II 466b, *ad* Add. 23556 I [collated in 1095/1684]), and Dāneshpazhūh, presumably on the authority of a MS, gives "abū l-Fatḥ" (Meshkāt III (2) 755, 13).
29. Al-Ḥasan in Shahrazūrī (*Zakhīrä*, ed. Eʿtemādī et al., I, introduction p. 22, -8), Yāqūt (II 54, 3), and in some MSS. In numerous other MSS, *Tārīkh-e Gozīdä* (p. 686, -7), and *Ḥabībo s-siar*, his father's name is given as Ḥosain.
30. His grandfather's and great-grandfather's names in this order in Yāqūt (II 54, 3) and MSS; in some other sources the order is reversed (cf. Blochet II 84, no. 820), or a Maḥmūd is listed as grandfather or great-grandfather (*Tārīkh-e Gozīdä*, p. 686, -7; Meshkāt III (2) 755, 14).
31. This *nisba* only in ebn-e Esfandyār, p. 86 bottom, no. 2.
32. Again, presumably on the authority of the MS discussed, Dāneshpazhūh in Meshkāt III (2) 755, 15.
33. All MSS and other sources are in agreement that Jorjān is Esmāʿīl's home (see references in preceding notes).
34. Preface to *Zakhīrä*; see **MS 1**, fol. 3b.
35. To my knowledge, the only evidence that Esmāʿīl was his student is his being accorded the title *khwājä* and the eulogy *raḥimahū llāh* (see also note 8 above); cf. Meshkāt III (2) 756, 2.
36. See note 10 above.
37. He died at Ṭūs in 463/1072.
38. II 54, 6. A certain theological interest on Esmāʿīl's part is shown by his remarks on Allah's wisdom in creating the ear (**MS 4**, fol. 114a, 7), in creating the lips (**MS 4**, fol. 132a, -3), and in letting man derive pleasure from sexual activity (**MS 4**, fol. 371b). Other, similar passages could easily be found.
39. In the preface to his Arabic translation of *Zakhīrä* (Meshkāt III (2) 759, 19).
40. It is not without interest to note the official titles and honorific epithets Esmāʿīl gives Qoṭboddīn in his *Zakhīrä* (ed. Eʿtemādī et al., I 1, 4–8, with cataloguer's emendation):

خداوند خوارزمشاه العالم العادل المؤيّد المظفّر المنصور
قطب الدين نصرة الإسلام والمسلمين قاهر الكفرة والمشركين
عماد الدولة فخر الأمّة يمين الملوك والسلاطين أمير الأمراء
تاج المعالي ارسلان تكين أبو الفتح محمّد ابن يمين الدين
معين أمير المؤمنين

On these titles cf. cataloguer, "Zur Titulatur der Ḫwārezm-Šāhe aus der Dynastie Anūštegīns," *Archäologische Mitteilungen aus Iran,* N.F. 9 (1976), 179–205. On Qoṭboddīn see *Cambridge History of Iran* V (1968), 107, 120, 140, 143 [Bosworth].

41. His own statement at the end of *bakhsh/ketāb* 9 of *Zakhīrä* (Meshkāt III (2) 759, 16).
42. IAU II 32, 1.
43. Died after 560/1165, worked at the ʿAḍudī hospital in Baghdād (see Ullmann, p. 163; EI² II 111b–113a [Pines]).
44. Died in 560/1165, also worked at the ʿAḍudī hospital in Baghdād (see Ullmann, p. 163; EI² III 956b–957a [Meyerhof]).
45. *Rasāʾil al-Waṭwāṭ* I 64, 66.
46. Ruled 522–551/1128–1156 (see EI² I 750a–b [Barthold/Spuler]). See also notes 61 and 64 below.
47. Shahrazūrī (in *Zakhīrä,* ed. Eʿtemādī et al., Introduction p. 22) and Yāqūt (II 54, 5).
48. Shahrazūrī (see note 47).
49. Shahrazūrī (see note 47), Yāqūt (II 54, 7), and Ḥājjī Khalīfa (I 368, 8, no. 987), resp. (In III 162, 10, no. 4738 and VI 507, 6, no. 14444, Ḥājjī Khalīfa gives 530/1135 as the date of Esmāʿīl's death.)
50. See below, note 56.
51. *Tatimmat Ṣiwān al-ḥikma* I 172; *Tatimma Persice,* p. 100, no. 107.
52. Yāqūt II 54, 7. Samʿānī was born at Marv in 506/1112, traveled far as a young man, and returned to Marv in 538/1143 (GAL I 329, no. 2; Supp. I 564, no. 2).
53. Failasūfo d-dowlä ʿAbdo l-Ḥosain Khān Zonūzī Tabrīzī mentions this book as written in 495/1101 (*Maṭraḥo l-anẓār* I 206). It is not clear whether its language was Arabic or Persian. No MSS are known.
54. This work is unknown to all the sources quoted here; the only reference to it is found in *Mūjez-e Kommī* (see **No. 161 : MS 18**). It cannot at present be determined whether or not it is identical with one of Esmāʿīl's known books. A tempting guess would be to relate its title, "Auspicious Gift," to Atsız's ascent to the throne (cf. **No. 86 : MS 57 III**).
55. Baihaqī, *Tatimma* I 173; *Tatimma Pers.,* p. 100, -1.
56. Esmāʿīl nowhere states that he wrote *Zakhīrä* in 504, only that he came to Khwārezm that year. But since he compiled *Khoffī* in 506, after *Zakhīrä,* and states in the preface to his Arabic translation of *Zakhīrä* (see next note for reference) that he was seventy years old when he composed (*jamaʿtu*) it in Persian, it appears reasonably safe to argue that he was born in or around 434/1042.
57. In the preface to his Arabic translation of *Zakhīrä,* Meshkāt III (2) 759, 16 to 760, 2.
58. Ibid.
59. Stewart, p. 106f., no. II; quoted by Rieu II 475a (*ad* Add. 23560 III) and Ḥosain, Shīrānī, p. 388, no. 2106.
60. Ibn al-Athīr XI 138, 12.
61. His titles as given in the preface of *Khoffī* read as follows (see **MSS 7 II** and **9 II** with cataloguer's emendation):

خداوند زاده أمير اسفهسالار أجلّ كبير بهاء الدين
عمدة الإسلام علاء الدولة والدين ضياء الأمّة نجم الملّة
مؤيّد الملك تاج الملوك والسلاطين نظام المعالي قزل ارسلان
وليّ العهد أبو المظفّر اتسز ابن خوارزمشاه حسام
أمير المؤمنين

(See note 40 above for bibliography on this titulature.) According to ibn al-Athīr X 182, 12, Atsız had led the Khwarezmian army even during his father's reign and conquered Minqıshlāq for Khwārezm. On Atsız see *Cambridge History of Iran* V (1968), Index, p. 716b, s.v. [Bosworth].

62. See **Nos. 9** and **10 : MSS 8** and **7 II**, Incipit.
63. In *Rasāʾil al-Waṭwāṭ* (II 12) there is a letter possibly addressed to this vizier; it is titled *kitābun ilā sh-shaikhi l-imāmi Majdi d-Dīni Ḥujjati l-ḥaqqi Ṣāḥibi l-Bukhārī.* Baihaqī has a short note on *al-imām aṣ-ṣāḥib* ibn Muḥammad al-Bukhārī, not containing any historical information (*Tatimma* I 146, no. 91; *Tatimma Pers.,* p. 90, no. 91).
64. See note 46 above. *Aghrāż* is not directly dedicated to Atsız, but the titles accorded to him in the preface clearly show that he was shāh at the time of composition:

خداوند وخداوندزاده ملك عالم عادل ولي نعمت
كريم الطرفين نصرة الدين علاء الدولة فخر السلاطين
أبو المظفّر اتسز ابن خوارزمشاه حسام أمير المؤمنين

This wording is taken from the MS Teheran Univ. Lib., no. 4856, without collation with other copies (see facsimile ed., p. 3, 5–7.

65. See **No. 14 : MS 11.**

66. It is not known whether this treatise was written in Arabic or in Persian; no MS of it has yet been discovered. In a Teheran library a *majmūʿa* exists including works by ar-Rāzī, Ḥunain, abū Sahl al-Masīḥī, and ibn at-Tilmīdh; the description does not name the author of a tract *aṭ-Ṭibb al-mulūkī* contained in this MS (ar-Rāzī wrote a work of this title). See RIMA III (1) 50, no. 147 II.

67. Baihaqī, *Tatimma Pers.*, p. 100, -1.

68. Meshkāt III (2) 761, 10.

69. In this work, Esmāʿīl discusses the theoretical part of medicine (*al-juzʾ al-ʿilmī min aṭ-ṭibb*); cf. the tables of contents in Moattar, p. 44f., no. 7, and Rahāvard, p. 240, no. 123. In at least some MSS, it is written in the form of tables (Shabbūḥ, p. 98, no. 125), conforming to Ḥājjī Khalīfa's testimony (III 537, 2, no. 6815). Moreover, the known copies differ on the number of *maqāla* (subdivided into *bāb*) in this book, between six, seven, and ten. See references in this note, GAL Supp. I 889 f., no. 15, 6, and Ullmann, p. 161, note 1.

    A Persian medical treatise is identified as Esmāʿīl's *Zobdato ṭ-ṭebb* by a note on one of the flyleaves in a Paris MS of the eighteenth century (Edgar Blochet, *Catalogue des manuscrits arabes . . . offerts à la Bibliothèque Nationale par M. J.-A. Decourdemanche* [Paris 1909], p. 87, no. Supplément persan 1748), and another Persian work, *Zobdä-ye qavānīn-e ʿelāj*, is ascribed to Esmāʿīl in Charminar, p. 242, no. 162. Since no more details are given in either place, it cannot be determined what kind of relationship exists between these texts and Esmāʿīl's Arabic *Zubda.*

70. Baihaqī, *Tatimma Pers.*, p. 101, 1–2. No MS known.

71. Ibid. No MS known.

72. Baihaqī, *Tatimma* I 173. No MS known.

73. Quoted by Baihaqī, ibid. (*Tatimma Pers.*, p. 101, 5 to 102, 7), and Shahrazūrī; for MSS see GAL I 486, no. 15, 5; Supp. I 889f., no. 15, 5.

74. GAL I 486, no. 15, 3–4; in the MS (Escorial I 422, no. 612, 9–10) only al-Jurjānī is given as the author's name, but since the date of transcription is 667/1269, as-Sayyid ash-Sharīf ʿAlī b. Muḥammad al-Jurjānī (cf. EI[2] II 602b–603a [Tritton]) is to be ruled out as the author.

    Aside from the works by Esmāʿīl here listed, ebn-e Esfandyār mentions a Persian translation of Avicenna's *Qānūn* done by Esmāʿīl (p. 86 bottom, no. 2), and Baihaqī adds to his list of medical works *kitāb ākhar fī l-ḥikma* without giving its title (*Tatimma* I 173; *Tatimma Pers.*, p. 101, 1). It seems likely that other smaller treatises transmitted under Esmāʿīl's name are extracts from his larger books; e.g., 1) *al-Aurām wa-l-buthūr*, 2) *al-Ḥummayāt wa-anwāʿhā*, 3) *Risāla fī amrāḍ al-ʿain* (all three in Munajjid, RIMA V 295, nos. 307–309), and 4) *K. dar ʿelm-e tashrīḥ* (PL II 210, no. 361 (3)). Hamarneh mentions, in addition to these, a didactic poem *al-Urjūza aṭ-ṭibbīya* (*Ẓāhirīya*, p. 361, -4), without giving references to MSS.

75. *Čahār maqālä*, pp. 110, 4, 7; 112, 2.

76. GAL I 486, no. 15, 1; Paris Ar. 2955 (p. 528a–b). For other rulers with the title al-Malik al-Ashraf, see Lane-Poole, *Dynasties*, index, and Bosworth, *Dynasties*, pp. 59–62 (Ayyūbids), 63–66 (Mamlūks), 76–77 (Rasūlids).

77. GAL Supp. I 889f., no. 15, 7.

78. He was the son of Idrīs Bidlīsī, the well-known Ottoman historian (see EI[2] I 1207b–1208b [V. L. Ménage]), and himself a historian of note (cf. Franz Babinger, *Die Geschichtsschreiber der Osmanen und ihre Werke* [Leipzig 1927], pp. 95–97, no. 77); his translations from Persian into Ottoman Turkish include *Mavāheb-e ʿAlīyä*, a commentary on the Koran by Ḥosain b. ʿAlī Vāʿeẓ Kāshefī (Ethé, *Ind. Off.* II 893, s.v. Abû al-Faḍl Muḥammad b. Idrīs).

79. Paris, Bibl. Nat., Cat. MSS Hébreux, p. 214b–215a, no. 1169. There is no indication as to the period of translation, but a probable *terminus ad quem* appears to be the fifteenth century A.D. (ibid., p. v).

80. PL II 209, no. 361.

81. *The* Ráhat-uṣ-Ṣudúr wa Áyat-us-surúr . . . *by Muḥammad ibn ʿAlí ibn Sulaymán ar-Ráwandí*, ed. Muḥammad Iqbál, "E. J. W. Gibb Memorial" Series, n.s. II (London 1921), Index, p. 571, s.v. *Zakhīrä-ye Khwārezmshāhī.*

82. Several of the sources confound the rulers who were patrons of Esmāʿīl, Qoṭboddīn Moḥammad and ʿAlāʾo d-dowlä Atsız, and later Khwārezm-Shāhs such as Il Arslān, Tegish, ʿAlāʾoddīn Moḥammad, or even others. See the sources listed here

in the preceding notes and cf., especially for the confusions, GAL I 486, no. 15, 1; *Tārīkh-e Gozīdā*, 686, -7; *Ḥabībo s-sīar* II 641, -8; *Haft Eqlīm*, quoted by Ethé I 464, no. 724–26, 1156; Ḥājjī Khalīfa I 368, no. 987; III 162, no. 4738; III 330, no. 5794; VI 507, no. 14444.

PL II 207, no. 361; Monzavī I 538a, nos. 4977–5065; Panjāb P.L., p. 318, nos. 245–46; al-Khāliṣī, p. 258, nos. 3–5; al-Mauṣil, p. 180, no. 161 [the section on anatomy from *Zakhīrā*; six illustrations]; Charminar, p. 242, nos. 159–61; Kekelidze, p. 117, no. 132 (P K 96); Konya, p. 34, no. (248) 145 [library of Yusuf Ağa]; Manisa, p. 4, no. (33) 1771; Meredith-Owens, pp. 27–28, nos. Or. 5317, Or. 5841, Or. 5863, Or. 6390; Miklukho-Maklaĭ, p. 230, no. 1675; Osmania Univ., p. 52, no. 25; Pizzi, p. 314, no. 24 [*ketāb* 6, *goftār* 3, on ophthalmology]; Tashkent VII 284, no. 5443 (8263 I); ibid., IX 276–79, nos. 6427–32 (9747, 3485, 3505, 3510, 3492, 11030); ibid., IX 280, no. 6434 (2275 IV) [section on pediatrics].

Esmāʿīl's Arabic translation of his *Zakhīrā*: Maḥfūẓ, *Īrān*, p. 76, no. 53 [Teheran Med. Fac.]; Meshkāt III (2) 761, 10.

Esmāʿīl's other Arabic works:

1. *Zubdat aṭ-ṭibb*: Ḥamārina, p. 360, no. 77 t (old number 4727); Shabbūḥ, p. 98, nos. 125–26; Maḥfūẓ, *Īrān*, pp. 23, 25, 76, nos. 72, 106, 56, resp.; [al-Munajjid], *Baʿtha*, p. 332, no. 1274; al-Munajjid, *Nawādir*, p. 74, no. 4231; Bibl. Nat., Vajda, p. 734, no. Ar. 5851; Rampur I 482, no. 106.
2. *aṭ-Ṭibb al-mulūkī*: Maḥfūẓ, *Īrān*, p. 50, no. 147 II.
3. *al-Aurām wa-l-buthūr*: al-Munajjid, *Maṣādir*, p. 295, no. 307.
4. *al-Ḥummayāt wa-anwāʿhā*: al-Munajjid, *Maṣādir*, p. 295, no. 308.
5. *Risāla fī amrāḍ al-ʿain*: al-Munajjid, *Maṣādir*, p. 295, no. 309.

No. 3 : MS 2

Zainoddīn Esmāʿīl b. al-Ḥosain al-Jorjānī

Zakhīrā-ye Khwārezmshāhī

ذخيرهٔ خوارزمشاهى

MS 2 (ex Coll. Min.), 318 fols., 247 x 187 mm

Bound in burgundy-colored leather over thick, stiff cardboard; simple blind-tooled borders; spine of brown leather; inner covers pasted with yellow paper; two flyleaves in front, one in back, of medium-thick, off-white European paper. Binding heavily rubbed, stained, faded; not original. Written on burnished, beige Eastern paper of varying thickness; stained, worn; some margins torn and mended. On lacunae see below.

20 lines, 155 x 115 mm, on blind-ruled frame and lines; grey to black with red overlinings and rubrics; medium-sized, fair *naskh*. Catchwords. Blank fols. separate the different *ketāb*: fols. 75b, 76, 77a; 152b, 153a; 278b, 279, 280, 281a; 317b.

Collations by scribe and two readers.

Anonymous, undated copy; ca. 1100/1700.

Readers' entries on inner covers, flyleaves, and fol. 318b, in both Arabic and Persian.

On fol. 1a *tamlīk* by ʿArab Qarīn (?), Rafīʿā-ye Yahūdī, Shemʿōn al-Yahūdī Baghdādī (*sic*), and one Moḥammad. On back inner cover two *tamlīk* by the same owner, Yōsēf ben Elʿāzār Kōhēn, written once in Hebrew and once in Arabic characters.

Owner's stamp of the above-mentioned Moḥammad on fols. 1a, 153a, 259a, 316a.

Incipit, fol. 1b

بسمله. كتاب نخستين از ذخيره خوارزمشاهى اندر
شناختن حد طب و منفعة ان ... واين كتاب شش
گفتار است گفتار اول ...

Explicit, fol. 317a, 9

واگر علامتهای بد نه اندر چنین وقتها که یاد کرده آمد
پدید آید کمتر باید پرسید واگر اندرین وقتها
ظاهر شود حکم باید کرد که بخواهد مرد والله اعلم
بالصواب والیه المرجع والماب تم هذا الکتاب ...

The MS contains *ketāb* 1-4 of *Zakhīrā-ye Khwārezmshāhī* by Esmāʿīl Jorjānī; the text of *ketāb* 1 begins without any preface. Within *ketāb* 3, *bakhsh* 1, there are two major omissions by the copyist: *jozv* 2 of *goftār* 3 (fol. 178a, 11; cf. **MS 1**, fols. 160a, -3 and 183b, 12), and *goftār* 7 (fol. 193a, -9; cf. **MS 1**, fols. 197b, -8 and 203a, 9). The collations do not take note of these omissions. In this MS, a detailed table of contents is given only for *ketāb* 2 and 4.

No. 4 : MS 3

Zainoddīn Esmāʿīl b. al-Ḥosain al-Jorjānī

Zakhīrā-ye Khwārezmshāhī ذخیرهٔ خوارزمشاهی

MS 3 (ex Coll. Min.), 147 fols., 263 x 155 mm

Bound in black leather over stiff cardboard; simple blind-tooled borders, three-medallion design with blind-stamped floral scrolls; spine and corners covered with black cloth; inner covers pasted with yellowish glazed paper, serving also as flyleaves. Binding faded, much worn; not original. Written on Eastern paper, medium thin to medium thick, slightly rough, cream-colored; worn, stained; edges of first and last fols. torn and mended; upper half of fol. 1 torn out, replaced by blank leaf. For lacunae see below.

24 lines, 195 x 100 mm, on blind-ruled frame and lines; black with red overlinings and rubrics. I. fols. 1b-70b, 110a-147b: medium-sized, neat *naskh*. II. fols. 71b-109b: medium-sized, even *nastaʿlīq*, rubrics in *naskh* of I; the same scribe as I. Catchwords throughout. Fol. 71a blank.

Collations by scribe.

Copied, and dated (fol. 70b) 15 Rajab 1078/31 October 1667, by Ṣūfī Kamāloddīn b. Ṣūfī Shamsoddīn Jahromī.

Marginal and interlinear notes by readers.

Beginning of *ketāb* 2, *bāb* 1, on fol. 1a, -7 (see below)

باب نخستین اندر شناختن تن درستی و بیماری [
بباید دانست که تن درستی مطلق آنست که
مزاج هر اندام از اندامها یکسان معتدل باشد ...

Explicit, fol. 147b, -2

وهرگاه که خون گرم شود بسببهای ضعیف بجوشد
همچون آتش برافروزد واگر نه آن باشد که
قوّت اسهال کردن داروی مسهل فزود ترشد]

End of *ketāb* 2, fol. 70b, 8

وقسطا بن لوقا میگوید که من دیدم مردیرا که بشتاب
برخواست [کذا] تا نعلین درپوشد وفرو بود تا دیگر
نعلین راست کند اندر فرو بودن بیفتاد وهلاک شد
تمام شد کتاب دوم از ذخیره بعون الله ....

Beginning of *ketāb* 3, fol. 71b

بسمله. کتاب سیوم که کتاب حفظ الصحه است.
آغاز کتاب سیّم از ذخیره خوارزمشاهی اندر حفظ الصّحة
واین چهارده گفتارست باید دانستن که اندرین کتاب
سیم تدبیر نگاه داشتن تندرستی وتدبیر هواها
وشناختن آبها وتدبیرهای طعام وشراب وتدبیر
خواب وبیداری وتدبیر حرکت وسکون وتدبیر
کسوتها وعطرها واستفراغها از هرگونه ...

The MS contains *ketāb* 2-3 of *Zakhīrä-ye Khwārezmshāhī* by Esmāʿīl Jorjānī. The text is incomplete in the following places: since part of fol. 1 is missing (see above), the table of contents prefixed to *ketāb* 2 is lost, as well as part of *bāb* 1 of *goftār* 1 in the same *ketāb.* The MS breaks off on fol. 147b within *bāb* 11, *jozv* 2, *goftār* 1, *bakhsh* 2, *ketāb* 3 (cf. **MS 1**, fol. 217b, 3). Within *ketāb* 3, there are four lacunae due to the scribe's negligence (?): A) within *bakhsh* 1: 1) fol. 126b, -7 (cf. **MS 1**, fols. 185a, 7 and 192b, -2), from within *goftār* 4, *bāb* 4 to within *goftār* 5, *bāb* 1; 2) fol. 133a, -1 (cf. **MS 1**, fols. 197a, -7 and 203a, -4), from within *goftār* 6, *bāb* 5 to within *bakhsh* 2, *goftār* 1, *jozv* 1, *bāb* 1; B) within *bakhsh* 2: 3) fol. 142a, 6 (cf. **MS 1**, fols. 210a, 7 and 210b, -8), from within *goftār* 1, *jozv* 2, *bāb* 1 to within *bāb* 4 of the same *jozv*; 4) fol. 143a, -7 (cf. **MS 1**, fols. 212a, 10 and 214a, -2), from within *goftār* 1, *jozv* 2, *bāb* 6 to within *bāb* 11 of the same *jozv.* Apparently the scribe copied this MS from a defective copy without noticing the lacunae.

No. 5 : MS 4

Zainoddīn Esmāʿīl b. al-Ḥosain al-Jorjānī

Zakhīrä-ye Khwārezmshāhī ذخيرۀ خوارزمشاهى

MS 4 (ex Coll. Min.), 434 fols., 278 x 203 mm

Bound in plain blackish-brown leather over stiff cardboard; inner covers pasted with red, worn paper, underneath it a medallion with stamped floral scrolls; binding stained, worn, discolored. Binding not original. Written on medium-thick, burnished, beige Eastern paper; stained, worn in places; some margins torn, mended, especially of the first and last fols.

21 lines, 190 x 118 mm, on blind-ruled frame and lines; black with red overlinings and rubrics; medium-large, vigorous copperplate *naskh*. Catchwords.

Collations by reader.

Copied, and dated Tatta, 27 Shavvāl 956/18 November 1549, by Shehāboddīn b. Fakhroddīn.

Medical notes on fol. 434b and in margins.

On fol. 434a two *tamlīk* by Ḥosain an-Nakhaʿī.

Illegible stamps, some of them erased, on fols. 1a, 211b, 425a, 429b, 434a.

Incipit, fol. 1b

بسمله. الحمد لله رب العالمين حمد الشاكرين و الصلوة
والسلام على رسوله محمد واله الطيبين الطاهرين كتاب
ششم اندر علاج ...

Explicit, fol. 434b

وطبيخ كرسنه ضماد برنهادن نيز سود دارد والله
اعلم بالصواب

The MS contains *ketāb* 6, on treatment of diseases *a capite ad calcem*, of *Zakhīrä-ye Khwārezmshāhī* by Esmāʿīl Jorjānī. In the preface (fol. 1b, 3) it is said that this *ketāb* is divided into 21 *goftār*, grouped in three *bakhsh*, of two, eight, and eleven *goftār* resp. The first two *bakhsh* are preceded by detailed tables of contents (fols. 1b, 5 to 2b, -7 and fols. 112a, -2 to 114a, 6), but not the third (fol. 239a, 5). In *bakhsh* 1, *goftār* 2, *jozv* 7, the fifth *bāb*, on the effects of chill on the eye, is left out (cf. **MS 5**).

No. 6 : MS 5

Zainoddīn Esmāʿīl b. al-Ḥosain al-Jorjānī

Zakhīrä-ye Khwārezmshāhī ذخیرۀ خوارزمشاهی

MS 5 (ex Coll. Min.), 231 fols., 205 x 125 mm

Bound in dark brown leather over stiff thick cardboard; simple blind-tooled borders, three-medallion design inlaid with thin leather, stamped with floral scrolls, white on black; inner covers pasted with faded light blue paper; two front flyleaves, the corresponding back leaves torn out. Binding worn; not original. Written on two varieties of Eastern paper: 1) body of MS: unevenly burnished, cream-colored, of varying thickness; 2) substituted fols. 1-9, 78, 128, 168-169, 176, 217-228, medium thick, glazed, off-white; some fols. stained; margins of last fols. repaired; MS trimmed down to present size.

10 lines, 135 x 76 mm, on blind-ruled frame and lines (slightly larger written surface on some of the substituted fols.); black with red rubrics. I. body of MS: large, vigorous *naskh*; II. fols. 1-9, 78, 128, 168-169, 176, 217-228: large, neat *naskh*; two different hands? (cf. fols. 1-9 with fols. 217-228). Catchwords throughout.

Collations by scribe in original parts.

Original MS copied, and dated 28 Shaʿbān 1058/17 September 1648, by ebn Zainoddīn ʿAlī Moḥtashem al-Ḥosainī; substitutions anonymous and undated, thirteenth/nineteenth century.

Medical notes in margins; recipes and verses on inner covers and flyleaves, some of them dated, e.g., 27 Ṣafar 1291/ 15 April 1874; in a *tārīkh*, dāro s-salṭanä-ye Eṣfahān is mentioned.

Illegible stamps of former owners throughout the MS; on fols. 82b, 91b, etc., the stamp of Zain ad-Dīn ʿAlī.

Incipit, fol. 1b

بسمله. و به نستعین. گفتار دوم در احوال بیماریهاء
چشم و اسباب و علامات و علاج آن و این
گفتار هشت [کذا. یعنی هفت] جزو است
جزو نخستین در شناختن ... و این جزو هفت بابست ...

Explicit, fol. 231b

واب وان نگاه کردن و شودمان [؟ یعنی شادمان ؟]
بودن سودمند بود انشاء الله تعالی وحده العزیز و صلی
الله علی محمد خیر خلقه و آله اجمعین والحمد لله رب العالمین
قد تم ...

The MS contains *ketāb* 6, *goftār* 2, on ophthalmology, of *Zakhīrä-ye Khwārezmshāhī* by Esmāʿīl Jorjānī (cf. **MS 4**, fols. 63a, -10 to 112a, -2). In this MS, the rubrications are often left out.

No. 7 : MS Ar. 60 IV

Zainoddīn Esmāʿīl b. al-Ḥosain al-Ḥosainī al-Jorjānī

Zakhīrā-ye Khwārezmshāhī ذخيرۀ خوارزمشاهى

MS Ar. 60 (ex Coll. Min.), 56 fols., 254 x 167 mm; binder's collection of one Arabic and three Persian works. *Zakhīrā-ye Khwārezmshāhī* on fols. 52–56, margins.

For the description of the MS see **No. 157 : MS Ar. 60 II.**

Incipit, fol. 52b

كتاب چهارمين از ذخيرۀ [كذا] خوارزمساهى در معرفة
بحران واين كتاب چهار مقاله است بايد دانست كه
اندرين كتاب چهارمين بيان كردن استخراج الامر
الامراض [كذا] خواهد بودن يعنى شناختن ...

Explicit, fol. 56b

واگر نضج ناقص بود هفت نوبت آن تب بدارد
وطبيب بايد كه در فرق ميان نضج ناقص ونضج تمام
نگاه كند]

This MS contains the beginning of *ketāb* 4 of *Zakhīrā-ye Khwārezmshāhī*, on the days of crisis (*boḥrān*). Cf. **Nos. 2–3 : MSS 1–2.**

No. 8 : MS Ar. 73 V

[Zainoddīn Esmāʿīl b. al-Ḥosain al-Jorjānī]

Three *bāb*, numbered 19–21, on urine

MS Ar. 73, 250 x 150 mm; collection of medical treatises in Arabic.
A noteworthy Persian extract on urine on p. 669.

Written on medium-thick, burnished, beige Eastern paper.

31 lines, 210 x 120 mm, on blind-ruled frame and lines of different measures; black with red overlinings; small careful *naskh*, leaning to *nastaʿlīq*; not fully punctuated with diacritical dots, but marked with *ihmāl* signs.

Copied by Yaḥyā b. ʿAbdo l-Vahhāb al-Kayzaqānī[1](?); undated. Another short excerpt by the same scribe is dated 850/1446 (p. 666).

Incipit

باب نوزدهم اندر شناختن حالهاى بيمار
از بوي بول هرگاه كه بول بيمار را بوي نه بود دليل
سردي مزاج وخامي ماده بود واندر بيماريهاى حاده عدم
رايحه دليل با بال شدن حرارة غريزى باشد...

Explicit, third line from bottom

بول خداوند درد پشت ودرد مفاصل سفيد وغليظ
بود واندرن شيشه ثفل سفيد همچون نعبه بار كرده [؟]
باشد [كذا] اين جمله انيست اندر بيشتر حالها
كونه باشد والله اعلم حرره العبير...

This excerpt from a larger work on medicine includes three *bāb* on urine, numbered 19 to 21. On the beginning of *bāb* 19 see Incipit; *bāb* 20 begins in line 10: اندر فرق ميان بول زنان ومردان , and *bāb* 21 in line 16: اندر ياد كردن ثمره بابها گشته . A comparison with the corresponding chapters in *ketāb* 2, *goftār* 5, of Esmāʿīl Jorjānī's *Zakhīrä-ye Khwārezmshāhī*[2] proves these sections here to be an abridgment of Esmāʿīl's *bāb* 26, 28, 29 (see *Zakhīrä, ketāb-e dovvom*, ed. Moṣṭafavī, *Sels. Entesh. Anjoman-e Āṣār-e Mellī* 76 [Tehrān 1349], pp. 196, 198–99).

1. A village and village district in the province of Sabzevār (*Farhang-e Joghrāfyāʾī-ye Īrān* IX 356a).
2. See **Nos. 2–6 : MSS 1–5.**

No. 9 : MS 8

Zainoddīn Esmāʿīl b. al-Ḥosain al-Jorjānī

Khoffī-ye ʿAlāʾī خفى علائى

MS 8 (ex Coll. Min.), 164 fols., 178 x 70 mm

Bound in black leather over thick, stiff cardboard; simple blind-tooled borders; inner covers pasted with brownish-beige European paper; one flyleaf each in front and back of the same sheet. Binding stained and worn; not original, of the recent past. Written on two varieties of Eastern paper: 1) body of MS: medium thick, slightly brittle, unburnished, light brown; 2) substituted fols. 33, 94, 96–98, 109, 153–154: medium thick, brittle, glazed, beige; stains, tears, holes; some fols. badly worn; margins and folds partly mended; trimmed down to present size; fols. 55–88 in one piece broken out of binding. On lacunae see below.

I. Body of MS: 15 lines, 143 x 38 mm; dark brown with red, or red over brown, rubrics; medium-large, vigorous old *naskh* of high distinction. Originally no catchwords, but later added at random, often wrong. II. Substituted fols. (see above): 15 lines, 143 x 38 mm, on blind-ruled frame and lines; black with red rubrics; medium-large, neat but academic *naskh*. Catchwords.

Collations by scribe I.

Anonymous, undated copy (end missing); the style of handwriting and the orthography, e.g., *b* for *p*, *f* for *bh*, suggest a date around 600/1200; this may be confirmed by the cut of this MS, following the specifications of the preface that *Khoffī* was written in two oblong volumes so that it could always be carried in the shafts of riding boots.[1] The substitutions in this MS date from the twelfth/eighteenth century.

Notes and scribbles in margins, partly in Hebrew characters.

This MS contains Esmāʿīl Jorjānī's "Bootbook for ʿAlāʾ [o d-dowlä]," *Khoffī-ye ʿAlāʾī*[2] (the title is vocalized on fol. 149a, -6). The copy is incomplete and misbound; the correct order of fols. is as follows: beginning missing (*bakhsh* 1, *maqālä* 1, *bāb* 1-3), 1–10, lacuna (from within *bāb* 6 to within *bāb* 7), 113–147, lacuna (part of *bāb* 13), 11–26, lacuna (*maqālä* 2, from within *bāb* 1 to within *bāb* 3), 27–32, lacuna (*bāb* 4), 160–164, lacuna (from within *bāb* 5 to within *bāb* 7), 148–159, lacuna (*bakhsh* 2, *maqālä* 2, part of *bāb* 1), 33–62, lacuna (part of *bāb* 5), 63–85, lacuna (from within *bāb* 9 to *bāb* 15), 86–87, lacuna (from within *bāb* 16 to within *bāb* 18), 88–112, lacuna (from within *maqālä* 4 to the end, i.e., *maqālä* 5–7). *Bakhsh* 2, on practical medicine, begins on fol. 149a, 9 with a new *basmala*, introduction, and a table of contents.

1. See **No. 10 : MS 7 II**, Incipit, and PL II 210, note 2. The anonymous author of *Mūjez-e Kommī* probably took his cue from Esmāʿīl in naming his work "Abridgment for the sleeve" (see **Nos. 161–62 : MSS 18–19**).
2. For a table of contents see Rieu II 475b, *ad* Add. 23560 III, quoted in Fonahn, p. 35, no. 39.

PL II 210, no. 361 (4); also ibid., 209 center; Monzavī I 526b, nos. 4860–73; Shīrānī II 388, no. 2106; Kekelidze, p. 128, no. 144 (P K 108); Osmania Med. Coll., p. 112, no. 32; Rampur, p. 130, no. 320 ["*fehrest-e . . . Khoffī*"]; Tashkent IX 279, no. 6433 (3334 XII).

No. 10 : MS 7 II

Zainoddīn Esmāʿīl b. al-Ḥosain al-Jorjānī

Khoffī-ye ʿAlāʾī خفّیِ علائی

MS 7 (ex Coll. Min.), 214 fols., 176 x 105 mm; binder's collection of two medical texts in Persian. *Khoffī-ye ʿAlāʾī* on fols. 109–214.

For the description of the MS see **No. 137 : MS 7 I**.

Incipit, fol. 109b

بسمله . و به نستعین . الحمد لله رب العالمین والعاقبه للمتقین
والصلوة علی محمد واله اجمعین چون مصنف این کتاب
سید اسمعیل جرجانی از تالیف ذخیرهٔ خوارزمشاهی
فارغشده بر لفظ بزرگوار امیر اسفهسالار اجل ... علاء الدولة
والدّین ابو المظفر قزل ارسلان ابن خوارزمشاه حرس الله
دولته برفت که ... کتاب مختصر بایستی که هر وقت در
ساق موزه توان نهاد ...

Explicit, fol. 214b

پیه بز و نمك بهم سرشته ضماد کردن پادزهر همه
جانوران گزنده است والله اعلم بالصواب
تمت الکتاب [کذا] ...

In this MS of Esmāʿīl Jorjānī's *Khoffī-ye ʿAlāʾī* (see Incipit) there are several lacunae: between fols. 156 and 157, 158 and 159, 167 and 168 one fol. each is missing; between fols. 123 and 124 two leaves are lost. Another lacuna, fol. 149a, -1 (cf. **MS 9**, fol. 30b, -7 to -2) results not from mechanical damage to this MS but from the scribe's negligence or a lacuna in the copy from which it was transcribed.

No. 11 : MS 9 II

Zainoddīn Esmāʿīl b. al-Ḥosain al-Jorjānī

Khoffī-ye ʿAlāʾī خفّی علائی

MS 9 (ex Coll. Min.), 85 fols., 235 x 125 mm; scribe's collection of three Persian texts; no. I (fols. 1-4b, -8), on calligraphy, not catalogued here. (See also **No. 191 : MS 9 III**.)
Khoffī-ye ʿAlāʾī on fols. 4-47, 64-84.

Bound in greyish-green, lightly dotted paper over stiff cardboard; spine of brown cloth; inner covers and one flyleaf each in front and back of one sheet of European paper each; watermark: Webster 1833; one additional flyleaf each in front and back of the same paper. Binding not original. Written on medium-thin, slightly coarse, beige Eastern paper; first and last fols. stained, foxed; some margins torn, most of them repaired; text sometimes pasted over or cut off by restoration; MS trimmed down to present size. For lacunae see below.

I. A) Fols. 1-47: 21 lines, 180 x 80 mm, on blind-ruled frame and lines; greyish-black with red overlinings and rubrics; simple cartouches for the title of *Khoffī* on fol. 4b and of *bakhsh* 2 on fol. 34b (empty); small neat *naskh*. Catchwords. B) Fols. 48-63: 160 x 80 mm, 9 x 5 fields in tables, on blind-ruled frame; mostly diagonal lines of alternating direction, forming fishbone pattern; same style of handwriting as A. Catchwords. II. Fols. 64-84; 18-19 lines, varying written surface; blackish with red and crimson rubrics; varying styles of *nastaʿlīq* in different sizes, less careful than I. Catchwords.

Interlinear and marginal collations by a reader.

Anonymous, undated copy (end missing); eleventh/seventeenth century.

Many marginal notes, one from *Sharḥ-e Nafīsī*;[1] fols. 84b, 85a filled with recipes and calligraphic exercises, each in a different hand, in black and red ink.

On fol. 85a a *tamlīk* by Muḥammad ʿAlī.

Incipit, fol. 4b, -6

بسمله. چون خادم دعاگوی اسمعیل بن الحسین
الحسینی الجرجانی از جمیع [کذا] کتاب ذخیرهٔ
خداوند خوارزمشاهی فارغ شد بر لفظ عالی خداوند
زادهٔ امیر اسفهسالار بهاء الدین عمدة الاسلام عماد الدولة
والدین ... نظام المعالی قزل ارسلان ابو المظفر اتسز ابن
خوارزمشاه حسام امیر المومنین حرس الله دولته رفت که...

Explicit, fol. 84a

ونمك وسدین بز بهم سرشته ضماد کردن پادزهر همه
جانوران است گزیدن [کذا] این همه مختصر بیش
از این احتمال نکند وداروهای دیگر در کتاب ذخیره
خوارزمشاهی باید جست تمام شد کتاب...

In this MS of *Khoffī-ye ʿAlāʾī* by Esmāʿīl Jorjānī, there is a long lacuna in *bakhsh* 2, *maqālä* 2. The text breaks off on fol. 47b within *bāb* 4; fols. 48-63 contain a totally different text (see **No. 191 : MS 9 III**), and on fol. 64a, *Khoffī* resumes within *bāb* 13 of the same *maqālä*. *Bāb* 11, on diseases of the anus, follows after *bāb* 17, on gynecology, on fol. 69b, 9. The missing parts are thus *bāb* 5-10, 12, and parts of *bāb* 4 and 13. In **MS 7 II**, *bāb* 13 and 15 discuss diseases of the spleen and dropsy, resp.; here, the order is reversed. In *maqālä* 3-7, the order of paragraphs is disrupted: *maqālä* 3, "on fevers," begins with this heading on fol. 72b, -4, but the paragraphs on *ḥommī-ye yowm* and *tab-e deqq* precede it (fol. 72a, 11 to 72b, -4). *Maqālä* 4, on tumors, sores, and wounds, occupies fols. 78b, -3 through 81a, but the paragraphs on *sūkhtegī-ye ātesh* and *dāḥes* follow on fol. 82a,

–8 to –1; *qūbā*ʾ is not discussed in this MS. *Maqālä* 5 follows on fols. 81b, 1 to 82a, 11, and *maqālä* 6 on fols. 82b, –8 to 83a, –5, but part of it occupies fol. 82a, –2 to 82b, –8; paragraphs on *kalaf* and *namash* are missing. Fol. 83a, –5 through fol. 84a are taken up by *maqālä* 7.

1. This could mean either of Nafīs b. ʿIwaḍ al-Kirmānī's two works, *Sharḥ al-Asbāb wa-l-ʿalāmāt*, or *Sharḥ Mūjiz al-Qānūn*; see Ullmann, pp. 170, 173.

No. 12 : MS 10

Zainoddīn Esmāʿīl b. al-Ḥosain al-Jorjānī

Khoffī-ye ʿAlāʾī خفّی علائی

MS 10 (ex Coll. Min.), 21 fols., 213 x 145 mm

Bound in flexible plain brown leather; inner covers bare; one flyleaf each of medium-thin, glazed, cream-colored Russian paper. Binding stained, worn, not original. Written on medium-thin, burnished, light brown Eastern paper; stained, worn; all edges mended with paper like that used for flyleaves. On lacunae see below.

20–22 lines, ca. 147 x 90 mm, on blind-ruled frame and lines; greyish-black with red overlinings; small ordinary *nastaʿlīq* leaning to *naskh*. Catchwords.

Collations by scribe.

Anonymous, undated copy; ca. 1100/1700.

Notes in margins and on fol. 20b; interlinear glosses, many giving *Farhang* as the source.

On fol. 20a a note saying that Navvāb-e ʿālī Tīmūr Pasha presented *kamtarīn* with this book, the *Sharḥ-e ʿAqāʾed-e Nasafī*, etc.

On fol. 20a a partially illegible stamp, reading "Aḥmad" and "Saʿdī," dated 1188/1774; was the owner named in this stamp the writer of the note just mentioned?

Incipit, fol. 1b

باب اول از مقاله اول در تدبیر هوا باید دانست
که اسباب صحت و بیماری شش نوع است . . .

In this MS of Esmāʿīl Jorjānī's *Khoffī-ye ʿAlāʾī*, the text begins without any preface or introduction (cf. **MS 7**, fol. 111a, 7); the copy contains all of *bakhsh* 1, but in a shorter version than that represented in **MS 8** (see *bāb* 4 and 7 in *maqālä* 1). In *bakhsh* 2, *maqālä* 1, on the physician's duties, is left out in this MS. *Bāb* 1 of *maqālä* 2, on diseases of the head, is shorter again than in **MSS 7** and **8**: paragraphs on *laqvä, sar gashtan, kābūs, tashannoj* are missing (cf. **MS 8**, fols. 43b, 1 to 47b, –4). The MS breaks off, on fol. 20a, 7, within *bāb* 2 of *maqālä* 2, on diseases of the eye, at the end of the paragraph on *sabal* (cf. **MS 8**, fol. 51b, 4). The later notes are written closely below the text. On fol. 20b, there is an excerpt from *maqālä* 3, on smallpox and measles, *jodarī* and *ḥaṣbä*, in the hand of the scribe (cf. **MS 8**, fols. 105a, –3 to 108a, 5).

No. 13 : MS 6

Zainoddīn Esmāʿīl b. al-Ḥosain al-Jorjānī

Al-aghrāżo ṭ-ṭebbīyä va-l-mabāḥeṣo l-ʿalāʾīyä

الاغراض الطبية والمباحث العلائية

MS 6 (ex Coll. Min.), 191 fols., 245 x 190 mm

Bound in black cloth over stiff cardboard; spine of moss-green leather; inner covers pasted with cream-colored paper; binding broken, one fol. loose; fol. 1 bound in upside down. Binding not original, of the recent past. Written on two varieties of Eastern paper: 1) body of MS: thick, burnished, cream-colored; 2) 45 substituted fols.: medium thick, slightly coarse, cream-colored; foxed, stained, worn; legibility sometimes impaired; many edges repaired; deep tears, recent mouse-eating. On lacunae see below.

I. Body of MS: 23 lines, 195 x 140 mm, on blind-ruled frame and lines; grey to black with red rubrics and overlinings; medium-large, good, old *naskh*. II. Substituted fols., except fols. 1, 2b, and 3a, 1-7: varying number of lines on varying written surface; black with red rubrics; medium-sized careless, uneven *naskh* leaning to *nastaʿlīq*. III. Fols. 1, 2b and 3a, 1-7: black with red rubrics and overlinings; medium-small, ordinary *naskh*. Catchwords throughout.

Old collations, marked in red *balagha*.

Anonymous, undated copy (end missing); certain features of orthography, such as the aspirated postvocalic *d* and كى for كه appear to suggest a date no later than 700/1300; substituted fols. much more recent, ca. 1100/1700.

Medical notes on fols. 1a, 3, 75b and in margins.

Two *tamlīk* on fol. 1a, one by ʿAbdo l-Jalīl b. ʿAbdo l-Vakīl, and the other by his son (?) Moḥammad Zakī b. ʿAbdo l-Jalīl al-M . . . ī [illegible] al-ʿAqīlī.

On many pages traces of a big round stamp with concentric inscriptions in gold ink, illegible.

The identification of this MS with Esmāʿīl Jorjānī's *al-Aghrāżo ṭ-ṭebbīyä va-l-mabāḥeṣo l-ʿalāʾīyä* rests on its comparison with the facsimile edition of a MS in Teheran University Library.[1] In the UCLA manuscript, the contents are divided into three *qesm*, and these into *goftār* and *bāb*.[2] The first two *qesm* correspond to *jeld* 1 and 2 of *bakhsh* 1 in the India Office copy, and *qesm* 3 equals *bakhsh* 2. In its present condition, this MS begins, on fol. 2a, with *bāb* 9 of *goftār* 3 of *qesm* 2, *andar naqīʿhā va-maṭbūkhhā*, and ends on fol. 191b, within *bāb* 1 of *goftār* 26 of *qesm* 3, on bone fractures. There are lacunae between fols. 8 and 9 (within the same *bāb*) and between fols. 188 and 189, from within *bāb* 1 to within *bāb* 4 of *goftār* 25 of *qesm* 3. Fol. 1 contains part of *bāb* 17 of *goftār* 3 of *qesm* 2 and corresponds to fols. 15b-16a.

The known MSS of *Aghrāż* differ[3] as to the number and names of their subdivisions and the arrangement of the subjects discussed in the text. In the above-mentioned facsimile edition, the book is divided into five *bakhsh*, the last two of which deal with simple and compound drugs, resp. In the UCLA manuscript, these are discussed in *goftār* 2 and 3 of *qesm* 2.[4]

1. No. 4856, copied in 789/1387. For a table of contents see there and Rahāvard, pp. 35-41.
2. This corresponds to Sepāhsālār MS no. 795 (*Cat.* III 175); cf. Rahāvard, pp. 35-41, no. 20.
3. In two *bakhsh*: Blochet II 120f., no. 880 III and Tashkent VIII 101, no. 5682; in three *bakhsh* (on theoretical medicine, simple drugs, and diseases *a capite ad calcem*): Tashkent VIII 100, no. 5681.
4. A detailed table of contents in Ethé I 1243-45, no. 2286. See **No. 2 : MS 1** on the place of *Aghrāż* among Esmāʿīl's works.

PL II 209, no. 361 (2); Monzavī I 473b, no. 4373-91; Shīrānī II 384-85, nos. 2085-86; Hadw, p. 69, no. 14; Bursa, p. 15, no. (61) 1145 [Harraççıoğlu library]; Charminar, p. 237, nos. 2-3; Eilers-Heinz, pp. 81, 233, nos. 91 and 301, resp.; Inst. Hist. Med., New Delhi I 1, no. MMS 11964; Meredith-Owens, p. 28, no. Or. 9580; Miklukho-Maklaĭ, pp. 51-52, nos. 159-60; Osmania Med. Coll., p. 110, no. 12; Tashkent VIII 100-101, nos. 5681-82 (7273 and 9253, resp.).

No. 14 : MS 11

Zainoddīn Esmāʿīl b. al-Ḥosain al-Jorjānī

Yādgār یادگار [؟]

MS 11 (ex Coll. Min.), 33 fols., 197 x 96 mm; binder's collection of two Persian works; no. II (fols. 28–33), a short Arabic-Persian glossary, not catalogued here.
Yādgār on fols. 1–24.

Bound in slightly flexible, plain brownish-black leather; inner covers pasted with thin paper, foxed and warped; a leaf from a German guidebook on Istanbul has been pasted in at the end instead of a flyleaf. Spine mended with piece of velvet; binding worn and faded; not original, too small for the size of fols.; spine too narrow for original extent. Written (fols. 1–27) on medium-thin, burnished, white European paper; watermarks: 1) in a four-lobed frame, a lamb passant, a staff with two triangular flags leaning against its shoulder; 2) a coat of arms (escutcheon party per pale, three bends dexter reduced, one bend sinister reduced, and one mullet in sinister base); 3) stylized monogram "VPH"; 4) a pair of crossed staves. First and last fols. stained; occasional wormholes; edges repaired; MS trimmed after being transcribed, but before marginal notes were written; a blank was pasted on fol. 1a and torn off again. On lacunae see below.

Fols. 1–3: 15 lines, ca. 130 x 60 mm; fols. 4–25: 17 lines, 150 x 60 mm, all on blind-ruled bicolumnar frame and lines (prepared for the transcription of poems); black with red rubrics and overlinings. Fols. 1–3: medium-sized neat *nastaʿlīq*; *ḥadīth* quotations and rubrics in *naskh*; fols. 4–25: medium-sized neat *naskh*. Catchwords throughout.

Collations by scribe.

Copied, and dated in a village of Dailamān 9 Jomādā I 1170/1 March 1757, by Āqā Moḥammad; he transcribed the MS from a copy done by ebn Ḥasan al-Kharkāmī in Dāro s-sorūr-e Lāhūr, in the service of

مسیح الانامی جالینوس الزمانی امیر سید حسین الحکیم گیلانی

Marginal notes by readers; on inner front cover and fols. 1a, 26a–27a, recipes; on fols. 24b–25b an excerpt *dar bayān-e khāṣṣīyat-e zāgh*, on the magic properties of vitriol, in the scribe's hand; on fols. 26a–27a quotations from *Zakhīrā(-ye Khwārezmshāhī?)* by reader; on fol. 27a a recipe following Aflāṭūno z-zamānī Ḥakīm abū l-Qāsem.

Incipit, fol. 1b

بسمله. سپاس و ستایش مر خدای را عز و جل که منزه
است از هر جسد که خلق در ضمایر و ترکیب و صورت
و امتزاج عناصر و وصفش درجه و چون و چند نیاید...

[۲ الف] پس این مقدمه را دعاگوی ضعیف
اسمعیل بن حسن بن محمد بن احمد العلوی
الحسینی احسن الله توفیقه از جمله کتاب ذخیره
[و] استنباطی کرد مشتمل بر نکتهای و دقایق

بسیار که کتابهای بزرگ ازاین دقایق قواعد خالی
نیست پس ترتیبش بر پنج بخش نهاده شد...

Explicit, fol. 24a

جهت گزیدن پشه علاج انست که خیر بوا بر
گزیدگی پشه نهند تا نیک شود ودیگر علاج
حاجت نیست باذن الله تعالی تمت الکتاب [کذا]
المسمی بالخفی خفی الاعلای [کذا]...

The identification of this incomplete MS as a copy of Esmāᶜīl Jorjānī's (fol. 2a) *Yādgār* rests on a comparison with his *Khoffī*, showing that the two texts are not identical (against the Explicit, see above), and its division into five ***bakhsh***.[1] However, the beginning of the preface is different in the UCLA manuscript from the other known MSS containing a preface; they begin (quoting as much as the catalogues give): (Ivanow 1533) الحمد لله... اما باید دانست که عنایت همه انست... and (Ivanow 1534) الحمد لله... سید اسمعیل بن حسن... In another MS, the text is divided into 137 chapters; its Incipit reads as follows:[2]

الحمد لله رب العالمین حمد الشاکرین والصلوة
والسلام علی النبی المصطفی محمد واله الطاهرین
باید دانست که عنایت بزرگ ان نیست که
کسی را چیزی بخشند...

It appears that these three MSS all represent the same version; the Explicit of the last reads[2]

واگر غذا خورند سپستان باید خورد تا بسیاری غذا...
چیز...

It will be noted that the introductory eulogies are the same as in *Zakhīrä* (cf. **No. 2 : MS 1**), suggesting that this may be the original wording of the preface of *Yādgār*. The heading of *bakhsh* 1 in the UCLA manuscript (fol. 2a, -1; see below) corresponds to a version represented in three MSS in Teheran Medical Faculty,[3] lacking a preface and beginning directly with the table of contents, but the text ends differently there:

وطعام غلیظ وشور وسخت درشت نخورد ورگ [و] نزند
والله اعلم تم

In the UCLA manuscript, the following are the subdivisions of the text and its topics:

1. *bakhsh* (in table of contents, fol. 2a, -1), in 18 *bāb*

اندر قواعد علمی که اندر علم طب بکار آید

2. *bakhsh* (fol. 2b, -1), in 30 *bāb* — اندر علاج بیماریهای سر تا پای

3. *bakhsh* (begins on fol. 11a, 6), 1 *bāb* — اندر تب و آبله و حصبه

4. *bakhsh* (begins on fol. 15b, 9), in 11 *bāb* — اندر آماسها و جراحتها و ریشها

5. *bakhsh* (begins on fol. 20a, -1), in 3 *bāb*

اندر علاج زهرها [یعنی علاج شکستگی و زینت و زهرها]

The contents of *Yādgār* are very similar, and sometimes identical, in their wording to *Khoffī-ye ʿAlāʾī,* but here therapy, i.e., prescriptions, takes up much more room.

This MS is badly fragmented: between fols. 2 and 3, two fols. are missing, including the continuation of the table of contents and the beginning of *bāb* 1 of **bakhsh** 1; this same *bāb* breaks off on fol. 3b, and the following 17 *bāb* of **bakhsh** 1 and the first 21 *bāb* of **bakhsh** 2 are wanting. *Bāb* 22 of this **bakhsh** begins on fol. 4; after another lacuna, fol. 5 begins within *bāb* 26 of **bakhsh** 2. The rest of the text is preserved.

1. See Ivanow, p. 715, no. 1533.
2. Amritsar, p. 100, no. 247 E (cf. Madras I 439, no. 391 [and, copied from this, ibid., p. 440, no. 392]). Stewart, p. 107, lists a MS of *Yādgār* in 14 chapters, "to which is added an extensive Pharmacopoeia."
3. Nashrīyä III 323b–324a.

PL II 211, no. 361 (5); Monzavī I 610a, nos. 5685–88; Nūrbakhsh I 78, no. 54 IV [? titled *Darmān wa-dārū*]; Amritsar, p. 100f., no. 247 (S. H. R. 2267); Leiden III 274, no. 1388 (Cod. 604 (3) Warn.); Osmania Med. Coll., p. 110, no. 6 [?].

No. 15 : MS 84

Amīno d-dowlä al-Ūtājī

[*Taqvīmo ṣ-ṣeḥḥä*] — [تقویم الصحّة]

MS 84 (ex Coll. Min.), 16 fols., 145 x 100 mm

Modern brochure, flexible, light blue, fading cardboard; one flyleaf in front of Eastern paper, thin, burnished, beige, and two flyleaves in back of Eastern paper, thick, burnished, greyish. Brochure broken in spine, some fols. partly torn out. Written on Eastern paper, medium thick, slightly coarse, cream-colored; some stains and spots, edges trimmed and restored; misbound. On lacunae see below.

Fols. 1b-2a: 12 lines; fols. 2b-16: alternating diagonal lines in 8 x 5 fields, 113 x 73 mm, borders and divisions blind-ruled; tables divided and framed in red; black with red rubrics; small, fair *nastaʿlīq*. Catchwords trimmed off when MS was restored. Old foliation.

Anonymous copy, dated 11 Jomādā I 996/8 April 1588.
On fol. 1a an illegible stamp; on fol. 16b a stamp reads "Muḥammad ʿAlī."

Incipit, fol. 1b

بسمله . وبه نستعين . الحمد لله رب العالمين والصلوة والسلام
على نبيه محمد واله اجمعين اما بعد بدان اسعدك الله
في الدارين كه اين كتاب خواص نباتات وغيره است
تصنيف حكيم فاضل امين الدولة الاوتاجي چون
حكم فرمان جهان گشاى پادشاه روى زمين ارغون
بران جمله نقاد [كذا] يافت كه كمترين اوتاجى
در هرگونه ...

Explicit, fol. 16b

سادج گرم وتر است دل را قوة دهد واز اجزاى [كذا]
قلبى باشد آواز را ضرر رساند دفع ان زعفران ونبات
كند والسلام

The MS is a misbound (fol. 4 after 13, and 10 after 12) and incomplete (fol. 5 is missing) copy of an untitled work on the medicinal properties of fruits, vegetables, animals, drinks, and clothing materials. In a copyist's sentence prefixed to the text, its title is given as *K. khavāṣṣ-e nabātāt* and the author's name as Amīno d-dowlä al-Ūtājī (fol. 1b, 3-5). In the preface he calls himself simply Ūtājī (fol. 1b, 6). He wrote this short treatise at the command of the Īlkhān Arghūn (683-90/1284-91)[1] and set it up in tables of five columns: 1) name, 2) nature (*ṭabīʿat*), 3) virtue (*manfaʿat*), 4) negative effect (*mażarrat*), 5) antidote (*dafʿ-e mażarrat*).

During the course of transmission of this text, considerable confusion has arisen as to the author's and dedicatee's names and the title of the treatise: in some MSS the author is called Amīno d-dowlä va-d-dīn [b.] Khwājä Rashīdoddīn Ūtājī,[2] in another only Amīno d-dowlä,[3] or just Ūtājī as in the UCLA copy. In the majority of copies, the dedicatee is Arghūn,[4] but Ghāzān's name appears too.[5] The UCLA manuscript does not have a title (see above);[6] in other copies, the treatise is called *Taqvīmo ṣ-ṣeḥḥä*[7] or *Nozhato l-molūk*, as in **No. 16 : MS 61 II.**[8] Further study will have to determine whether all of the MSS derive from the same text, or whether there were different versions from the beginning.

1. See note 4 below.
2. See PL II 217, no. 373; Monzavī I 551b, no. 5154.
3. Monzavī I 458a, no. 4218; cf. PL II 217, no. 373.
4. See preceding two notes for reference.
5. PL II 217, no. 373.
6. Cf. Monzavī I 551b, no. 5154.
7. PL II 217, no. 373.
8. See next catalogue entry and Monzavī I 458a, no. 4218.

See notes 2 and 3 above for references in PL and Monzavī.

No. 16 : MS 61 II

Amīno d-dowlä al-Ūtājī

Nozhato l-molūk نزهة الملوك

MS 61 (ex Coll. Min.), 247 fols., 215 x 150 mm; scribe's collection of three works. *Nozhato l-molūk* on fols. 182–198.

For the description of the MS see **No. 41 : MS 61 I.**

Incipit, fol. 182a

بسمله . وبه ثقتي . الحمد لله رب العالمين والصلوة والسلم
على خير خلقه محمد واله اجمعين وبعد چون حكم
جهان مطاع قرار يافت كه فقير حقير نسخه در معرفت
خواص الاشياء كه خلاصه علم طبّست از علم طب
استخراج ...

Explicit, fol. 198a

وبعضى درانها خطها كشيده بود بسيار دران كار
تسكين غم اورد وخوابهاى پريشانه نمايد [كذا.
يعنى نشاند] وبچگانرا گرم اورد   تم الكتاب ...

The MS contains an anonymous treatise *Nozhato l-molūk* (fol. 182a, 11) on the medicinal properties of fruits, vegetables, animals, pearls, gemstones, etc. In the short preface the author calls himself only *faqīr-e ḥaqīr* (fol. 182a, 3). It reads very much like Amīno d-dowlä's *Taqvīmo ṣ-ṣeḥḥä* (see **No. 15 : MS 84**); the list of sources—Plato, Aristotle, Hippocrates, Galen, ibn Sīnā, "and others"—is the same, except that here, ibn Sīnā is added. The relationship between the two texts has to be determined by close comparison. In this MS, there is no clear division into sections. Some paragraphs are headed *faṣl*; a *maqālä* 1 begins on fol. 191a, 1.

No. 17 : MS 20

Najmoddīn Maḥmūd b. Faqīh Elyās Shīrāzī

Ghīāṣīyä غیاثیّه

MS 20 (ex Coll. Min.), 229 fols., 166 x 105 mm

Bound in burgundy-colored leather over stiff, thick cardboard; on front and back simple blind-tooled borders and three-medallion design with blind-stamped floral scrolls; inner covers pasted with dyed paper; three flyleaves of thin, lilac-colored cardboard in front, three of thin off-white cardboard and one of thick brownish paper in back. Binding, including flyleaves, not original. Written on European paper of two varieties: 1) body of MS: medium thin to medium thick, glazed, and dyed turquoise; of watermark only the date remains legible: 18·9; 2) fols. 124–127, 130–137: softer and paler dyed than 1; of the watermark the date 1818 is legible. Legibility of text sometimes impaired by stains and ink smears; MS trimmed down for present binding. One fol. in front is missing (see below, Incipit).

9 lines, 110 x 55 mm, on blind-ruled frame and lines; black with red rubrics and punctuation; medium-small, uneven *nastaʿlīq* with rubrics in neat *naskh*. Catchwords.

Collations by scribe.

Anonymous copy, dated Sunday, 6 Jomādā II 1236/10 March 1821.

Marginal notes; fol. 225b filled with verses and recipes; on fols. 211a, 5 to 225a, 6, prescriptions for various diseases, titled *fāʾedä*; they are not part of *Ghīāṣīyä*, but were copied by the same scribe.

Incipit, fol. 3a, 1 (one [?] fol. with eulogies is missing)

اما بعد در این مدت که دعاگوی مخلص محمود بن الیاس
از واردان شبهه موهم[؟] وزایران سدة منیع امیر کبیر مفخر
بینظیر ملك الامرا افتخار العجم و الترك مظهر الانصاف
و العدل تسیدر[آیا یعنی یسیدر؟] ابن الامیر العادل
جهان پهلوان خسرو توران جرغوطای انکه ... اشارت
فرمود دعاگوی مخلص را تا کتابی مختصر در علم طب
بزبان فارسی ترکیب و تالیف کند ...

Explicit, fol. 210b, -3

با یکدیگر بجوشانند وسررا به بخار آن فرود ارند والله اعلم...

The treatise *Ghīāṣīyä* (fol. 10a, -2) by Maḥmūd b. Elyās (fol. 3a, 1) is divided into four *maqālä*: 1) in 17[1] *bāb* on theoretical medicine, 2) in 59 *bāb* on therapeutics, 3) in 28 *bāb* of alphabetical order on simple drugs, 4) in 22 *bāb* on compound drugs. The known MSS of *Ghīāṣīyä* differ on the name of the dedicatee and on the author,[2] but they all seem to contain the same text. An acephalous Teheran MS[3] calls the dedicatee [Maẓharo l-enṣāf] va-l-ʿadl Ghīāṣo d-dowlat va-d-dīn Yesüder b. . . . Jarghūṭāy, giving the same text as the UCLA manuscript, with the addition of the Islamic *laqab*. The title of the treatise being *Ghīāṣīyä*, a *laqab* formed with the element *ghiyāth* can be expected to be included in the dedicatee's names. Here, it appears as alien, however, among the dedicatee's and his father's Mongol names and their titles that represent the pre-Islamic Iranian ideal of a ruler—*khosrav-e ʿādel, kūy-e javānmardī*—and evoke memories of the *Shāhnāmä*: *khosrav-e Tūrān*. The terms in which these non-Muslim invaders are extolled here can be seen as reflecting an attempt to integrate them somehow into the traditional Iranian view of history. The absence of Islamic given names also points to a date relatively soon after the Īlkhāns established their rule in Persia.

The name Jarghūṭāy appears in different spellings: an *amīr-e hazārä* Jarghūṭāy and his brother Yesüder[4] are mentioned by Rashīdoddīn under the year 683/1284;[5] a Čarghādāy was, as one of Baydū's intimates, killed by Ghāzān in 694/1295.[6] It is not clear whether the two are identical. Vaṣṣāf[7] reports that a Yesüder was sent to Yazd towards the end of Arghūn's rule[8] to apprehend its *atābeg*, the Hazāraspid Yūsofshāh,[9] because he was in arrears with his tribute. Instead, Yūsofshāh killed him, allegedly because Yesüder had not treated Yūsofshāh's mother with due respect.[10] If this Yesüder is to be identified as the dedicatee of *Ghīāṣīyä*, the treatise cannot have been composed later than 687/1288.[11]

Najmoddīn Maḥmūd b. Ṣāʾenoddīn Elyās[12] b. Shīr-e Bārīk[13] Shīrāzī was a prominent *faqīh* ("Faqī [*sic*] Najm")[14], physician, and medical author at the time when Rashīdoddīn was vizier. Rashīdoddīn appointed him head of the *atābegī* hospital in Shīrāz and appropriated a generous salary for him.[15] In the printed edition of Muʿīn ad-Dīn Junaid ash-Shīrāzī's *Shadd al-izār*, the best biographical account on Maḥmūd b. Elyās, the date of his death reads 6 · · ,[16] but in a MS of the same work the date is given as 720/1320.[17] Muʿīn ad-Dīn Junaid also lists Maḥmūd's works:[18] 1) *K. al-ḥāwī fī ʿilm at-tadāwī*, in Arabic, his best known book;[19] 2) *Sharḥ al-fuṣūl li-Buqrāṭ*, of which no MSS are as yet known; 3) *K. at-tashrīḥ*, also in Arabic;[20] 4) *K. asrār an-nikāḥ*, in Arabic;[21] 5) *K. al-aghdhiya wa-l-ashriba*, no MSS known; 6) *ar-Risāla ath-thaljīya*, Arabic;[22] 7) "*Sharḥ ar-Rashīdīya*," Arabic; it appears likely that this is identical with both the *Laṭāʾif ar-Rashīdīya* mentioned by Rashīdoddīn himself,[23] and with *al-Asʾila ar-Rashīdīya*, preserved in a MS at Tabrīz.[24] Absent from this list in *Shadd al-izār* are Maḥmūd's works in Persian: *Ghīāṣīyä* and *Toḥfato l-ḥokamā*.[25]

1. In the Bankipore MS, the first *maqālä* has 18 *bāb* (*Cat.* XI 39, no. 1012). For a detailed table of contents see Rahāvard, pp. 338-40, no. 282 II.
2. PL II 218, no. 375.
3. Nashrīyä III 44a, no. 95 II; cf. Monzavī I 558a, s.v. *ṭebb—dar čahār maqālä*.
4. On these names see Blochet II 104, no. 860.
5. *Tārīkh-e Abāghā Khān . . . va-Arghūn Khān*, ed. Jahn, p. 53, -2.
6. *Tārīkh-e Ghāzān Khān*, ed. Jahn, p. 95, 2; Amīr Qutlughshāh married a daughter of Jarghūṭāy, ibid., pp. 37a, 7 and 38b, 8.
7. Lithograph ed. (Bombay 1269/1852-53), p. 253, 3.
8. *dar ākher-e ʿahd-e Arghūn Khān*, ibid.; see also note 11 below. Arghūn reigned 683-90/1284-91.
9. Cf. EI[2] III 336b-337b, s.v. *Hazāraspids* [Spuler].
10. See *Tārīkh-e Yazd*, p. 26, 15, and *Tārīkh-e jadīd-e Yazd*, pp. 75-76.
11. After Yūsofshāh had killed Yesüder, punitive action was taken against him and an expeditionary force sent to Yazd, on whose approach Yūsofshāh fled to Sīstān; see preceding two notes for references. Cf. also ʿAbbās Eqbāl, "Ketāb-e Ghīāṣīyä dar ṭebb," *Yādgār* III 3 (1325), pp. 65-67.
12. This is the correct form of his father's name and *laqab* (see Blochet II 104, no. 860; Īraj Afshār, "Maḥmūd-e bn-e Elyās-e Ṭabīb," *Majallä-ye Mehr* VIII 3/4 (1331), pp. 158-60, 234-36; Meshkāt III (2) 740. Often the name of Maḥmūd's father is given simply as Faqīh Elyās.

13. *Shīr-e bārīk*, "slim lion," is first attested as a sobriquet of the Ṣaffārid emir of Sīstān Ṭāher b. Khalaf (fl. ca. 400/1010, see Bosworth, pp. 103–05, no. 43; *Tārīkh-e Sīstān*, ed. Maleko sh-shoʿarāʾ Bahār [Teheran 1314 *h.sh.*], p. 345, 8). In Muḥammad b. Aḥmad an-Nasawī's *Sīrat as-Sulṭān Jalāl ad-Dīn Mankubirtī*, it is mentioned no longer as a mere nick-name, but as a regular *ism*: Bahāʾoddīn Moḥammad b. Shīr-e Bārīk (Persian translation, ed. M. Mīnovī [Teheran 1344], pp. 252, 7f. and 389, -2f. [*Entesh. Bongāh-e Tarj. va-Nashr* 214. *Majmūʿä-ye Motūn-e Fārsī* 19]; in the Arabic edition by Ḥāfiẓ A. Ḥamdī [Cairo 1953], the name is garbled). From approximately the same period as an-Nasawī reported on, the name Bahāʾoddīn Moḥammad-e Shīr-e Bārīk is transmitted as a legend to one of the fighting horsemen on the large *mīnāʾī* bowl in the Freer Gallery of Art (see Esin Atil, *Ceramics from the World of Islam* [Washington, D. C., 1973], pp. 112–15, no. 50 [illus.]).
14. See note 15 for reference.
15. See *Mokātabāt-e Rashīdī*, p. 62, 1–4, and note 1 (*resālä* 19), and pp. 252–56 (*resālä* 41); cf. Afshār (note 12 above), pp. 160, 234.
16. Edd. Moḥammad Qazvīnī and ʿAbbās Eqbāl (Tehrān 1328), p. 278, 1. In *Fārsnāmä-ye Nāṣerī* II 141, 18, his death is similarly dated in the decade 690–700/1291–1300, but both dates are evidently incorrect: in *Mokātabāt-e Rashīdī* (note 15 above), *resālä* 19, Maḥmūd is listed among scholars to be honored by stipends, etc. This letter cannot have been written before 699/1299, since a campaign in Syria is mentioned in it.
17. Quoted in Bankipore IV 101–103, no. 67.
18. Edd. Qazvīni/Eqbāl (note 16 above), p. 277, 8ff.; quoted also in Bankipore IV 101–103; Afshār, pp. 235–36; Rahāvard, p. 316, no. 183.
19. See Ullmann, p. 178.
20. Meshkāt III (2) 740, no. 448 V.
21. Tabrīz, Mellī, no. 3433 (see Nashrīyä IV 285); is this the same treatise as *Risāla fī l-bāh* in Mōṣul (p. 34, no. 154 IV)?
22. See GAL Supp. II 299, no. 3 (a MS in Rāmpūr).
23. See note 15 above for reference.
24. Mellī, no. 3433 (Nashrīyä IV 285).
25. Horn, ZDMG 54 (1900), p. 326, no. 526 (MS Nuruosmaniye, no. 3469).

PL II 217, no. 375, and 318, no. 584 (74); Monzavī I 570a, nos. 5310–18; note 3 above; cf. Bodleian I 971, no. 1614; cf. also Monzavī I 569a, no. 5303, s.v. *ʿElājo l-amrāż* (a treatise on diseases *a capite* in 58 *bāb* by an anonymous author, who dedicated his work to the Timurid Jalāloddīn Eskandar [see **No. 40 : MS 24 VIII**]; it appears possible that these 58 *bāb* were excerpted from the second *maqālä* of Najmoddīn Maḥmūd's work); Inst. Hist. Med., New Delhi I 55, no. MMS 9465; Tashkent IX 339, no. 6511 (3334 III).

Maḥmūd's works in Arabic:
1. *Asrār an-nikāḥ*: Tabrīz I 56, no. 37 (*shomārä-ye daftar* 3433); al-Mauṣil, p. 34, no. 154 IV [?].
2. *Tashrīḥ*: Tabrīz I 269, no. 209 (*shomārä-ye daftar* 3452).
3. *al-Asʾila ar-Rashīdīya*: Tabrīz I 55, no. 36 (*shomārä-ye daftar* 3433).

No. 18 : MS 20a

Najmoddīn Maḥmūd b. Faqīh Elyās Shīrāzī

Ghīāṣīyä غياثيه

MS 20a (ex Coll. Min.), 19 fols., 185 x 122 mm

Modern brochure of thin, flexible, fading green cardboard; one flyleaf each in front and back, of thin, smooth, white paper, added when rebound. Written on Eastern paper, medium thick, slightly transparent, burnished, off-white. On lacunae see below.

16 lines, 143 x 80 mm, on blind-ruled frame and lines; black with red rubrics and overlinings; medium-sized, fine *nastaʿlīq*. Catchwords.

Collations by scribe.

Anonymous, undated copy (fragment); twelfth/eighteenth century.

This MS contains fragments of Najmoddīn Maḥmūd's treatise *Ghīāṣīyä* (cf. **No. 17 : MS 20**); they are parts of *maqalä* 2 (from within *bāb* 33 to within *bāb* 49) and of *maqalä* 4 (from within *bāb* 1 to within *bāb* 15). The copy is misbound; the correct order of fols. is as follows: lacuna, 13–17, 19, 18, lacuna, 1–12, lacuna.

No. 19 : MS 56 II

Maḥmūd b. ʿUmar al-Jaghmīnī

al-Qānūnja fī ṭ-ṭibb القانونجة في الطبّ

MS 56 (ex Coll. Qāʾenī), 129 fols., 210 x 122 mm; scribe's collection of one Persian and one Arabic medical text. *al-Qānūnja fī ṭ-ṭibb* on fols. 90–117.

For the description of the MS see **No. 134 : MS 56 I.**

Incipit, fol. 90b

بسمله . الحمد لله رب العالمين والصلوة والسلام على خير
خلقه محمد وآله اجمعين اعلم ان الطب علم يعرف
منه احوال بدن الانسان من جهة ما يصح ويزول
عنها ليحفظ الصحة حاصلة ويستر وزايله [؟]
امّا بعد فهذا مختصر مشتمل على زبدة ما يجب
استحضاره من صناعة الطب انتخبته من كتب المتقدمين
ورتبه [كذا] على عشرة مقالات [كذا]...

Explicit, fol. 117b, 9

واللبنيات باردة غليظة والغذاء المتخذ من المياه المعصرة
كماء الحصرم والرمان والسماق فقوتها مثل قوة عصارتها
واما الحلو فالعسلي معين للهضم والعجين مولد للسداد
تمت الكتاب [كذا]...

The identification of this anonymous, untitled treatise on medicine as al-Jaghmīnī's[1] well-known *Qānūnja* rests on a comparison with other MSS of the same work of its Incipit and the organization of its subjects in ten *maqāla*.[2] The ten discourses are titled as follows in this MS:

maqāla 1. (begins on fol. 90b, 7) in 5 *faṣl* في امور الطبيعة

2. (begins on fol. 94b, 9) in 7 *faṣl* في التشريح كل اعضاء [كذا]
3. (begins on fol. 97b, 8) in 5 *faṣl* في احوال البدن الانسان [كذا] واسبابها و علاماتها وعلامات الدالة
4. (begins on fol. 101a, -6) in 4 *faṣl* في النبض و التفسرة
5. (begins on fol. 104b, 1) in 10 *faṣl* في تدبير الاصحاء و في علاج المرضى على وجه كلّي
6. (begins on fol. 107b, 4) in 13 *faṣl* في امراض الراس
7. (begins on fol. 110a, 10, wrongly titled *al-maqāla ar-rābiʿa*) in 18 *faṣl* في امراض بواقي الاعضاء من الصدر الى اسفل السرة
8. (begins on fol. 112b, -3) in 9 *faṣl* في امراض بقية الاعضاء
9. (begins on fol. 114a, 11) in 8 *faṣl* في علل الظاهرة [كذا] في ظاهر البدن و الحميات
10. (begins on fol. 116a, 4) in 3 *faṣl* في قوة الاطعمة والاشربة المالوفة

1. By listing *al-Qānūnja* here, it is suggested that the date of al-Jaghmīnī's death is 745/1344, as indicated in a Gotha MS of *al-Qānūnja* (see Pertsch, Gotha, Arab. III 468, no. 1928; cf. EI[2] II, s.v. al-Djaghmīnī [Suter/Vernet]). Following the testimony of various manuscripts, it appears most likely that the author of *al-Mulakhkhaṣ fī l-haiʾa* and other works on related subjects is not identical with Maḥmūd b. ʿUmar al-Jaghmīnī, if the latter did indeed write *al-Qānūnja* (see Sellheim, pp. 159–60, no. 46).
2. See Dietrich, p. 85, no. 31.

PL II 219, no. 377; cf. Monzavī I 504a, nos. 4667–68; Ullmann, p. 154, note 4.

No. 20 : MS 36

Zainoddīn ʿAlī b. Ḥosain Anṣārī "Ḥājjī Zaino l-ʿAṭṭār"

Ekhtīārāt-e Badīʿī اختيارات بديعى

MS 36 (ex Coll. Min.), 297 fols., 252 x 172 mm

Bound in plain black leather over stiff cardboard; inner covers pasted with beige paper; back cover broken off; stained, cut, worn; a third of the MS is out of binding; loose leaves. Binding not original. Written on two varieties of Eastern paper: 1) fols. 1–286: medium thick, burnished, cream-colored; 2) fols. 287–297: medium thin, burnished, cream-colored; first and last fols. repaired; stained, foxed, worn. For lacunae see below.

I. Fols. 1-284: 21 lines, 160 x 104 mm, on blind-ruled frame and lines; black with red rubrics; medium-sized, fluent, open, fine *nastaʿlīq*, not fully punctuated with diacritical dots. II. Fols. 287-296: 23 lines, 160 x 120 mm, on blind-ruled frame and lines; black and red; medium-sized, careful but inelegant *naskh*. Catchwords throughout. Fols. 285-286, 297 blank.

Collations by scribe and readers.

I. Copied by Saifoddīn Aḥmad b. Moḥammad b. Moḥammad al-Kowsūnī, known as Saifā; he dated *maqālä* 1 on the last Thursday of Rabīʿ II 907/11 November 1501 (fol. 257a, -8) and *maqālä* 2 on Sunday, 13 Rajab 907/Saturday, 22 January 1502 (fol. 284b, -7). II. Anonymous, undated, copy, later than I; ca. 1000/1600.

Medical notes in margins throughout MS; among them quotations from Dioscorides,[1] ibn Sīnā, and ibn Jazla.[2]

On fol. 1a several notes, partly illegible, partly clear: by ʿAbdo r-Raḥīm al-Ḥosainī; . . . (illegible) b. amīr Moḥammad Jaʿfar al-Ḥosainī; ebn Zaino l-ʿĀbedīn Moḥammad Yūsof; verses on the death of one Moḥammad ʿAlī, dated 1100/1688. Another note on fol. 1a is dated 25 Daimāh, corresponding to 10 Jomādā II 1074: 25 Daimāh [i.e., A. Galāl. 585] corresponds to *30 Jomādā I* 1074/30 December 1663; 10 Jomādā II 1074/9 January 1664.

Five effaced stamps on fol. 1a and two on fol. 296a; the date of 1143/1730 on one stamp each on fols. 1a and 296a; on fol. 296a one stamp reading: Muḥammad Ṣādiq.

Incipit, fol. 1b

بسمله . و به نستعين . امداد حمد بى حد واعداد
سپاس بى قياس مبدعى را كه اثار ابداع او بر هر
ورقى از اوراق و شجرى از اشجار سمت وضوح يافته
و بر هر ثمرى از اثمار و زهرى از ازهار انوار ايجاد او
تافته بيت ...

Explicit, fol. 284b, -11

و در هاون كند و چند نوبت باب شيرين نشويد و بعد
ازان داروهاى سوده بران افشاند و بمبالغه بسايد
و ديگر بار نشويد و استعمال كند نافع باشد والله اعلم
بالصواب واليه المرجع والماب تم تمام شد مفردات
و مركبات احسارات بديعى ...

Maqālä 1 ends on fol. 257a, -12

يتمه [كذا] نبايست كه نشراري منبل دارو خوانند و در
جراحتها مستعمل كنند و رحمهاى تازه والسلام
والله اعلم بالصواب واليه المرجع والماب تم كتاب
مفردات احسار البديعى [كذا] على يد ...

Maqālä 2 begins on fol. 257b

بسمله. وبه سسعس. بد انك اس معالهٔ دوم ار احسارات
بدىعى كه دكر خواهم كرد در مركبات مستعمل است
باب الاول فى المفرحات مفرح ياقوتى...

Beginning of Persian-Arabic index, fol. 287b

بسمله. وبه نستعين. چنين گويد مولف اين كتاب كه چون
درين ديار زبان عجم متداولست ودرين كتاب اسامى
ادويه وَغيره بلغة عرب نوشته شده اين فهرست نهاديم...
[سـ ٥] باب الالف اطليلال [كذا] آب آب نمك...
م م ماء الملح

End of Persian-Arabic index, fol. 294a, 13

باب الياء ياسمين صحرايى ياسم ياقوت يبروح
طيان [يعنى طيّان] ياسمون م م
يتوع يربوع يشب يقطين ينبوت [كذا] ينتون
م م جرالبشن م خرنوب تافيتا [كذا]
تمت الفهرست [كذا]

The MS contains the well-known *materia medica* and dispensatory *Ekhtīārāt-e Badīʿī* (fol. 2b, 7) by [Zainoddīn] ʿAlī b. Ḥosain al-Anṣārī *al-moshtaher be*-Ḥājjī Zaino l-ʿAṭṭār (fol. 2a, 4) in two *maqālä*; the first discusses *materia medica* in 28 *bāb* in alphabetical order, following the *abtath*-alphabet, and the second comprises 16 short *bāb* on compound medicines according to their preparation, in the following order:

1. (begins on fol. 257b, 3) *mofarreḥāt*
2. (begins on fol. 260a, 8) *maʿājīn*
3. (begins on fol. 265b, 8) *jovāreshnāt*
4. (begins on fol. 268b, 3) *eṭrīfalāt*
5. (begins on fol. 269a, 1) *morabbayāt*
6. (begins on fol. 270a, 10) *ashrebä va-robūb*
7. (begins on fol. 273b, 9) *laʿūqāt*

8. (begins on fol. 274a, -7) *safūfāt*
9. (begins on fol. 275a, 10) *ḥobūb*
10. (begins on fol. 276b, 12) *aqrāṣ*
11. (begins on fol. 279b, 2) *īārajāt*
12. (begins on fol. 280b, 1) *adhān*
13. (begins on fol. 281b, 1) *teryāqāt*
14. (begins on fol. 283a, 6) *sanūnāt*
15. (begins on fol. 284a, 4) *shīāfāt*
16. (begins on fol. 284a, 9) *marāhem*[3]

In the first *maqālä,* the author discusses the simple drugs under their Arabic names—or rather, one of their Arabic names—but he also lists them under their various other names with cross-reference to the main entry (e.g., fol. 150b, -10 to ult.). After completing his work, he compiled a Persian-Arabic index to this first *maqālä* in order to facilitate its use even more (see above).

Ḥājjī Zaino l-ᶜAṭṭār dedicated his book *Ekhtīārāt-e Badīᶜī* to ᶜEṣmato d-Donyā va-d-Dīn Badīᶜo l-Jamāl (fol. 2a, -3) and dated it 770/1368 (not in this MS; cf. **MS 38**, fol. 3a, 12) at the end of the introduction. The dedicatee is introduced with the following titles:

بلقيس زمين وزمان ملكه تخت نشين سلطان نشان
سلطان خواتين جهان بيت... عصمة الدنيا والدين...

and her name is followed by these eulogies:

خلّد الله أيام سلطنتها وأبّد آثار معدلتها

(fol. 2a, -7 to -2). These formulations render it likely that Badīᶜo l-Jamāl was active in affairs of state and not leading a life of seclusion in the *ḥarim.* In *Tārīkh-e Gozīdä,* a *khānzādä* Badīᶜo l-Jamāl is mentioned as married to Mobārezoddīn Moḥammad Moẓaffarī, father of Shāh Shojāᶜ, and trying to secure the throne for her own son by Mobārezoddīn, Solṭān Bāyazīd.[4] This was shortly before Mobārezoddīn's death in 765/1363, though. Further references to Badīᶜo l-Jamāl's activities could not be found.

The main source for details of Ḥājjī Zaino l-ᶜAṭṭār's life is an untitled[5] work by a son of his, presumably called Ḥājjī Aḥmad[6] b. ᶜAlī b. al-Ḥājj Jamāloddīn Ḥosain al-Anṣārī, on the "lives and sayings of philosophers." According to him,[7] Jamāloddīn Ḥosain, a physician of Eṣfahān, had moved to Shīrāz in 715/1315; in 730/1329, a son was born to him in the same city, who was named ᶜAlī. This ᶜAlī, later known as Ḥājjī Zaino l-ᶜAṭṭar (see above), became the favorite physician of Shāh Shojāᶜ (reigned 760-86/1358-84) and for sixteen years was in constant attendance on him. ᶜAlī died in 806/1403. Besides *Ekhtīārāt-e Badīᶜī,* his works include *Meftāḥo l-khazāyen,* on simple and compound drugs and *succedanea* in three *maqālä,*[8] *Toḥfato s-salāṭīn, Toḥfato l-khavānīn,*[9] and a *Resālä dar ṣefat-e mardān va-zanān.*[10]

Another son of ᶜAlī's, Ḥosain, wrote a treatise on the exact vocalization and declension, according to the rules of Arabic grammar, of those drug names occurring in the first *maqālä* of his father's *Ekhtīārāt.*[11] In the introduction to this book, in the MSS variously titled *Ṣeḥāḥo* or *Eṣḥāḥo l-advīä,*[12] he writes that he was prompted by the request of friends to undertake this work.[13] In all likelihood, it was he who made additions to the text of *Ekhtīārāt,* introduced by *ebn-e moᵓallef gūyad,* that are contained in this and some other MSS,[14] and finally, his book *Dastūro l-aṭebbāᵓ ᶜan qavāᶜedo l-ḥokamāᵓ* discusses very similar subjects (see **No. 31 : MS 45**).

1. It cannot now be determined whether the quotations from Dioscorides were taken by the author from b. al-Baiṭār's *Jāmiᶜ*, containing the text of Dioscorides in its entirety (see Ullmann, p. 282), or from a Persian version of Dioscorides (cf. Ullmann, p. 262).

2. See Ullmann, pp. 160, 274; PL II 206, no. 360.
3. This second *maqālä* is also preserved in two different enlarged versions, of 30 and 33 *bāb*, resp.; see Bodleian I 956, nos. 1583 and 1584 (PL II 222).
4. "E. J. W. Gibb Memorial" Series, XIV 1, pp. 679, 19 and 682, 2.
5. The MS itself is untitled (Brit. Mus., Or. 165 IV), but in the list of the author's works given in it, a *Dastūro s-soᶜadā* "on the sayings of sages" is mentioned. Since the subject is the same as in the untitled book itself, it might be possible to identify the two writings as the same, too. (See Rieu II 873a, quoted ibid., 469a, and PL II 220, no. 380).
6. The name is misspelled حا حمد (Rieu II 873a, *ad* Or. 165 IV, fol. 108b).
7. Brit. Mus., Or. 165, fol. 108 (Rieu II 469a, *ad* Add. 16748).
8. Composed in 767/1365 and preserved in an autograph copy of 769/1367 (Bodleian I 955, no. 1579; PL II 221, no. 380 (1)); it appears to be in effect some kind of first draft for *Ekhtīārāt* and was actually largely superseded by the later book in the further course of transmission (see Monzavī I 599b, nos. 5598–5614).
9. It is not clear whether or not these two titles refer to the same book (see Rieu II 469a and III 1088b ad loc.). No MS is known of either.
10. It appears likely that the *Resālä dar bāh* listed in PL II 223, no. 380 (3), is identical with this work.
11. PL II 223 top.
12. Cf. **No. 31 : MS 45**, note 4.
13. Rahāvard, p. 17, 2 to 18, 5; cf. **MS 45.**
14. Cf. **Nos. 22–23 : MSS 38** and **38a**. During the last years of his father's lifetime, he copied *Ekhtīārāt* (dated 805/1402–03; Ethé I 1251, no. 2289). In the light of these activities, it does not seem rash to attribute to him the additions to his father's text, although he did not sign them with his name.

PL II 221, no. 380 (2); Monzavī I 464b, no. 4260, and 465b, nos. 4276–4338; for the Arabic-Persian glossary see Monzavī I 571b, nos. 5321–24; cf. ibid., 482a, nos. 4460–62 (?), and 572b, no. 5331; for an enlarged version of *maqālä* 2 see Monzavī I 465b, no. 4275, and Panjāb P.L., p. 313, no. 241.

Panjāb P.L., p. 337, no. 254; Tabrīz I 37, no. 20 (*shomārä-ye daftar* 3482); Shīrānī II 382, nos. 2078–79; al-Mauṣil, pp. 107, 275, nos. 99 and 54 III, resp.; Aziz Pasha, p. 55, no. II; Bursa, p. 14, no. (48) 1139 [Harraççıoğlu library]; Charminar, p. 238, no. 58; Eilers-Heinz, pp. 207, 261, nos. 263 and 335, resp.; Katrak, p. 25f., no. 101; Kekelidze, pp. 61, 71, nos. 41 (P K 7) and 61 (P K 27), resp.; Luzac, p. 29, no. 220; Miklukho-Maklaĭ, p. 37, nos. 33–39; Naniana II 243, no. CXIII; Osmania Med. Coll., p. 111, no. 20; Osmania Univ., pp. 52–53, nos. 27, 45, resp.; Rampur, p. 138, no. 342; Tashkent V 290, no. 3958 (3507); ibid., IX 350–52, nos. 6521–25 (3503, 3620, 7518, 9687 I, 3496, resp.).

Meftāḥo l-khazāyen: Kekelidze, p. 61, no. 41 (P K 7); Miklukho-Maklaĭ, p. 558, no. 4174.

No. 21 : MS 37

Zainoddīn ᶜAlī b. Ḥosain Anṣārī "Ḥājjī Zaino l-ᶜAṭṭār"

Ekhtīārāt-e Badīᶜī اختيارات بديعي

MS 37, 145 fols., 242 x 165 mm; Persian-Arabic index on fols. 1–10 added later, written in different hand.

Bound in dark brown waxed cloth over slightly flexible cardboard; inner covers pasted with cream-colored paper. Binding modern, twentieth century. Written on two varieties of Eastern paper: 1) fols. 1–10, medium thick, burnished, cream-colored; 2) fols. 11–145, thick, burnished, cream-colored. Margins water-stained; some wormholes; edges trimmed when binding was done. For lacunae see below.

I. Fols. 1–10a: 24 lines; black and red; medium-small ordinary *naskh*, leaning to *nastaᶜlīq*. II. Fols. 10b–145: 21 lines, 160 x 100 mm, on blind-ruled frame and lines; black with red rubrics; medium-sized, energetic, open, fine *nastaᶜlīq*, not fully punctuated; lemmata partially vocalized. Catchwords.

Collations by scribe.

No. II (fols. 10b–145) is anonymous and undated (end missing), but a *terminus ad quem* is furnished by a note on fol. 10a, written by the scribe of I (fols. 1–10a); it is dated in the "imperial army-camp," *ordū-ye homāyūn*, at Bāghābād in the province, *velāyat*, of Nasā, 5 Zū l-qaᶜdä 913/7 March 1508.

On fol. 9b, beginning of a table of contents with foliation, containing the entries *āṭrīlāl* to *akhīnūs*; Turkish glosses on fols. 14–17 and 188b.

On fol. 10a several *tamlīk* erased and pasted over; on fol. 1a two legible *tamlīk*, one by al-Ḥājjī ʿAlī, the other by ʿAbdo r-Raḥmān b. Maḥmūd aṣ-Ṣeddīqī.

On fols. 1a, 10a, 66a, erased stamps; one partially legible stamp on fol. 10b, reading: Ṣāliḥ.

Incipit (beginning of index), fol. 1b

بسمله. چنین گوید مؤلف این کتاب که چون درین
دیار زبان عجم متداولست ودرین کتاب اسامی ادویه
وغیره بلغت عرب نوشته شده بود این فهرست
نهادیم ونام چیزها بپارسی وعربی نوشته شد...
باب الالف   اطریلال   آب
آب نمك   آب گوشت   آب دهن
ماء الملح   ماء اللحم   لعاب ...

End of index, fol. 9a, -4

یاقوت   یبروح   یبوع   یربوع   یشب
حجر الشیب [؟ آیا یعنی البشن ؟]
یفطیش [کذا. یعنی یقطین]   ینوث [یعنی ینبوت]
یسون [یعنی ینسون]   تم الفهرست بعون الملك
باقی

Beginning of text, fol. 10b

بسمله. وبه نستعین. امداد حمد بی عدد واعداد
سپاس بی قیاس مبدعی را که...

Explicit, fol. 146b, -1

وبدان [یعنی زبده] حقنه کردن وورمهای صلب حار
که در رحم وامعاء ‹و› اشس [کذا] باشد سود دهد]

This MS contains the first part of *Ekhtīārāt-e Badīʿī* (fol. 11b, 7) by ʿAlī b. al-Ḥosain al-Anṣārī *al-moshtaher be-*Ḥājjī Zaino l-ʿAṭṭār (fol. 11a, 5) and the author's own Persian-Arabic index to *maqālä* 1. The text breaks off within the section on *zobdä* (cf. **MS 36**, fol. 110b, -4), and in the index there is one fol. missing between fols. 1 and 2.

No. 22 : MS 38

Zainoddīn ʿAlī b. Ḥosain Anṣārī "Ḥājjī Zaino l-ʿAṭṭār"

Ekhtīārāt-e Badīʿī

اختیارات بدیعی

MS 38 (ex Coll. Min.), 224 fols., 240 x 161 mm

Bound in black leather over stiff thick cardboard; simple blind-tooled borders, three-medallion design with blind-stamped floral scrolls; inner covers pasted with beige paper; two flyleaves in back of European paper, medium thin, glazed, cream-colored; watermark: six-pointed star, shield showing a crowned lion rampant, "B G". Binding not original, of the recent past. Written on three varieties of Eastern paper: 1) body of MS: medium thick, burnished, beige; 2) substituted fols. 25–32, 65–72, 122–129, 149–150: medium thin to thin, slightly transparent, burnished, beige; 3) fol. 1: medium thin, burnished, cream-colored; MS loose in binding, sewing loose; margins of first fols. repaired; stained, worn; ink smears. For lacunae see below.

I. Body of MS: 23 lines, 170 x 100 mm, on blind-ruled frame and lines; black with red rubrics; medium-small, dense, slow-moving, very neat, fine *nastaʿlīq*. II. Fols. 197–198, 209, 216–217: equally fine as I, but smaller, written with a narrower pen, and sparsely punctuated with diacritical dots; by the same scribe as I. III. Substituted fols. 25–32, 65–72, 122–129, 149–150: in overall appearance like I, but much less neat and much less distinguished. Catchwords in I–III. IV. Fol. 1, table of contents later prefixed to MS: medium-large, careful, but inelegant *nastaʿlīq*. Secondary foliation in MS.

Collations by scribe with signs *ṣaḥḥa* and *nuskha*.

Copied by Moḥammad Yūsof b. ʿAbdo l-Laṭīf Kaḥḥāl; he dated *maqālä* 1 early on Tuesday, 28 Zū l-qaʿdä 922/23 December 1516.

Marginal notes throughout the MS; on fol. 2a, a metrological extract from the *Aqrābādhīn* by al-Qalānisī and a *qeṭʿä* on the treatment of *soʿāl* by Mowlānā Ḥakīmoddīn, both written by an owner whose name was erased.

Two notes on fol. 1a give the date of 12 Rabīʿ I 1166/17 January 1753; on fol. 2a there are several notes; the names of two owners have been erased, one *tamlīk* by al-Ḥosain b. Ḥaidar al-Ḥosainī and one by Moḥammad Ṣāleḥ Kaḥḥāl-e Kāshānī are preserved.

On fol. 1b several stamps: 1) Tāj ad-Dīn Muḥammad, 1166; 2) a pious formula dated 1166/1752; 3) Muḥammad Mīrzā, [1]166; on fol. 2a a stamp of one (abū?) al-Muẓaffar ʿAlī, 1038/1628.

Incipit, fol. 2b

بسمله. امداد حمد بی عد واعداد سپاس بی قیاس
مبدعی را که...

Explicit, fol. 222b, margin (see below)

و دیگر بار بشوید واستعمال کند نافع باشد

End of *maqālä* 1, fol. 195a

ینمه نباتیست که بشیرازی منبل دارو خوانند ودرجراحتها
مستعمل کنند و زخمهای تازه والله اعلم تم...

Beginning of *maqālä* 2, fol. 195b

بسمله. امّا بعد بدانکه این رساله ایست از کتاب اختیارات
بدیعی درمرکّبات مستعمل است والله الموفّق...

The MS contains *Ekhtiārāt-e Badīʿī* (fol. 3a, -10) by ʿAlī b. al-Ḥosain al-Anṣārī *al-mashhūr be-*Ḥājjī Zaino l-ʿAṭṭār (fol. 2b, -4). There are lacunae between fols. 89 and 90 (according to the secondary foliation 15 fols. are missing), 209 and 210, 221 and 222, and after fol. 222 (one fol. missing); the end of the text was later supplied in the margin of fol. 222b. Another fol. is missing before fol. 1, containing the beginning of the table of contents. All *bāb* of the two *maqālä* are listed in it with the number of the fol. where they start.

The text of this MS incorporates the additions by *ebn-e moʾallef*; see, e.g., the article on *amlaj*.

No. 23 : MS 38a

Zainoddīn ʿAlī b. Ḥosain Anṣārī "Ḥājjī Zaino l-ʿAṭṭār"

Ekhtiārāt-e Badīʿī اختیارات بدیعی

MS 38a (Ar. 113; ex Coll. Min.), 280 fols., 250 x 157 mm; binder's collection of one Persian and one Arabic medical text. *Ekhtiārāt-e Badīʿī* on fols. 1–240.

Bound in burgundy-colored leather over stiff cardboard, flap; simple blind-tooled borders, three-medallion design with blind-stamped floral scrolls and peacock on covers and flap; inner covers pasted with beige paper. No. I (fols. 1–240) written on Eastern (?) paper, medium thin, burnished, beige; first and last fols. damaged, partly torn out, soiled; upper half of fol. 240 torn out; some repair. On lacunae see below.

19 lines, 175 x 90 mm, on blind-ruled frame and lines; black with red rubrics; medium-sized, driving, sometimes very dense *shekastä-āmīz*. No catchwords (trimmed off?).

Collations by scribe.

Copied, and dated Ḥaidarābād on Sunday, 6 Rabīʿ I 1046/Friday, 6 August 1636, by ebn-e Ḥasanʿalī Qāsemʿalī as-Sarbadārī al-Besṭāmī.[1]

Entries by readers on fol. 1a, in margins throughout, and on inner covers.

On fol. 1a and back inner cover each a *tamlīk* by Saifollāh.

Incipit, fol. 1b

بسمله. امداد حمد بیعد واعداد سپاس بیقیاس مبدعی را
که آثار ابداع او...

Explicit, fol. 240b, -6

بتمه[کذا] نباتی است که آنرا بشیرازی منبل دارو خوانند
و در جراحتها استعمال کنند و زخمتهای تازه والله اعلم
بالصّواب والیه المرجع والمآب تمت الکتاب[کذا]...

The MS contains *maqālä* 1 of *Ekhtīārāt-e Badīʿī* by Ḥājjī Zaino l-ʿAṭṭār; title and author's name are not mentioned in this copy, since there is a long lacuna between fols. 1 and 2, comprising most of the preface and *bābo l-alef* to within the section on *asārūn* (ca. 12 fols. are missing); fol. 2a, 1 reads

بسیار بود وآن نوع بود غلیظ ورقیق وازیك بیخ
ریشهای بسیار بود...

This MS represents the version by *ebn-e moʾallef.*

1. It appears possible that he is a descendant of the Sarbadār dynasty of Khorāsān; see John Masson Smith, *The History of the Sarbadār Dynasty 1336–1381* . . . , Columbia University Publications in Near and Middle East Studies, Series A, 11 (The Hague 1970).

No. 24 : MS 39

Zainoddīn ʿAlī b. Ḥosain Anṣārī "Ḥājjī Zaino l-ʿAṭṭār"

Ekhtīārāt-e Badīʿī اختیارات بدیعی

MS 39 (ex Coll. Min.), 218 fols., 240 x 178 mm

Binding patched together from different fragments: front and back cover not matching, pasted together with black cloth; front cover: dark brown leather over stiff cardboard, three-medallion design with corresponding corners, blind-stamped floral scrolls; back cover: pink cloth over stiff cardboard. Binding worn, not original. Written on Eastern paper, thin to medium thick, burnished, beige; stained, worn, but quite clean overall. For lacunae see below.

15 lines, 185 x 125 mm, on blind-ruled frame and lines; black with red rubrics; large, energetic, inelegant *naskh*. Catchwords.

Collations by scribe.

Anonymous, undated copy (end missing); eleventh/seventeenth century.

Incipit, fol. 1a

دروی به بندند [یعنی درونج را] وازمیان هر دوران زن
بیاویزند که حامله بود...

Explicit, fol. 218b

وحرارت وی [یعنی قدید] کمتر از نمکسود بود قوة
بدن بدهد ومستسقی [..]

This is an incomplete copy of *maqālä* 1 of *Ekhtīārāt-e Badīʿī* by Ḥājjī Zaino l-ʿAṭṭār; the beginning of the text on fol. 1a (within the section on *dorūnaj*) corresponds to **MS 38**, fol. 74b, 13, and its end on fol. 218b (within the section on *qadīd*) to **MS 38**, fol. 144b, 5. Fols. 24–29 are misbound; they include the sections *ḥennā* to *khobz* (cf. **MS 38**, fols. 60a, 12 to 62a, -4).

No. 25 : MS 40

Zainoddīn ʿAlī b. Ḥosain Anṣārī "Ḥājjī Zaino l-ʿAṭṭār"

Ekhtīārāt-e Badīʿī اختیارات بدیعی

MS 40 (ex Coll. Min.), 333 fols., 284 x 187 mm

Bound in grey and black marbled paper over stiff cardboard; corners and spine of plain black leather; endpapers brown; two flyleaves in back of medium-thin, cream-colored European paper. Binding not original, of the recent past. Written on two varieties of European paper: 1) fols. 1–273: thin, transparent, burnished, white; watermarks obscure; 2) fols. 274–333: medium thin, slightly transparent, burnished, beige; no watermark; edges, where torn, carefully mended; some stains, on the whole rather clean. On lacunae see below.

21 lines, 220 x 120 mm, on blind-ruled frame and lines; black with red rubrics; I. fols. 1–273: medium-large, very even but unattractive *naskh*; II. fols. 274–333: medium-small, careful *naskh*. Catchwords throughout.

Collations by scribe.

Anonymous copy, dated 20 Moḥarram 1181/18 June 1767.

Notes by scribe and readers throughout MS.

On fols. 315b and 333b, notes by Ḥosain *valad-e ʿābedain* (?); on the last flyleaf in back a note in the name of Mīrzā Ḥosain Khān, son of Lashkarnevīsbāshī, written by Moḥammad ʿAlī, known as . . . [illegible] aṭ-Ṭabīb on 4 Rajab 1311/ 11 January 1894.

Incipit, fol. 1a

دسمو[؟] میکند واگر دماغ وی
با گوشت با سرکه ...

Explicit, fol. 333b, 9

وچند نوبت باب شیرین بشوید واستعمال کند والله اعلم
بالصواب تمت [کذا] مجلد الثانی من کتاب ...

End of *maqālä* 1, fol. 315b, 4

ینمه بپارسی نباتی است که انرا اسره ومیل دارو [کذا]
خوانند ودرجراحتها کنند [کذا] وزخمهای تازه ازان
نیك شود تمام شد ...

The MS contains *Ekhtīārāt-e Badīʿī* by Ḥājjī Zaino l-ʿAṭṭār, but the text is incomplete in a few places: the preface and first part of *bāb* 1 of *maqālä* 1 are missing (cf. **MS 38**, fols. 1-6a, -4); there is a lacuna between fols. 23 and 32 (cf. **MS 38**, fols. 15 and 20, resp.). Fols. 24-31 are misbound; they belong between fols. 63 and 64.

No. 26 : MS 41

Zainoddīn ʿAlī b. Ḥosain Anṣārī "Ḥājjī Zaino l-ʿAṭṭār"

Ekhtīārāt-e Badīʿī اختیارات بدیعی

MS 41 (ex Coll. Min.), 313 fols., 256 x 135 mm

Bound in plain black leather over stiff cardboard; front endpaper European, unburnished, dyed, pale aquamarine; watermark: galleon and "181" (date with fourth digit not visible?); two blank fols. each in front and back added when present binding was done, of cream-colored Russian (?) paper. Binding worn, back cover broken off; not original. Written on three varieties of European paper: 1) body of MS: medium thin, burnished, beige; watermark: cross in medallion; 2) substituted fols. 1-18, 251-260, 278-312: medium thin, burnished, white; watermark: coat of arms with geometrical symbol in shield and name VALLARINO; 3) fol. 313: same as front endpaper (see above), but with different watermark: hunting horn and "8" (part of date?). In original fols. of MS many stains; foxed; some edges repaired.

19 lines, 185 x 75 mm, on blind-ruled frame and lines; black with red rubrics; I. body of MS: medium-small, fluent, fine *nastaʿlīq*; II. fols. 1-18, 251-260, 268-313: medium-small, neat *naskh*. Catchwords throughout.

Collations by respective scribes.

Anonymous copies; I undated (not preserved); II dated Behbehān, 2 Zū l-qaʿdä 1230/6 October 1815.

Marginal notes throughout.

On fol. 1a one illegible stamp.

Incipit, fol. 1a

این کتاب اختیارات بدیع [کذا] است .
بسمله . امداء [کذا] حمد بی عدو اعداد سپاس بی قیاس ...

Explicit, fol. 313a, 6

بعد ازان داروها سوده بران افشانند و بشایند وبشویند
واستعمال کنند [کذا] والله اعلم بالصواب تمت [کذا]
الکتاب ...

A complete, if restored, copy of ***Ekhtīārāt-e Badīʿī*** (fol. 2a, -3) by ʿAlī b. al-Ḥosain al-Anṣārī *al-moshtaher be-*Ḥājjī Zaino l-ʿAṭṭār (fol. 1b, -10).

No. 27 : MS 42

Zainoddīn ʿAlī b. Ḥosain Anṣārī "Ḥājjī Zaino l-ʿAṭṭār"

Ekhtīārāt-e Badīʿī — اختيارات بديعی

MS 42 (ex Coll. Min.), 519 fols., 203 x 147 mm

Bound in rust-colored leather over stiff cardboard; simple blind-tooled borders, three-medallion design with gilt-stamped floral scrolls; one flyleaf each in front and back of European paper, medium thin, burnished, beige; watermark obscure. Binding not original. Written on two varieties of European paper, one medium thin, burnished, brown, and the other medium thick, burnished, white; first and last fols. worm-eaten; edges torn, foxed; overall clean. On lacunae see below.

14–15 lines, 145 x 85 mm, on blind-ruled frame and lines; greyish-black with red rubrics; different styles of medium-sized, clear, but unattractive *nastaʿlīq* leaning to *naskh* (one scribe?). Catchwords.

Occasional collations by scribe.

Copied, and dated Sunday, (?) Ṣafar 1117/31 May–21 June 1705, by ebn-e abū l-Ḥasan Hedāyatollāh al-Ḥasanī al-Ḥosainī aṭ-Ṭabāṭabāʾī.

Some marginal notes on the first fols.

On front flyleaf a *tamlīk* by Navvāb . . . [illegible] Shāhzādā Ḥātem (?) and another by ʿAbdo l-Mobdī (?).

Incipit, fol. 1a

حوادث ومفتح اسباب کامرانی ...

Explicit, fol. 519a, -4

ینمه نباتیست که بشیرازی منبل دارو خوانند در
جراجتها [کذا] وزخمها بکار دارند بکار دارند [کذا]
والله اعلم بالصّواب وَاِلیه المرجع والمآب

The MS contains the first *maqālä* of *Ekhtīārāt-e Badīʿī* by Ḥājjī Zaino l-ʿAṭṭār; title and author's name are not preserved in this copy, since two leaves are missing before fol. 1 (cf. the beginning of the text here with **MS 38**, fol. 3a, 9).

No. 28 : MS 43

Zainoddīn ʿAlī b. Ḥosain Anṣārī "Ḥājjī Zaino l-ʿAṭṭār"

Ekhtīārāt-e Badīʿī اختيارات بديعى

MS 43 (ex Coll. Min.), 263 fols., 206 x 147 mm

Bound in crimson leather over stiff cardboard; simple blind-tooled borders, three-medallion design with blind-stamped floral scrolls; spine of brown leather; one flyleaf each in front and back of medium-thin, unburnished, white European paper. Binding worn, stained. Written on two varieties of European paper: 1) fols. 1, 3–263: thin, slightly transparent, burnished, white; watermark: Latin cross in shield; 2) fol. 2: medium thin, burnished, cream-colored; no watermark. Some wear and tear throughout; fol. 2 later substituted for damaged or missing leaf.

22 lines, 140 x 80 mm, on blind-ruled frame and lines; black with red rubrics; medium-small, even, but undistinguished *nastaʿlīq*. Catchwords.

Collations by scribe.

Anonymous, undated copy; a note on fol. 1a, dated 1187/1773, provides a *terminus ad quem* (see below); twelfth/eighteenth century.

Medical notes in margins and on back flyleaf.

On fol. 1a a note giving the birth dates of father and son: Mīrzā Moḥammad Jaʿfar, Sunday, 6 Moḥarram 1187/*Tuesday*, 30 March 1773, and Mīrzā Khalaf, Saturday, 4 Rajab 1212/23 December 1797; the note was written by Moḥammad b. Ḥājjī Bāqer.

On fol. 1a an erased stamp.

Incipit, fol. 1b, and Explicit, fol. 263a, correspond to **No. 20 : MS 36**, Incipit, and end of *maqālä* 1, resp.

This MS contains *maqālä* 1 of *Ekhtīārāt-e Badīʿī* by Ḥājjī Zaino l-ʿAṭṭār.

No. 29 : MS 30 II

Zainoddīn ʿAlī b. Ḥosain Anṣārī "Ḥājjī Zaino l-ʿAṭṭār"

Ekhtīārāt-e Badīʿī اختيارات بديعى

MS 30 (ex Coll. Min.), 85 fols., 185 x 110 mm; scribe's collection of two works.
Ekhtīārāt-e Badīʿī on fols. 15–26, etc. (see below).

For the description of the MS see **No. 66 : MS 30 I.**

Incipit, fol. 15a, 1

سه مثقال بوزیدان سه مثقال بنج بابونه پنج مثقال فرنجمشك
پنج درم خسك مربی ...

Explicit, fol. 84a

و دیگر بار بشویند و استعمال کنند که درین باب نیکو
باشد والله اعلم بحقایق الاشیا تم المجلد الثانی ...

This MS is an incomplete copy of *maqālā* 2 of Zaino l-ᶜAṭṭār's well-known pharmacopoeia. The text begins here within *bāb* 2 on electuaries (*maᶜājīn*), and the correct order of fols. is: beginning missing, 15–26, lacuna of one (?) fol., 27, 61–84.

No. 30 : MS 44

Zainoddīn ᶜAlī b. Ḥosain Anṣārī "Ḥājjī Zaino l-ᶜAṭṭār"

Ekhtīārāt-e Badīᶜī اختیارات بدیعی

MS 44 (ex Coll. Min.), 124 fols., 150 x 100 mm

Bound in strong flexible plain black leather. Written on European paper, medium thin, burnished, white; watermark obscure; especially the first and last fols. are worn and browned; many spots and stains; original white color of paper rarely preserved. On lacunae see below.

11–13 lines, 100–110 x 60–70 mm, on blind-ruled frame and lines; borders of a single red hairline; black with red rubrics; medium-small, open, clear, but undistinguished *nastaᶜlīq* leaning to *naskh*. Catchwords.

Anonymous, undated copy; thirteenth/nineteenth century.

Recipes in different hands on fols. 1–13; on fols. 14–20 excerpts on *mālīkhūlīā* (*sic*) from different books; on fols. 29b–30 prescriptions in various hands. On fols. 21–29a see below.

Incipit, fol. 31a

بسمله. الحمد لله ربّ العالمین والصّلوة والسّلیم [کذا]
علی نبیّه وخیر خلقه محمّد واله اجمعین امّا بعد بدانکه
این مقالهٔ دوّیم است از رسالهٔ سیّوم مفاتیح الخزاین
که ذکر کرده در مرکبات مستعمل ...

Explicit, fol. 124b, -1

وصافی کنند ونیمن روغن کنجد بازیت برسر آن
کنند وبجوشانند تا روغن نماند]

Fols. 31–124 of this MS contain *maqālä* 2 of *Ekhtīārāt-e Badīʿī* by Ḥājjī Zaino l-ʿAṭṭār, not "the second *maqālä* of the third *resālä*" of *Mafātīḥo l-khazāyen*, as is stated at the beginning of the text (see Incipit). This copy is incomplete at the end, breaking off within *bāb* 15 on *rowghanhā* (cf. **MS 38**, fol. 222a, 12). Fols. 21–29a of this MS include excerpts from *maqālä* 1 of *Ekhtīārāt*; there are sections on the following drugs: 1) *beṭṭīkh-e zeqqī*, 2) *beṭṭīkh*, 3) *halīlaj*, 4) *tamar-e hendī*, 5) *tamar*, 6) *shaljam*, 7) *rībās*, 8) ʿ*adas*, 9) *laban*, 10) *khormā*, 11) *anār-e shīrīn*, 12) *anār-e torsh*, 13) ʿ*enab*, 14) *fostoq*.

No. 31 : MS 45

Ḥosain b. ʿAlī b. Ḥosain al-Anṣārī al-ʿAṭṭār

Dastūro l-aṭebbāʾ ʿan qavāʿedo l-ḥokamāʾ دستور الاطبّاء عن قواعد الحکماء

MS 45, 252 fols., 223 x 130 mm

Bound in dark brown leather over stiff thick cardboard, flap; simple blind-tooled borders, central medallion with corresponding corners, blind-stamped floral scrolls, also on flap; inner covers pasted with modern white European paper; three flyleaves in front, one in back; one each of thick coarse brown paper, the other two in front of light beige and cream-colored paper respectively. Binding stained and worn; not original, spine too narrow for MS. Written on three varieties of Eastern (?) paper: 1) thin, burnished, cream-colored (fols. 1–6, etc.); 2) medium thin to thin, burnished, light brown (body of MS); 3) medium thin, burnished, beige (fols. 75–83, etc.). Badly worm-eaten; surface of paper often roughened by water; some margins torn, cut, repaired; MS trimmed down from original size.

23 lines, 144 x 75 mm, on blind-ruled frame and lines; black with red rubrics, occasionally left out; medium-sized, copperplate *naskh*. Catchwords.

Anonymous, undated copy; eleventh/seventeenth century.

Readers' notes on flyleaves, and throughout the MS marginal and interlinear notes and glosses in Arabic, Persian, and Turkish; quotations from Galen and Avicenna; the recipe for a *mofarreḥ-e yāqūtī* taken from Khwājä Fakhroddīn Ṣāʾen.

Incipit, fol. 1b

شکر نامحدود وسپاس نامعدود خالقی را که هر ذره
از ذرات کاینات برهستی ذات او دلیلی واضح
وهر نوعی از انواع موجودات بر تحقیق صفات او
حجتی قاطع شعر ...

Explicit, fol. 252b

باب الیا سمرع [؟ آیا یعنی بروح؟] سکبینج [؟ آیا یعنی شابیزج؟]
والله اعلم بالصواب

Ḥosain b. ʿAlī b. Ḥosain al-Anṣārī al-ʿAṭṭār (fol. 1b, -2) divided his ***Dastūro l-aṭebbā*ʾ** *ʿan qavāʿedo* ***l-ḥokamā*ʾ** (fol. 2a, -1) into thirty *faṣl*; the first two give an introduction to anatomy and therapy in general, in *faṣl* 3–27 the treatment of diseases is discussed in the usual order, and in the last three *faṣl*, nomenclature, examination, and substitution of drugs are the topics. On fol. 2b, 2 a detailed table of contents begins, listing all thirty *faṣl*:

1. (begins on fol. 2b, -7) در تشریح بدن انسان بطریق اختصار
2. (begins on fol. 19a, 9) در معرفه امراض
3. (begins on fol. 39a, 9) در امراض دماغ
4. (begins on fol. 49a, -5) در صداع وشقیقه
5. (begins on fol. 53a, 1) در امراض چشم
6. (begins on fol. 65a, 5) در امراض گوش
7. (begins on fol. 69a, 2) در امراض دهان وحلق وحنجره
8. (begins on fol. 78a, -3) در امراض سینه وشش وسرفه وذات الجنب وغیره
9. (begins on fol. 87a, 1) در امراض دل
10. (begins on fol. 91a, 7) در امراض جگر
11. (begins on fol. 96b, -1) در امراض معده
12. (begins on fol. 106a, -4) در امراض سپرز
13. (begins on fol. 109a, -7) در امراض روده
14. (begins on fol. 115b, 11) در امراض مقعد
15. (begins on fol. 119a, 9) در امراض گرده ومثانه
16. (begins on fol. 128b, 11) در امراض قضیب وباه

17. (begins on fol. 135b, -2) در امراض زنان وانچه بریشان تعلق دارد

18. (begins on fol. 144a, 3) در مفاصل ونقرس وعرق النسا

19. (begins on fol. 161a, 2) در بهق وبرص وداء الثعلب وداء الحیه

20. (begins on fol. 166a, -6)

در جذام وجمره واکله واورام وطاعون وسرطانات ودمامیل وخنازیر

21. (begins on fol. 175a, 11)

در جراحتها وبصول [؟ آیا یعنی عرض مانند قروح با
تفرق الاتصال ؟] وشوك وكسر وجبر

22. (begins on fol. 183b, 2) در بثور وثاليل وجرب وقوبا وغيره

23. (begins on fol. 189b, 11) در گزندگی جانوران

24. (begins on fol. 200a, -6) در ادویه قتاله

25. (begins on fol. 206a, 2)

در مسهلات وقايقات [؟ آيا يعني مقيّئات ؟]

26. (begins on fol. 218a, -2) در تبها

27. (begins on fol. 221b, 1) در متفرقات

28. (begins on fol. 228a, 9) در اسامی ادویه وطبایع ان برموز

29. (begins on fol. 242b, -5) در اصلاح ادویه

30. (begins on fol. 248a, 1) در ابدال ادویه

Apart from the first two *faṣl,* the text is little more than a list of medications, simple and compound, arranged according to their indication. In each chapter, the simple drugs are listed first in alphabetical order (*abtath*), then the compound medicines κατὰ γένη, without regard to alphabetical order. The main sources of the book are Esmāʿīl Jorjānī[1] for the generally medical part, and Ibrāhīm b. Muḥammad as-Suwaidī[2] for *materia medica.*[3]

The author of ***Dastūr,*** Ḥosain b. ʿAlī b. Ḥosain al-Anṣārī al-ʿAṭṭār, was a son of Zainoddīn ʿAli, called Ḥājjī Zaino l-ʿAṭṭār, the author of ***Ekhtīārāt-e Badīʿī.***[4] Ḥosain has so far been known mainly for his ***Ṣeḥāḥo l-adviā.***[5] At the request of friends who missed indications of vocalization and *iʿrāb* of the drug names in ***Ekhtīārāt,*** he composed it as a supplement to his father's work.[6] In later centuries, Ḥosain's work was used by Nūroddīn Moḥammad b. ʿAbdollāh Shīrāzī in his *Alfāẓ-e adviā*[7] and by Moḥammad Ḥosain b. Khalaf Tabrīzī "Borhān" in his *Borhān-e qāṭeʿ.*[8] ***Faṣl*** 28 of *Dastūr* closely resembles *Ṣeḥāḥ* in its subject.

Ḥosain b. ʿAlī wrote *Dastūr* in 839/1435 (fol. 2b, 1) and apparently intended to dedicate it to one of the rulers of his time. In this MS, however, *laqab, kunya, ism,* and patronymic of the dedicatee are omitted (without blank space); only a wealth of honorific titles is given in the preface (fol. 2a).

The UCLA manuscript of *Dastūr* is the only one now known of this work.

1. See **MS 1**, etc.
2. See Ullmann, p. 284.
3. For Ḥosain's indebtedness to his father cf. the initial doxologies in both *Ekhtīārāt* and *Dastūr*.
4. See **MS 36**, etc.
5. See PL II 223, under no. 380 (2); Nashrīyä III 301b, s.v. *Esḥāḥo l-advīä*; the title varies in the MSS and later testimony. It appears probable, however, that by choosing this title the author meant to allude to al-Jauharī's famous *aṣ-Ṣiḥāḥ*.
6. See Nashrīyä III 301b. On Ḥosain's editorial work on his father's *Ekhtīārāt* see **No. 20 : MS 36.**
7. See **MS 105**, fol. 3a, -6.
8. See Blochmann, p. 5, no. 32; Rieu II 500a.

Not in PL or Monzavī; Gujarat I 230, no. 146 (titled [?] *Mofradāt wa-morakkabāt*, identical with **MS 45**?).

No. 32 : MS 12

Manṣūr b. Moḥammad b. Aḥmad b. Yūsof b. Faqīh Elyās

Kefāyä-ye Mojāhedīyä کفایۀ مجاهدیه

MS 12 (ex Coll. Min.), 109 fols., 266 x 170 mm

Bound in dark brown leather over stiff cardboard; three-medallion design with blind-stamped floral scrolls on front and back; flyleaves of European paper, in front two blue, in back three white leaves; watermark of blue paper: 1863; binding worn and torn, MS loose. Written on Eastern paper of two varieties: 1) fols. 1–100: medium thick, burnished, tan; 2) fols. 101–109: thin, brittle, burnished, light brown; worn and torn, wormholes, stains. For lacunae see below.

21 lines, 215 x 110 mm, on blind-ruled frame and lines; black with red rubrics; medium-large, very even, clear *naskh*. Catchwords.

Collations by scribe.

Copied, and dated 19 Ẕū l-ḥejjä 1096/16 November 1685, by Moḥammad Raḥīm b. Moḥammad Moqīm Tabrīzī.

Notes on flyleaves and in margins.

One illegible stamp in *ṭughrā* shape on the last back flyleaf, verso.

Incipit, fol. 1b

بسمله. و به نستعین. شکر و سپاس مر خالقی را که در
خلقت انسان دقایق حکمت بی پایانست . . .

Explicit, fol. 109a, 7

واگر کبابه با حلتیت در دهن گیرند و بخایند واب در
قضیب بمالند همین عمل کند والله اعلم بحقایق الامور
تمت . . .

Lacunae between fols. 60 and 61, 61 and 62, 80 and 81, 81 and 82, 107 and 108.

Manṣūr b. Moḥammad b. Aḥmad b. Yūsof b. Faqīh Elyās (fol. 2a, 11) dedicated his well-known medical compendium *Kefāyä-ye Mojāhedīyä* (fol. 2a, -2) to Mojāhedoddīn Zaino l-ᶜābedīn b. Shāh Shojāᶜ, Moẓaffarid ruler of Fārs, 786–89/1384–87.[1] Apparently Manṣūr descended from a Shīrāz family that had produced several generations of scholars before him:[2] Najmoddīn Maḥmūd, the author of *K. al-ḥawı fı ᶜilm at-tadawı* and of *Ghıāṣıyä,*[3] was the son of one Faqīh Elyās, who was in all likelihood Manṣūr's great-great-grandfather as well. Both authors lived in Fārs, Maḥmūd being director of the *atābegī* hospital in Shīrāz,[4] and Manṣūr dedicating his two works, *Kefāyä* and his anatomy,[5] to rulers of the area. Manṣūr's grandfather is probably Jalāloddīn Aḥmad b. Yūsof b. Elyās Shīrāzī, mentioned as a physician and author of a *dīvān* in Persian and Arabic; he died in Shīrāz in 744/1343.[6] There appears to be no difficulty of chronology.[7]

1. Bosworth, p. 161, no. 62; the *laqab* Mojāhedoddīn is to be found in Mīrkhwānd, *Rowżato ṣ-ṣafāᵓ*, ed. Ketābkhānä-ye Khayyām (Tehrān 1339), IV 572, -7.
2. Junaid ash-Shīrāzī does not mention Manṣūr in his *Shadd al-izār,* but his entries on Najmoddīn Maḥmūd and Jalāloddīn Aḥmad follow one another, and a comparison of their ancestors' names with those of Manṣūr's argues in favor of their identity (*Shadd al-izār,* pp. 277–79, nos. 201–202; see esp. p. 279, note 4).
3. See **No. 17 : MS 20.**
4. See Rashīdoddīn Fażlollāh, *Mokātabāt,* pp. 62, 252–56.
5. See **No. 38 : MS 17.**
6. Junaid ash-Shīrāzī, p. 278–79, no. 202; *Fārsnāmä-ye Nāṣerī* II 134, 4–8.
7. Cf. Īraj Afshār, "Maḥmūd-e bn-e Elyās-e Ṭabīb," *Majallä-ye Mehr* VIII 3 (1331/1952–53), p. 159, 2–6.

PL II 225, no. 384 (1); Monzavī I 585a, nos. 5458–94; Panjāb P.L., p. 785, no. 580; Shīrānī II 390, nos. 2165–66; Mashhad, Honar, p. 78; Nūrbakhsh I, pp. 15, 38, nos. 12 and 29 II, resp.; Bursa, p. 15, no. (59) 1137 [Haraççıoğlu library]; Charminar, p. 238, nos. 61–64 [?]; Eilers-Heinz, p. 306, no. 392; Madras IV 1150, no. 964 (b); Miklukho-Maklaĭ, p. 440, no. 3416; Naniana II 225, no. CIII; Rampur, p. 132, nos. 324–25; Tashkent IX 284–86, nos. 6437–38 (5536 and 11665 VIII, resp.).

No. 33 : MS 13

Manṣūr b. Moḥammad b. Aḥmad b. Yūsof b. Faqīh Elyās

Kefāyä-ye Mojāhedīyä کفایهٔ مجاهدیّه

MS 13 (ex Coll. Min.), 244 fols., 140 x 90 mm

Bound in green cardboard (leaves of a Hebrew book pasted together with thin green cardboard); spine, burgundy cloth; two flyleaves in front, three in back; edges of binding worn, some leaves loose. Written on European paper, thin, burnished, cream-colored; watermark obscure; first fols. torn, repaired; heavy wear and tear.

16–20 lines, 100 x 60 mm, on blind-ruled frame and lines; black with red rubrics; small, ordinary *nastaᶜlīq.* Catchwords.

Copied, and dated Friday, 3 Shaᶜbān 1210/12 February 1796, by ebn Moḥammad Reżā-ye Najafābādī.

On flyleaves, Persian notes in Hebrew and Arabic characters; marginal notes in Arabic script throughout the MS, in Hebrew script only through fol. 188b.

On first front and last back flyleaves *tamlīk* by Ḥakīm Dāvūd b. Ḥakīm Hārūn b. Ḥakīm Ebrāhīm b. Mollā Raḥīm (?); his stamp: ᶜabduhū Dāvūd, passim.

Incipit, fol. 1b, as in **No. 32 : MS 12.**

Explicit, fol. 244b, 10

وچون خشك میشود دیگری بر میدارند ومکرر همین
عمل کند که ذکر بزرگ شود والله اعلم بالصواب
تمت ...

No. 34 : MS 14

Manṣūr b. Moḥammad b. Aḥmad b. Yūsof b. Faqīh Elyās

Kefāyä-ye Mojāhedīyä کفایهٔ مجاهدیّه

MS 14 (ex Coll. Min.), 239 fols., 210 x 153 mm

Bound in stiff cardboard, spine black leather; covers lacquered, three-medallion design with floral scrolls in colors on black; front cover lost. Written on Italian paper, medium thick, glazed, white; watermark: coat of arms, FIN PICARDO, and E FIGLI. Margins of first and last fols. torn, some spots.

15 lines, 150 x 90 mm, on blind-ruled frame and lines; black with red rubrics; medium-sized, very even *nastaʿlīq*. Catchwords. Fols. 238b and 239a blank.

Collations by scribe.

Anonymous copy, dated 1244/1828.

Notes on fols. 1b, 239b, and back inner cover, and a few in text.

On fol. 238a, a *tamlīk* by Moḥammad Bāqer Ḥājjī al-Yamīn (al Ḥaramain?); his stamp: yā imām Muḥammad Bāqir, passim.

Incipit, fol. 1b, 5, as in **No. 32 : MS 12.**

Explicit, fol. 238a, -6

واگر زنجبیل باسقمونیا باعسل بر ذکر طلا کنند همین
عمل کند والله اعلم بحقایق الامور...

No. 35 : MS 15

Manṣūr b. Moḥammad b. Aḥmad b. Yūsof b. Faqīh Elyās

Kefāyä-ye Mojāhedīyä کفایهٔ مجاهدیّه

MS 15 (ex Coll. Min.), 212 fols., 200 x 115 mm

Bound in dark brown leather over stiff cardboard; three-medallion design with blind-stamped floral scrolls on front and back; one flyleaf each in front and back of European paper; watermark obscure; edges of binding worn, spine repaired in black leather, partly loose. Written on Eastern paper of two varieties: 1) fols. 1-4, etc.: thin, brittle, burnished, beige; 2) body of MS: medium thick, burnished, off-white. First fols. torn along edges, partly repaired; extensive stains. For lacunae see below.

I. Fols. 1-115: 17 lines, 135 x 75 mm, on blind-ruled frame and lines; greyish-black with red rubrics; medium-sized, fair *nastaʿlīq*; II. fols. 116-212: 17-23 lines, 140-55 x 70 mm, on blind-ruled frame and lines; black with red rubrics; medium-sized, fair *shekastä-āmīz*. Catchwords throughout.

Collations by scribe.

Anonymous, undated copy (end missing); a *terminus ad quem* is provided by a *tamlīk* on the back inner cover, dated 1117/1705; MS not much earlier.

Notes by readers on fol. 1b and in margins.

Tamlīkāt and stamps effaced on fol. 1b; on note on the back inner cover see above.

Incipit, fol. 1b, 1, as in **No. 32 : MS 12.**

Explicit, fol. 212b, -1

واگر قضیب را بخرقه درشت بمالند بعد ازان
بزفت روغنی [...]

There is one fol. missing after fol. 212, containing the end of *Kefāyä*; other lacunae in this MS are: one fol. is missing between fols. 2 and 3, and there are missing leaves between fols. 15 and 16, and between fols. 105 and 106.

No. 36 : MS 16

Manṣūr b. Moḥammad b. Aḥmad b. Yūsof b. Faqīh Elyās

Kefāyä-ye Mojāhedīyä کفایهٔ مجاهدیّه

MS 16 (ex Coll. Min.), 107 fols., 210 x 145 mm

Bound in flexible olive-green leather; simple blind tooling; one flyleaf in front. Binding somewhat worn, not original. Written on Eastern paper, thin, burnished, cream-colored; first and last fols. torn along edges, a few spots and stains. For lacunae see below.

14 lines, 130 x 85 mm, on blind-ruled frame and lines; black with bold, overlined rubrics, also black; medium-sized, fair *nastaʿlīq*. Catchwords.

Collations by scribe and readers.

Anonymous, undated copy (end missing); ca. 1100/1700.

Incipit, fol. 1a, 1

اشتها شود واگر مفرط بود موجب صفرت ...

Explicit, fol. 107b, -1

با اسفاناج خورند وشراب خشخاش وریباس]

Beginning and end of the text are missing in this MS; its Incipit corresponds to **No. 32 : MS 12**, fol. 13a, -4 (within *fann* 1, *qesm* 1, *maqālä* 3, *bāb* 1), and its Explicit to **MS 12**, fol. 72a, 8 (within *fann* 1, *qesm* 2, *maqālä* 2, *bāb* 15).

No. 37 : MS 16a

Manṣūr b. Moḥammad b. Aḥmad b. Yūsof b. Faqīh Elyās

Kefāyä-ye Mojāhedīyä كفايۀ مجاهديّه

MS 16a, 20 fols., 190 x 130 mm

No binding, stitching partly lost, MS loose. Written on European paper, medium thin, slightly transparent, burnished, white; watermark obscure. Some stains, foxed. For lacunae see below.

21–24 lines, 140 x 90 mm, on blind-ruled frame and lines; black, with overlined rubrics, some repeated in crimson ink in margins; medium-sized clear, even *naskh* leaning to *nastaʿlīq*. Anatolian hand (?), see below. Catchwords.

Anonymous, undated copy (end missing); ca. 1200/1800.

On fol. 20b table of contents by scribe; on fol. 20a–b recipes in Turkish, partly in scribe's hand; recipes for amulets on fol. 1a.

Incipit, fol. 1b, 1

بسمله. اما بعد بدانكه اين نسخه ايست درباب حكمت
مشتمل بر پانزده فصل باب دويم در ترياقها در ترياق
كبير واورا ترياق فاروق گويند ...

Explicit, fol. 19b, -1

روغن بابونه بابونه تازه يكمن درچهارمن آب بجوشانند

On fol. 1b, the text is wrongly titled by the scribe رسالهٔ فیثاغورس (repeated on fol. 1a by reader). In reality, it represents a fragment of Manṣūr b. Moḥammad b. Aḥmad's *Kefāyä*: *fann* 2, *maqālä* 2, *bāb* 2 to within *bāb* 14, on compound drugs (cf. **MS 15**, fols. 180b, -4 to 200a, -5), with the difference that here *bāb* 10 discusses *safūfāt* instead of *maṭbūkhāt*.

No. 38 : MS 17

Manṣūr b. Moḥammad b. Aḥmad b. Yūsof b. Faqīh Elyās

[*Tashrīḥ-e badan-e ensān*] [تشریح بدن انسان]

MS 17 (ex Coll. Min.), 33 fols., 340 x 210 mm

Bound in blue, beige, and pink marbled paper over cardboard; spine of black cloth; one flyleaf each in front and back; edges worn. Binding not original. Written on European paper, medium thin, burnished, aquamarine; watermark: coat of arms and name in capitals, not clear. Fols. 27-30 loose, margins of several fols. torn; repaired, including text.

19 lines, 210 x 115 mm, on blind-ruled frame and lines; black with red rubrics; medium-sized ordinary *nastaʿlīq*. Catchwords. Fols. 1a, 32b, 33b blank.

Fünfbilderserie of anatomical illustrations on fols. 5a, 15a, 20b, 22b, 30a; room for illustrations remained unfilled on fol. 6a, 6b.

Collations by reader.

Anonymous copy, dated Eṣfahān, Monday, 4 Shaʿbān 1128/*Friday*, 24 July 1716.

Verses written by reader on fol. 33a.

Illegible stamp on fol. 33a.

Incipit, fol. 1b, 1

بسمله. شکر وسپاس پادشاهی را سزد وحمد وثنای بی قیاس خالقی را که درخلقت انسان دقایق حکمتش بی پایان است . . .

Explicit, fol. 32a, 8

لا جرم ناقص عقل و بی فهم وکم خرد افتاده است باشد [کذا] وچون [کذا] دراین سخن او ارادت فاعل مختار است واظهار قدرت شاملهٔ که مندرجست در تحت حکمت بالغه جل جلاله تمام شد . . .

Manṣūr b. Moḥammad b. Aḥmad (fol. 2a, 4) did not title his treatise on the anatomy of the human body (درتشریح بدن انسان , fol. 2a, 5). He dedicated it to the sultan Żīāʾoddīn Pīr Moḥammad Bahādor (fol. 2a, 11), in all likelihood Pīr Moḥammad b. ʿOmar Shaikh, the Timurid ruler of Fārs 796–812/1393–1409.[1] The text is divided into a *moqaddemä* درتعریف اعضا وتقسیمات او and five *maqālä*:

1. درذکر عظام وانچه متعلق است بدو
2. درذکر عصب واقسام او
3. درذکر عضل وکیفیت حدوث او
4. دربحث اورده وتشعّب او
5. درشرایین وانواع او

and a *khātemä* دراعضاء مرکب وکیفیت تولد جنین

1. See PL II 226, no. 384 (2).

PL II 226, no. 384 (2); Monzavī I 508b, nos. 4699–4716; MacKinney, p. 108, nos. 9.1–2 [National Library of Medicine, Bethesda, Md., MSS P. 18–19]; Tashkent IX 283, no. 6436 (3663 V).

No. 39 : MS Ar. 102 IV

Manṣūr b. Moḥammad b. Aḥmad b. Yūsof b. Faqīh Elyās

[*Tashrīḥ-e badan-e ensān*] [تشریح بدن انسان]

MS Ar. 102, 201 fols., 210 x 113 mm; scribe's collection of three medical texts in Arabic (ibn an-Nafīs's anatomy, *at-Tuḥfa al-ʿalāʾīya*, and *Bayān ayyām al-baḥārīn*) and one in Persian.
[*Tashrīḥ-e badan-e ensān*] on fols. 157–181.

Bound in plain brown leather over thick stiff cardboard; inner covers pasted with heavily foxed European paper (originally light blue?). Binding somewhat worn. Written on European paper, medium thin to medium thick, burnished, light greyish-blue; watermark: galleon in wavy water, other motifs and name in capitals obscure.

29 lines, 160 x 65 mm, on blind-ruled frame and lines; black with red rubrics, these sometimes in black instead; very small, neat, but unattractive hand, varying from near *naskh* to *shekastä-āmīz*, with *naskh* proper for *Qorʾānic* quotations, etc. Catchwords. Fols. 150–157a blank.

Collations by scribe.

Copied by Moḥammad Kāẓem valad-e marḥūm-e maghferat-panāh-e Mīrzā Mahdī al-Ḥosainī (*sic* on fol. 200b); no. I dated by him Wednesday, 17 Rabīʿ I 1235/*Monday*, 3 January 1820.

On fol. 1a, a note on the sale of medical books, *Qānūn* and زبد الحکمه ناصری.[1]

The scribe's stamp on fol. 197b: ʿabduhū r-rājī Muḥammad Kāẓim al-Ḥusainī, 1208/1793.

Incipit, fol. 157b

بسمله. شکر وسپاس بیقیاس پادشاهی را سزد وحمد وثنا خالقی را رسد که درخلقت انسان دقایق حکمتش بی پایان است...

Explicit, fol. 181a, 16

پس لا جرم ناقص عقل وبیفهم وکم خرد افتاده باشد
وحق درین سخن ارادت فاعل مختار است واظهار
قدرت شامله که مندرج است در تحت حکمةِ بالغه
وهو یخرج الحیّ من المیّت ومخرج [کذا] المیت من الحی
یفعل الله ما یشاء بقدرته وتحکم ما یرید بمشیته والله
اعلم واحکم تمت

In this MS the anatomical illustrations to which the scribe's title on fol. 157b, تشریح مصوّر, alludes, are left out; there are only a few small sketches of bones in black outlines. Fols. 164b (below line 8), 168a, 169b, 173a–b, and 175a were left blank, probably for larger illustrations.

The author's name appears as Manṣūr b. Moḥammad b. Aḥmad (fol. 157b, -5), and the dedicatee's as Amīrzādä Żīāʾoddīn Pīr Moḥammad Bahādor Khān (fol. 158a, 5).

1. Probably *Zobdato l-ḥekmä-ye Nāṣerī* by Dr. Polak; see PL II 294, no. 530 (5).

No. 40 : MS 24 VIII

Anonymous

[*Qarābāẕīn*] [قراباذین]

MS 24 (ex Coll. Min.), 156 fols., 182 x 128 mm; binder's collection of eight works.
Untitled treatise on compound drugs on fols. 121–152.

For the description of the MS see **No. 61 : MS 24 I.**

Incipit, fol. 127b, -4

وصلات صلوات مبارکات وتحف تحیات نامیات
زاکیات طیبات ...

Explicit, fol. 152b, -3

حب اصطمون [کذا. یعنی اصطماخقون] بدن را از
فضول مختلف پاک کند وبلغم غلیظ لزج وسودا براند

صفة ان حب بلسان چوب عود بلسان سليخه سنبل
اسارون دارچينى پنج ازل

The author of this untitled treatise (اين رساله, fol. 128b, -5) on compound medicines calls himself simply اين فقير حقير كه بضاعت افتاده (fol. 128b, 8). The drugs are listed in forty *bāb* according to their preparation and indication. The work is dedicated to Timur's grandson Jalāloddīn Eskandar b. ʿOmar Shaikh (fol. 128b, top margin), who reigned in Fārs 812-17/1409-14.[1] Two other works on medicine by unknown authors were inscribed to this ruler: *Shāfīä dar ʿelāj,*[2] on therapy, and *Āʾīnä-ye Eskandar,*[3] on ophthalmology. A book on sexual medicine written for him, *Manāfeʿo n-nās,*[4] is preserved in a MS giving the author's name as Yaḥyā b. Saʿd Ṭabīb. A world history compiled at his court[5] also lacks title and author's name. Aubin's studies[6] on Eskandar and his patronage of art and letters suggest the possibility that he appropriated to himself other authors' works by suppressing their names and even the titles of their books.

This MS must have been transcribed from a totally disordered copy: on fol. 121a, 1 the text begins abruptly within a list of ingredients for a prescription and continues with recipes for *maʿājīn* and *mofarreḥāt* until fol. 127b, -4. There this section breaks off, and eulogies on Mohammad, part of the preface, follow (see above, Incipit); the introduction and table of contents go through fol. 129a. *Bāb* 1 and 2 follow, equally disordered. *Bāb* 10 follows immediately after *bāb* 6 on fol. 141a, 1; *bāb* 7 begins on fol. 142b, 5; *bāb* 8 and 9 (fol. 143a, 2 to 143b, 5) are both titled *galangobīn*: one of them is probably missing. In the table of contents, *bāb* 7 and 9 are erased. On fol. 143b, 5 *bāb* 10 begins again: fols. 143b, 5 to 144b, 7 repeat fols. 141a, 1 to 142a, 2. Fols. 142a, 3 to 142b, 5 and 144b, 8 to 146a, -6 represent different parts of *bāb* 10. The text breaks off within *bāb* 16, and all the rest is missing. Since this MS is not defective here (see fols. 152–156), the copy it was transcribed from must have been incomplete.

1. See J. Aubin, "Le mécénat timouride à Chîrâz," *Studia Islamica* VIII (1957) 71–88. On his titles see Blochet (note 2 below).
2. Blochet II 97, no. 847.
3. Rahāvard, p. 1, no. 259 IX.
4. Teheran, Sénat, no. 2328 III (Nashrīyä II 238).
5. PL I 86, no. 115.
6. See note 1 above.

Not in PL or Monzavī.

No. 41 : MS 61 I

abū Zain Kaḥḥāl

Sharāyeṭ-e jarrāḥī شرايط جراحى

MS 61 (ex Coll. Min.), 247 fols., 215 x 150 mm; scribe's collection of three works. (See also **Nos. 16** and **148 : MSS 61 II** and **61 III**.)
Sharāyeṭ-e jarrāḥī on fols. 3–181.

Bound in flexible plain black leather, inner covers bare; somewhat worn. Written on European paper, medium thin, transparent, glazed, white; watermark: running deer with antlers and name in capital letters (illegible because bound in). First and last fols. foxed; attempt made to blot out marginal notes; trimmed down by binder.

17 lines, 145 x 85 mm, on blind-ruled frame and lines; on some fols. written surface extends into margins; greyish-black to black with pink rubrics; one scribe employing different styles of handwriting: small to large, fair *nastaʿlīq*; *naskh* leaning to *nastaʿlīq*; neat, but undistinguished *naskh*; elegant, even copperplate *naskh*. Catchwords. Fols. 1, 2, 111b, 199b, 200, 201a, 244b, 245-247 are blank. From here on the original foliation will be quoted: it begins on fol. 3, counted as fol. 2, and runs through fol. 199, counted as fol. 198.

Collations by scribe.

Copied by Sayyed Moḥammad Bāqer b. Moḥammad Ḥosain al-Ḥosainī al-Monajjem; no. II he dated Friday, 4 Jomādā II, omitting the year; second half of thirteenth century/ca. 1835-80.

Marginal notes throughout.

Incipit, fol. 3a

واین کتابرا برده مقالت نهادیم مقاله اول ...

Explicit, fol. 181b

اما جامه را نگاهداشتن از دیوچه افسنتین
وپودنه وپوست ترنج درجامه نگاهداشتن باشد
تمام شد...

The MS contains an acephalous copy of abū Zain Kaḥḥāl's book *Sharāyeṭ-e jarrāḥī* (fol. 3b, 7). The damage must have occurred in the copy from which this was transcribed, since two blank fols. precede the text here. The author dedicated his treatise to the Tīmūrid ruler Shāhrokh, who reigned 807-50/1404-46.[1] It consists of ten *maqālä*, subdivided into *sharṭ* (table of contents on fol. 3a-b):

1. (begins on fol. 3b, 8) in 22 *sharṭ*

درشناختن نسبت بدن وشناختن ارکان ومزاج واختلاط
وقوا واعضا وشناختن تشریح بطریق کلی

2. (begins on fol. 17b, 6) in 26 *sharṭ*

درشناختن فصد واداب ان از تدارك خطا واجب برفصد
ومنع از فصد وحضرت [؟] خون وشناختن نیش وحجامت
ومضرت ومنفعت ان

3. (begins on fol. 33b, -7) in 11 *sharṭ*

درشناختن ترکیب ادوّیه [کذا] وقوت بطریق سؤال
وجواب وصفت طلا وضمادها وروغنها ومرهمها

وداروها و ترکیب نمودن سنونها وادوّیه [کذا]
گوشت خورنده وبرارنده ولاذق [کذا] وداروهای گوش
وشیافها وغرغرها وداروهای مفرد

4. (begins on fol. 63b, -5) in 6 ***sharṭ***

اندر شناختن تفرق اتصال وسببهای ان واماس وسبب ان
ودرد و اسباب ان درد وابلها ونام هریک ودانستن
مسایلی چند که درین فن بکار اید

5. (begins on fol. 67b, 2) in 90 ***sharṭ***

درشناختن اسباب وعلامات هر بیماری

6. (begins on fol. 86a, -7) in 31 ***sharṭ***

اندر شناختن مرضها [یعنی ازسر تا پای. بیاض فی الاصل]

7. (begins on fol. 92b, 5) in 9 ***sharṭ***

درشناختن نبض واختلافات ان

8. (begins on fol. 96b, 9) in 98 ***sharṭ***

درمعالجات مرضها [بیاض فی الاصل]

9. (begins on fol. 154b, 1) in 15 ***sharṭ***, arranged in 2 ***bakhsh***

درشناختن علم بدن واین مقاله دوبخش باشد بخش اول درشناختن
وشکافتن وبریدن وبیرون اوردن خنازیر وبچه مرده وپیکان وامثال
ان از بدن بخش دوّیم درداغ کردن هرعضوی چنانکه باید

10. (begins on fol. 163b, 6) in 20 ***sharṭ***

درشناختن گزیدن بهایم وانسان وماران وطلاها وضمادها
وتریاقها که درین باب بکار اید

In this treatise on the "requirements of surgery," procedures properly to be called surgical are discussed in just one *maqālä*, no. 9; circumcision, castration, and extraction of vesical and renal calculi are the operations described first. The author appears to speak here from experience and repeatedly warns against carelessness and arrogance on the part of the surgeon (see fols. 155a, 7 to 156b, -4). Certainly this *maqālä* deserves close study as one of the few discussions of surgery in Persian medical literature.

1. See PL II 228, no. 388.

PL II 228, no. 388; Monzavī I 552a, no. 5158.

No. 42 : MS 21

Moḥammad ʿAlāʾoddīn b. Hebatollāh Sabzvārī "Ghīāṣo ṭ-Ṭabīb"

Zobdat-e qavānīno l-ʿelāj زبدة قوانين العلاج

MS 21 (ex Coll. Min.), 141 fols., 188 x 124 mm

Bound in crimson leather; simple blind-tooled borders; stained, worn. Binding not original. Written on Eastern paper, medium thick, layered, burnished, cream-colored; fols. 2 and 141 substituted later in different paper. Water stains especially in the first and last fols.; spots, torn edges, repairs; some fols. loose. On lacunae see below.

11 lines, 120 x 70 mm, on blind-ruled frame and lines; black with red rubrics; medium-large, good *naskh*; fols. 2 and 141 in later but similar hand. Catchwords.

Collations, with *ṣaḥḥa*, by scribe.

Anonymous, undated copy (last fol. of the original MS missing); eleventh/seventeenth century.

Marginal notes by different readers.

On fol. 1a several erased *tamlīk*, of one the date 115 (i.e., 1115/1703?) is left; in the place of an erased note a *vaqfīyä* in Persian is written by Moḥammad Jaʿfar b. Moḥammad aṣ-Ṣafī al-Fārsī, *khādim al-madhhab al-Jaʿfarī*, on 23 Rajab 1248/16 December 1832;[1] the beneficiaries of the *vaqf* were to be himself for his lifetime, and after his death his male descendants; his stamp reads ʿabduhū Muḥammad Jaʿfar b. Muḥammad Ṣafī and is dated 1238/1822; a dated entry on fol. 82a was written by Moḥammad Reżā Ḥājj valad-e ʿAlīqolī, on the evening of Wednesday, 15 (?) Ṣafar 1156/10 April 1743.

Incipit, fol. 1b

بسمله . الحمد لله الذى خلق الانسان وجعله اشرف
مواليد الاركان والصلوة على من خص باعدل الامزجة
وارسل الى الانس والجان طبيب قلوبنا وشفاء
الامراض وعيوننا محمد ...
اما بعد چون اشارة شريفه والتماس بعضى اعزه
واخوان ... مرة بعد اخرى بترتيب وتاليف مختصرى
در معالجات شرف صدور يافته بود امتثالا لاشارتهم ...

Explicit, fol. 141a

وطاب دهن زوردار سمر [؟] جميع حيوانات
است تمت [كذا] الكتاب ...

This incomplete MS contains an anonymous, untitled treatise on therapy and protection against noxious animals in fourteen *bāb*, subdivided into *faṣl*. There are three lacunae: between fols. 1 and 2, 124 and 125 of probably one fol. each, and between fols. 140 and 141 of several fols. (the catchword on fol. 140b has been altered to conceal the lacuna). A comparison with Ethé I 1259, no. 2302, and Rieu II 477b (Add. 23557 II) shows that this work is identical with a treatise by Moḥammad ʿAlāʾoddīn b. Hebatollāh Sabzvārī, called Ghīāṣo ṭ-Ṭabīb. The MSS give different forms of its title: *Zobdat-e qavānīno l-ʿelāj,*[2] *Qavānīno ṭ-ṭebb,*[3] and *Shefāʾo l-amrāż.*[4] It cannot now be decided which is the correct wording. According to the British Museum manuscript, the author finished his work in Rabīʿ I 871.[5] Another book of his, preserved in a Bodleian MS, is *Resālä fī vajaʿ-e mafāṣel.*[6] Elgood wrongly identifies Ghīāṣo ṭ-Ṭabīb with Ghīāṣoddīn b. Moḥammad Eṣfahānī, the author of *Merʾāto ṣ-ṣeḥḥä.*[7]

1. Another *vaqfīyä* of his in **No. 111 : MS Ar. 110.**
2. Rieu II 477b; Blochet II, no. 889.
3. In *Ḥajalato l-ʿarāyes*: see **No. 44 : MS 22 I.**
4. Meshkāt III (2) 786.
5. Rieu II 477b.
6. Bodleian I 959, no. 1588.
7. Pp. 355–56; see also PL II 229, no. 395.

PL II 228, no. 391; Monzavī I 476b, no. 4413; 548b, nos. 5136–38; 597b, no. 5584; cf. the title *Shefāʾo l-amrāż,* 553b; Miklukho-Maklaĭ, p. 303, no. 2166; Yale, Persian 207.

No. 43 : MS 77 V

Ghīāṣoddīn ʿAlī b. ʿAlī Amīrān al-Ḥosainī al-Eṣfahānī

Dāneshnāmä-ye jahān دانشنامهٔ جهان

MS 77 (ex Coll. Min.), 160 fols., 247 x 132 mm; scribe's collection in six sections, nos. I–V by the same scribe; nos. I–IV, VI (fols. 1–59, 146–160) non-medical, not catalogued.
Dāneshnāmä-ye jahān on fols. 59–142.

Bound in black leather over stiff thick cardboard; blind-tooled borders, three-medallion design with blind-stamped floral scrolls; inner covers pasted with European paper, dyed pink; two flyleaves each in front and back of original MS (before fol. 1 and fols. 144–145; fols. 146–160 bound with it later), of Eastern and European papers; watermark: galloping horse on ground and POLLERI; edges of binding worn, otherwise little wear. Binding not original. Written on Eastern paper, medium thin to medium thick, burnished, beige; fols. 146–160 of Russian paper; blind stamp: FALBSKOI FABRIKI and O M; little wear.

Fols. 1–143: 19 lines, 170 x 80 mm, on blind-ruled frame and lines; black with red and crimson rubrics, sometimes repeated in margins; medium small, dense, neat *nastaʿlīq*. Catchwords.

Fols. 1–143: copied, and dated (fol. 142b, 2) 1 Zū l-ḥejjä 1021/4 March 1612, by Darvīsh Moḥammad b. Loṭfollāh Dāmghānī.

Medical notes by scribe on fols. 142b–143b.

Owner's stamp on fol. 119a: yā ʿAbbās ʿalī.[1]

Incipit, fol. 59b, 9

بسمله. وبه نستعین. سزاوار ستایش وسپاس مبدعیست
که باقتضای ذاتی او که بلسان صاحب نوامیس الهی
بامر کن معبر گشته جوهر بسیط شریف مدرك بالذات ومنشاء
مکونات که بلسان حکیم باسم عقل کل خوانده شده تعین یافته ...

Explicit, fol. 142a, -3

وآن پردها منتسج می باشند از عروق صغاری که نابتند از
غصون رحم تمام باشد. تشریحات تمام اعضای ظاهری
وباطنی آدمی که خاتمه کتاب دانشنامه جهان مشتمل
بود. بران امید که ناظران را کمال فایده حاصل گردد بحق
محمد وآله اجمعین تمت الکتاب [کذا] ...

End of main section of text and beginning of *khātemä,* fol. 123a, 1

واحتیاط رسمی آنست که نسخ وکتب این فن را
مخبرند ودهند بیان مسایل فصول واصول ونتایج این
کتاب دانشنامه جهان برین وصیت ختم شد در شهور
سنه تسع وسبعین وثمانمائه بعد ازین شروع در خاتمه
کتاب نموده می شود بعون الله تعالی وحسن تیسیره
بسمله. این خاتمه کتاب دانشنامه جهانست
که کمترین خاندان علی عمران غیاث الدین علی ابن علی
امیران الحسینی الاصفهانی بر ترتیب آن اقدام نموده در
شهور سنه تسع وسبعین وثمانمایه در دیار پرانوار
بدخشان وبیان مقاصد این خاتمه در صدر کتاب
مقرر شده که متضمن تشریحات اعضای انسانست ...

Ghīāṣoddīn ᶜAlī b. ᶜAlī Amīrān[2] al-Ḥosainī al-Eṣfahānī (fol. 60a, 4) wrote his encyclopedia of natural sciences *Dāneshnāmä-ye jahān* (see above) at Badakhshān in 879/1474 (see above).[3] He dedicated it to the Timurid ruler of Badakhshān, Solṭān Maḥmūd Bahādor Khān,[4] according to a MS in Mashhad.[5] In the main section Ghīāṣ discusses various sciences,[6] whereas in the *khātemä* (fols. 123a, 3 to 142b, 1) his subject is the anatomy of the human body. The *khātemä* is divided into one *tabṣerä,* on the four elements, the basic qualities, etc., and into 32 *vaṣlä,* on the "simple and compound" parts of the body.[7]

1. Possibly identical with the first owner of **MS 66**; see **No. 194** below.
2. This appears to be the correct form of the name of the author's father (see Rieu II 439b, *ad* Add. 16829; Ethé I 1186, nos. 2173–74; Bodleian I 891, no. 1456; in Pertsch, p. 372, no. 353, the name is ʿEmrān).
3. On his work *Dorrato l-mesāḥat*, written for the instruction of two architects in 884/1479, see Monzavī I 171a, no. 1488; PL II 10, no. 22.
4. See EI^2 I 852b, s.v. Badakhshān (851b–855a [W. Barthold/ A. Bennigsen and H. Carrère-d'Encausse]).
5. See *Dharīʿa* VIII 46, 7 (no. 115).
6. A detailed table of contents is found in Pertsch (see note 2 above for reference).
7. Another work on medicine of his is extant in a manuscript at Punjab Public Library (Panjāb P.L., p. 336, no. 253 b). Its title is *Ḥefẓo l-badan* and it discusses the medicinal properties of drugs in tabular form, divided into sixteen *faṣl*; for similarly organized works cf., e.g., **No. 15 : MS 84.**

Monzavī I 422a, nos. 3903–16; Cambridge, *Supp.*, p. 80, no. 470 (p), King's, No. 187; Katrak, p. 139, no. 595 [Gujarati version by Aspandyarji].

No. 44 : MS 22 I

Sharafoddīn Ḥasan Shīrāzī

Resālä-ye yanbūʿ رسالهٔ ینبوع

MS 22 (ex Coll. Min.), 194 fols., 210 x 135 mm; in the margins of fols. 20b–22a another text in a different hand (see **No. 87 : MS 22 II**).

Bound in olive-green leather over thick, stiff cardboard; flap; simple blind-tooled borders, three-medallion design with blind-stamped floral scrolls; spine of black leather; inner covers pasted with blue, yellow, and pink marbled paper; front flyleaf of light yellow Russian (?) paper. Binding worn, corners damaged. Written on medium-thick, burnished, white European paper; watermark obscure; first and last fols. torn, repaired, and pasted back into MS; fol. 194 substituted later, of the same paper as front flyleaf; stained, worn throughout.

I. 15 lines, 138 x 95 mm, on blind-ruled lines; black with red rubrics and overlinings; medium-small, uneven, undistinguished *naskh* leaning to *nastaʿlīq*; fol. 194a substituted later, medium-small, ugly *shekastä-āmīz*. Fol. 1b has a *sarlowḥ*: multicolored floral scrolls on ultramarine and gold; title and author given in vocalized, ultramarine *thuluth* on gold (see below); fols. 1b and 2a have a fine *jadval* of black, gold, two black, blue lines; fols. 2b–193b have a border of a single blue hairline. II. Margins of fols. 20b–22a: diagonal and horizontal lines; medium-small, copperplate *naskh*.

Collations by scribe I.

Anonymous, undated copy (end missing); ca. 1000/1600. The substituted end of the text was copied, and dated in Moḥarram 1280/18 June–17 July 1863, by *khādemo l-aṭebbā* Mīrzā ʿAbdo r-Raḥīm Ṭabīb; according to his colophon, the *aṣl* was written in 931/1524 (does this refer to the MS from which he transcribed, possibly even the last damaged fol. of this MS? See also below.).

Medical notes on fol. 1a and in margins, among others from works such as *Khoffī-ye ʿAlāʾī*.[1]

On fol. 1a a *tamlīk* by one Aḥmad Kharkāmī and an effaced stamp.

Incipit, fol. 1b

کتاب ینبوع تصنیف مولانا شرف الدین حسن طبیب
بسمله. الحمد لله رب العالمین والصلوة والسلام علی رسوله
وحبیبه محمد وآله الطیبین الطاهرین بدانکه آدمی مرکبست
ازین جسد محسوس وروحی غیر محسوس که حکما آنرا نفس
ناطقه میگویند...

Explicit, fol. 194

طلا للحكة والقمل ميويزك وزرنيخ سرخ وزراوند طويل از هريك
يك جز واجزارا كوفته وپخته بزيت سرشته درو درحمام
بعد از عرق طلا كنند تمام شد كتاب رساله ينبوع الطب ...

Sharafoddīn Ḥasan (see Incipit)[2] divided his treatise *Resālä-ye yanbūʿ*[3] into twenty *faṣl,* of which the first eighteen deal with generalities on the human body and a short review of diseases in the usual order *a capite ad calcem* and general diseases (fols. 1b to 38a, 4). The last two *faṣl,* taking up by far the greater part of the book, give a detailed account of foodstuffs and simple and compound drugs. *Faṣl* 19, here numbered 18, discusses aliments; it is completed by a *khātemä* (begins on fol. 93b, 8) in three *jomlä,* on unguents (*adhān*), ophthalmic medicines, and salves (*marāhem*). *Faṣl* 20, here numbered 19, begins on fol. 95b, 3; it is divided into six *aṣl.* In the first four *aṣl,* generalities of *materia medica* and pharmacy are discussed (fols. 95b, 8 to 101a, -4). The fifth *aṣl,* in three *jomlä,* after two preliminary *jomlä* (fols. 101a, -3 to 101b, 9) lists, in the third *jomlä,* simple and compound drugs according to their indication in the usual order of diseases (through fol. 167a, 7). The sixth and last *aṣl,* finally, gives a survey of compound drugs according to their preparation, in nineteen *faṣl.*

Sālekoddīn Moḥammad Ḥamavī Yazdī[4] copied *Resālä-ye yanbūʿ* in 1006/1597 as part of his collection *Ḥajalato l-ʿarāyes*; he says that Sharafoddīn was an authority for Ghīāṣoddīn Manṣūr Dashtakī[5] and lived in the ninth/fifteenth century. His son, Najīboddīn ʿAbdollāh, was physician to Shāh Ṭahmāsp Ṣafavī and "Qoṭbshāh Dekkanī."[6] ʿEmādoddīn Maḥmūd Shīrāzī mentions Sharafoddīn along with his own grandfather as attending Solṭān Yaʿqūb Aq Qoyunlu.[7] These accounts are corroborated by internal evidence of the text itself: there is no mention of *āteshak* or another name designating syphilis. This strongly suggests a date of composition before 900/1494 and rules out the authorship of ʿEmādoddīn Maḥmūd, a physician well aware of this new disease.[8] Thus it appears certain that Shāh ʿAbbās's poet and boon companion Sharafoddīn Ḥasan "Shefāʾī" has nothing to do with *Resālä-ye yanbūʿ*.[9]

1. See **MSS 7–10.**
2. In *Ḥajalato l-ʿarāyes* he is called Sharafoddīn Ḥasan Shīrāzī; see below, note 6.
3. In the Incipit it is called *Ketāb-e yanbūʿ*; the substituted colophon has *Resālä-ye yanbūʿo ṭ-ṭebb,* and in *Ḥajalä,* it is simply *Yanbūʿ* (see note 6 below).
4. See PL II 255, no. 437; **No. 99** below (**MS 46 II**), notes; Leipzig, *Cat.*, p. 512, no. CCLXVII, 6.
5. Divine and philosopher, lived 900–948/1494–1541/2; see Rieu II 826a, *ad* Add. 16819 I (quotations from *Majāleso l-moʾmenīn*), and Ethé I 393, no. 204 (*Haft Eqlīm*).
6. Nashrīyä III, 15a, no. 8 (see no. 9 for the date); cf. Elgood, p. 356. Which ruler of the Qoṭbshāhī dynasty is meant is not clear; see EI[1] II 1254, s.v. Ḳuṭb Shāhī [T. W. Haig].
7. See **No. 102 : MS 46 III.**
8. See **MS 46 II**, etc. In the British Museum copy, a scribe's note names ʿEmādoddīn as the author of *Yanbūʿ*; cf. PL II 243f., no. 411 (12).
9. On Shefāʾī see Eskandar Monshī II 1082, 13; Ethé I 834, no. 1531; Browne, Lit. Hist. IV 256.

Monzavī I 611a, nos. 5692–94; cf. ibid., no. 5695; 576a, nos. 5369–70, s.v. *Favāyed-e aghzīä*; see PL II 244, no. 411 (12); cf. also Monzavī I 577a, no. 5193; Kekelidze, p. 59, no. 37 (P K 3) [?]; Tashkent IX 345, no. 6518 (8896 II).

No. 45 : MS 98

ibn an-Nafīs/ Qoṭb Moḥammad Ṭabīb [?]

Resālä-ye Sohailīyä رسالهٔ سهيليّه

MS 98, 112 fols., 207 x 110 mm

Bound in flexible plain black leather; inner covers bare; one flyleaf each in front and back, of European paper, in front glazed and dyed light greyish-green, in back glazed and cream-colored (watermarks obscure in both); binding worn and stained. Binding and flyleaves not original. Written on Eastern paper, medium thin, burnished, white; edges torn, repaired; worn; stains and spots. On lacunae see below.

19 lines, 163 x 63 mm, on blind-ruled frame and lines; black with red rubrics; medium-sized, good *nasta'līq*. Catchwords.

Anonymous, undated copy (end missing); twelfth/eighteenth century.

Medical notes on flyleaves, among them quotations from Mīrzā Moḥammad Mo'men Tonakābonī.

This is an incomplete copy of *Resālä-ye Sohailīyä* (fol. 34a, 5, in the title of *jomlä* 4). As far as preserved in this MS, it is divided into seven *jomlä*, on theoretical and practical medicine:

1. (beginning missing, starts on fol. 3a, 1) in 4 *bāb*, subdivided into *faṣl*, and partly further into *qesm*, on theoretical medicine.
2. (begins on fol. 13b, 3) in 2 *bāb*, subdivided into *faṣl* — در بیان علم عملی
3. (begins on fol. 21a, 7) in 2 *faṣl* — در بیان احکام ودوا وخاصیت دواهاء [کذا]
4. (begins on fol. 34a, 5) in 23 *faṣl* — در مرضها خاصة
5. (begins on fol. 97a, -2) in 3 *bāb*, subdivided into *faṣl* — در مرضها عامه
6. (begins on fol. 108a, -4) — در مرضهاء آینه
7. (begins on fol. 110b, -3) — در زهرها ودور بودن ازان

The text breaks off on fol. 111b within the section on "pesticides"; the order of fols. is to be rearranged as follows: beginning missing, fol. 2 (containing part of the table of contents), lacuna (of one fol.?), fol. 3 (within *faṣl* 2 of *bāb* 1 of *jomlä* 1), fols. 4–104, fol. 1, fols. 105–111, end missing.

Qoṭb Moḥammad Ṭabīb did a Persian version of ibn an-Nafīs's *Mūjiz al-Qānūn* for Neẓāmoddīn Shaikh Aḥmad Sohailī (died 907/1501-02);[1] it is titled *Sohailīyä* and is divided into a *moqaddemä* and seven *jomlä*.[2] Close examination of the two texts, Qoṭb's *Sohailīyä* and the UCLA manuscript, is needed to determine whether they are identical.

1. Ḥosain Vā'eẓ Kāshefī revised *Kalīlä va-Demnä* for him under the title *Anvār-e Sohailī* (see Rieu II 756a).
2. See Monzavī I 505b, s.v. *Sohailīyä*, nos. 4676–77; one of the two MSS listed was transcribed in 907/1501 (Majles, no. 5315).

Monzavī I 505b, nos. 4676–77; Tashkent X 4; ibid., 119, no. 6866 (11541); cf. PL II 201, no. 355 (5); Ullmann, pp. 154, 173.

No. 46 : MS 23

Shāh Bahā'o d-dowlä b. Shāh Qāsem b. Moḥammad Nūrbakhshī

Kholāṣato t-tajāreb — خلاصة التجارب

MS 23 (ex Coll. Min.), 336 fols., 304 x 187 mm

Bound in plain black leather over thick, stiff cardboard; inner covers pasted with yellow-green paper; binding worn, stained, faded, torn along edge of spine. Binding not original. Written on medium-thin, burnished, cream-colored Eastern paper; edges of first and last fols. torn, mended; many leaves loose in binding; MS trimmed down when restored.

25 lines, 217 x 117 mm, on blind-ruled frame and lines; black with red rubrics and overlinings (rubrics sometimes left out); medium-large, even *nastaʿlīq*. Catchwords.

Collations by scribe and readers.

Copied, and dated Saturday, 16 Moḥarram 1062/*Friday*, 29 December 1651, by Żīāʾoddīn Moḥammad b. Ḥājj Moḥammad al-Kāteb.

Rubrics often repeated in margins; on fols. 1a and 336 recipes, poems, prayers; on fol. 336b a horoscope, dated Tuesday, 12 Rabīʿ II 1204/*Wednesday*, 30 December 1789, for Mīrzā Moḥammad Ebrāhīm's birth.

On fol. 1a several *tamlīk* erased; on fols. 1a and 301a a *tamlīk* in a flamboyant calligraphy by ebn ʿAbdo l-Qāder Moḥammad Qāsem at-Tūnī; his stamp at the side is dated 1064/1653. On fols. 1a and 335b *tamlīk* by abū l-Ḥasan b. ʿAbdo l-Qāder ash-Sharīf aṭ-Ṭabīb, dated 1141/1728; his stamp is dated 1149/1736.

On fol. 1a a stamp reading: huwa ʿabdu l-ʿAlīyi abū l-Ḥasan, dated 1132/1719.

Incipit, fol. 2a, -11

بسمله. وبه نستعين. حمد بلا احصى حكيمى را سزد كه
بكمال حكمت و وفور عنايت و قدرت ماهيت اشرف
انسانى را از جمله خزانه جود خلعت وجود پوشانيد...
اما بعد چنين معروض ميدارد خادم فقراء الملة بهاء الدوله
هداه الله تعالى كه چون كلام حضرت سيد الانام عليه
التحيه والسلام كه من كتم علما نافعا الجمه الله تعالى يوم
القيامة بلجام من النار امر بود باظهار علم نافع مردين را بابدن...

Explicit, fol. 335a, 3

ورب عبارتيست از غليظ ساخته عصاره چيزها خواه
بافتاب بود وخواه باتش چنانكه در رب فواكه مقرراست
والله اعلم بالصواب تمت الكتاب [كذا]...

Kholāṣato t-tajāreb (fol. 2b, 1) by Bahāʾo d-dowlä (fol. 2a, -3) is divided into 28 *bāb*, on hygiene, pediatrics, fevers, diseases *a capite ad calcem*, other general diseases, compound medicines, and technical terms used in the field.[1] A detailed table of contents is prefixed to the text in this MS, on fols. 1b-2a. The author wrote his work as an act of piety, to communicate to his brethren the useful knowledge he had acquired (see above, Incipit), at the village of Ṭorosht in the province of Rāz (*sic*) in 907/1501-02 (fol. 2a-b).

Kholāṣato t-tajāreb merits detailed study as a late compendium of medicine that is not limited to a discussion of *materia medica* or compound drugs; it appears to be, at least in some parts, the sum of the author's personal practice and observations.[2] The concept of contagion is not alien to him, although it does not modify his notion of disease as an imbalance of the four humors and remains within the framework of the traditional theory of miasmata in the air. Two short paragraphs on syphilis may be quoted here to illustrate Bahāʾo d-dowlä's acumen as a clinical observer:[3]

ویك نوع دیگر [یعنی از بثور] ارمنی دانه است که اندر فرنگ
پیدا شد وازانجا بروم وعربستان رسید ودر سنه اربع وتسعمائه
دراذربایجان پیدا شد وبعد ازان اندر عراق وفارس وغیره
منتشر گشت واکثر مردم ازاین ممالك وغیرها برآوردند
وبرمی اورند...

(fol. 117a, 4-6)

واین مرض [یعنی ارمنی دانه که اندر خراسان بابله فرنگ
مشهور بود، ۱۲۱ ب، ۱۰-۱۱] ازجمله امراض مسری بود
ولیکن بسیار سریع السرایه نباشد وازمجامعه با اتشك دار
رود...

(fol. 122a, 3-4)

Bahāʾo d-dowlä was the son of Sayyed Moḥammad Nūrbakhsh's younger son Shāh Qāsem.[4] According to *Ḥabību s-sīar,* he went from [the Persian] ʿErāq to Herāt shortly before the death of Solṭān Ḥosain Baiqara, stayed at the *khānqāh* of Khwājä Afżaloddīn Kermānī, and won the sultan's favor. After Ḥosain's death, he went back to ʿErāq and Āẕarbaijān, and entered the service of Shāh Esmāʿīl Ṣafavī. Three years later he died. This account would fix the date of his death in the year 914/1508, or possibly 915/1509, approximately three years after Ḥosain Baiqara's death in 911/1505.[5]

In addition to *Kholāṣä,* Bahāʾo d-dowlä left a commentary on *arbaʿūn ḥadīthā,* titled *Hadīyato l-khair.*[6] No other work of his is known as yet.

The MSS of *Kholāṣä* and *Hadīyä* and the biographical sources are at variance with each other on Bahāʾo d-dowlä's, his father's, and his grandfather's names and *laqab.* In a MS of *Hadīyä,* the author is called Ḥasan b. Qāsem b. Moḥammad an-Nūrbakhsh,[7] and in two MSS of *Kholāṣä* his name is given as Moḥammad Ḥosain Nūrbakhshī,[8] but most commonly he is known by Bahāʾo d-dowlä.[9] His father's, Shāh Qāsem's, *laqab* is given as Qevāmoddīn by Ḥājjī Khalīfa[10] and some MSS of *Kholāṣä,*[11] but in *Ḥabību s-sīar, Haft Eqlīm,*[12] and Taqī Kāshī's[13] *taẕkerä* no *laqab* is found; in other MSS of *Kholāṣä,* Shāh Qāsem's *laqab* is Serājoddīn, and his father's, Moḥammad's, is given as Shamsoddīn.[14] Bahāʾo d-dowlä had at least two sons, Shāh Reżā[15] and Naṣro d-dowlä Aḥmad. A grandson of the latter, Neẓāmoddīn Aḥmad b. Qāsem, copied *Kholāṣä* in 984/1576.[16]

1. For a detailed table of contents see Bankipore XI 12-14, no. 971.
2. Cf. Elgood, pp. 353-55 and index.
3. Cf. also the other sections on *amrāż-e vabāʾī.*
4. See the following text and notes.
5. *Ḥabību s-sīar* IV 612, 5-15.
6. *Dharīʿa* VII 218, 6 (no. 1054). In the Bodleian Library is preserved a treatise on physiognomy, *Resālä dar ʿelm-e ferāsat,* the author of which is called Nūrbakhsh (*Cat.* I 1083, no. 1880; identical with ibid., 903, no. 1476 I?). It is not known whether Bahāʾo d-dowlä is the author of this tract.
7. See preceding note for reference.
8. Ethé I 1282, no. 2348; 1602, no. 2955.
9. In *Ḥabību s-sīar,* he is called Shāh Bahāʾoddīn (IV 612, 5).
10. III 164, 8, no. 4750.

11. Blochet II 101, nos. 852-53; Bursa, Haraççıoğlu, p. 15, (58) 1138 (F.).
12. Ethé I 458, nos. 724-26; nos. 1077-80.
13. Sprenger I 42, no. 570.
14. Browne, *Catalogue*, p. 186f., P. 24 (10); this MS was copied from the author's autograph at three removes; Bankipore XI 12, no. 971. Cf. also *Dharīʿa* VII 218, 3.
15. See note 13 above.
16. See note 11 above, on the Bursa MS.

PL II 230, no. 400; Monzavī I 527a, nos. 4874-93; Tabrīz I 463, no. 392 (*shomārä-ye daftar* 3479); Bursa, p. 15, no. (58) 1138 [Harraççıoğlu library]; Tashkent IX 287-91, no. 6440 (3664).

No. 47 : MS 25

Yūsof b. Moḥammad b. Yūsof "Yūsofī"

[*Majmūʿä dar ṭebb va-ghair-e ān*] [مجموعه درطب وغيران]

MS 25 (ex Coll. Min.), 120 fols., 195 x 98 mm; scribe's collection of eleven works: ten from Yūsofī's *Majmūʿä* and one anonymous text. Nos. I, V, and X non-medical, not catalogued. (See also **No. 192 : MS 25 XI**.)
Yūsofī's [*Majmūʿä dar ṭebb va-ghair-e ān*] on fols. 1–107.

Bound in stiff, lacquered cardboard, spine of black leather; covers green, with a pink rose in the center and red and gold borders. Written on Italian paper, medium thin, slightly transparent, glazed, tan; watermark: coat of arms (a cross in the shield), and GB and BELLANDO; part of fol. 9 torn off (text damaged).

18 lines, 135 x 45 mm, on blind-ruled frame and lines; fols. 92a (center) to 104b are written in three columns of verses: the two lateral ones in diagonal lines, the center one in vertical lines; fols. 105a–107a written in two columns to form a herringbone design, fols. 107b–115b in four columns of the same pattern; written surface the same throughout; black with crimson rubrics; medium-small, fine *nastaʿlīq*. Catchwords. Fols. 1, 2a, 116–120 blank.

Collations by scribe.

Copied, and dated Wednesday, 7 Ramażān 1242/4 April 1827, by Naṣrollāh.

A recipe is pasted onto fol. 120.

A stamp on fol. 115b reads lā ilāha illā llāhu l-maliku l-ḥaqqu l-mubīn, ʿabduhū Muḥammad Kāẓim and is dated 124· (fourth digit of date illegible)/1824–33.

Incipit, fol. 2b, 1

بسمله. مجموعهٔ در طب وغیر آن مشتمل بر انوار حکمت...
[۲ ب، ۷] قطعه آمد این مجموعهٔ زیبا رقم   تحفه بر شه
عالم پناه   افتاب آسمان سلطنت   داور دوران
همایون پادشاه ... [۲ ب، ۱-] یوسفی بر آستانش آمده
بندهٔ دیرینهٔ بی اشتباه

Explicit, fol. 107b

اهدا زخویشتن رود هوشش   هردو عالم شود فراموشش
تمت مجموعه مولانا یوسفی حکیم...

Yūsof b. Moḥammad b. Yūsof "Yūsofī" (fol. 22a, 9)[1] collected twelve of his works in this *majmūʿä* and dedicated it to the Mughal emperor Homāyūn (fol. 2b, 9). In the preface (fol. 2b, 2–7) he lists their titles:

1. *Anvār-e ḥekmat*
2. *Qaṣīdä dar ḥefẓ-e ṣeḥḥat*
3. *Qaṣīdä dar loghāt-e Hendī*
4. *Qaṣīdä dar asmāʾ-e ajnās-e advīä*
5. *Maṡnavī dar maẕammat-e bakhl va-bakhīl*
6. *Jāmeʿo l-favāyed*
7. *Settä-ye żarūrīyä*
8. *Dalāyelo n-nabż*
9. *Dalāyelo l-bowl*
10. *Favāyedo l-akhyār* (leg. *Favāyed-e akhyār*)
11. *Tadbīr-e maʾkūl va-mashrūb*
12. *Monājāt dar ṭalab-e ʿeshq va-maḥabbat*

Nos. 8 and 9 are missing in the text of this *majmūʿä*; the others are listed below by their actual number:

II. Fols. 15b, 8 to 17b, -2: *Qaṣīdä dar ḥefẓ-e ṣeḥḥat*

Incipit

قصیده در حفظ صحة. بعد از حمد حکیم دانا وتحیت زبده
رسل وانبیا... نموده می اید که این قصیده است مبیّنه
در حفظ صحت... [۱۶ الف، ۱] ایکه داری تندرستی از در
[حکمت درا
تا بعلتهای گوناگون نگردی مبتلا

Explicit, fol. 17b, -7

یوسفی را بکر معنی جلوه گر امد بفکر
تا مگر سویش گشاید پادشه چشم رضا
حامی شرع محمد پادشه بابر که هست
افتاب وماه را از روی او نور وضیا

زخدا امید دارم که گیرد هرزمان
دشمنش را انچنان دردی که نپذیرد دوا

This *qaṣīdä* deals with preventive medicine, i.e., diet and hygiene, in 42 verses, introduced by a prose preface and a dedicatory *maṣnavī* of five verses to the Mughal Bābar (fol. 15b, -2).

III. Fols. 17b, -1 to 19b, -8: *Qaṣīdä dar loghāt-e Hendī*

Incipit

قصیده درلغات هندی . نام هرچیزی بهندی بشنو ازمن [ای پسر]
خاصه نام هر دوائی نفع برداری مگر
بل تکلّم دان وبل برکر بگو یعنی سخن
شکر فرماید ترا انکس که گوید شکر گر
جیت وکن آمد زبان وگوش داری ریش دان
نوج را میخوان بر دکانه کور و مهر گر

Explicit

یوسفی بهرت درین ابیات کردست انچه ذکر
گر کنی از برترا هردم رسد نفع دگر
از ضرر دارد مدامت در پناه خویشتن
انکه درعالم بتقدیرش بود نفع وضرر

The *qaṣīdä* is a "Hendī"-Persian glossary of anatomical terms, drug names, victuals, etc., in 43 verses.

IV. Fols. 19b, -7 to 21a, 5: *Qaṣīdä dar asmāʾ-e ajnās-e advīä*

Incipit

قصیده دراسماء اجناس ادویّه [کذا] . گر کنی گوش سویم ازدل وجان
مشکلات ترا کنم آسان

کنم از بهر خدمت تو رقم   نام هر داروئی بکلك و بیان ...
[۱۹ ب، ۱۰-] سادج هندی آمده تیج   لعبت بربریّه سورنجان

Explicit

یوسفی این قصیده از بهرت   زد رقم بر صحیفه دوران
که چو خوانی وخط بری گوئی   که برو باد از خدا غفران
دارد امید مغفرت گرچه   نامه او سیه شد از عصیان

An Arabic-Persian glossary of *materia medica* in 47 verses.

VI. Fols. 22a, 2 to 85b, -1: *Jāmeᶜo l-favāyed*

Incipit

جامع الفواید. بسمله. حمد نامحدود حکیمی را که بقانون حکمت وکامل الصّناعت رحمت رافع انواع امراض... [۲۲ الف، ۸] وبعد چنین بندهٔ ضعیف وکمینه نحیف المستشفی بشفاء النافع المجیب یوسفی ابن محمد بن یوسف الطبیب...

Explicit

وغذا اکرا بشیر گاو خورند نافع باشد انشاءُ [کذا] اللّه تعالی باتمام واختتام انجامید تسوید این بیاض وترشیح این ریاض والحمد لله علی الأتمام [کذا] والصلوة والسلام علی محمد خیر الانام واله البررة الکرام تم...

Jāmeᶜo l-favāyed (fol. 22b, 2) is a treatise on treatment of diseases *a capite ad calcem*, written as a commentary to, and incorporating, the author's robaᶜīyāt *ᶜElājo l-amrāż*. In his own epilogue, he gives Herat, 917/1511, as place and date of composition (see **No. 62 : MS 26 I**).

VII. Fols. 86a to 92b, 4: *Settä-ye żarūrīyä*

Incipit

سته ضروریه . الحمد لله المنعم لحیوة النفوس وصحة الاجسام
والصلوة والسلام علی واضع قانون الشرع ومن تبعه الی یوم
القیام وبعد این نسخهٔ است موسوم بسته ضروریه . . .

Explicit

ولازم افراط احتباس بود سده وعفونت وسقوط شهوت
وثقل بدن والله اعلم خاتمه اینمحقر که باد فاید سند
همه آفاق را چه خاص وچه عام
یافت در سال نهصد وچل وچهار
سمط خط وصورت اتمام

This treatise discusses the six constituent factors of health or disease (climate and seasons, food and drink, exercise and rest, emotions, sleep and waking, evacuations) in a *moqaddemä,* six chapters, and a *khātemä,* all preceded by a preface and a dedicatory *maṡnavī* of nine verses to the Mughal Homāyūn (fol. 86a, 8). Yūsofī wrote this short tract in 944/1537 (see Explicit above).

VIII. Fols. 92a, 5 to 102a: *Favāyed-e akhyār*

Incipit

بدان چونکه گفتی سپاس ودرود
که در فن طبست این قطعها
فواید شدش نام وهرحرف ازوست
زدریای حکمت دری بی بها

Explicit

بدستیاری کلکم شد این رساله تمام
که آفتی نرسد زانقلاب ایامش

زخواندنش بفواید رسند چون اخیار
بود فواید اخیار سال اتمامش

According to verse 2, these *qeṭʿä* verses, groups of two or three on diet and therapy, are simply titled *Favāyed,* but in the preface to this *majmuʿä* they are called *Favāyedo l-akhyār.* This is certainly a mistake for the chronogram *favāyed-e akhyār* (see Explicit), which gives the date of 913/1507.

IX. Fols. 102b–106a (right half): *Tadbīr-e maʾkūl va-mashrūb*

Incipit, fol. 102b (top right)

رساله در تدبیر ماکول ومشروب . زبانرا چه در اوّل این کلام
زحمد وتحیت رساندی بکام
بدان ای خردمند روشن ضمیر
که گوید چنین یوسفی حقیر
که این نسخه بهر تو کردم رقم زتدبیر ماکول ومشروب هم

Explicit, fol. 106a (bottom right)

برآورد ازلطف خود حاجتم عطا کرد بیحد وعد نعمتم
زغمهای او باد سامان من فدای ره او دل <و> جان من

These 111 couplets of *maṣnavī* verses, including a *khātemä* of seven lines, were composed in 906/1500 (*khwosh* is the chronogram مرا سال تاریخ او خوش نمود, fol. 102b, -5 [right]).

1. **MS 30 I**, fol. 4b, 8, gives Yūsofī's name in its full form: Yūsof b. Moḥammad b. Yūsof aṭ-ṭabīb *al-moshtaher be*-Yūsofī. Most MSS of *Jāmeʿo l-favāyed* abbreviate this in one way or another. On Yūsofī see also **No. 86 : MS 57 III.**

Monzavī I 588a, no. 5502 (?); another collection of Yūsofī's medical works (the same as in **MS 25**, with the exception of **MS 25 IV**): Shīrānī II 394, no. 2134; in PL no *majmūʿä* is listed separately; see below under single titles.

MS 25 III, *Qaṣīdä dar loghāt-e Hendī*: PL II 239, no. 408 (10); Monzavī I 573a, nos. 5333–37.

MS 25 IV, *Qaṣīdä dar asmāʾ-e ajnās-e advīä*: PL II 239, no. 408 (11); Monzavī I 573b, nos. 5338–42.

No. 48 : MS 24 V

Yūsof b. Moḥammad b. Yūsof "Yūsofī"

Tadbīr-e maʾkūl va-mashrūb تدبیر مأکول ومشروب

MS 24 (ex Coll. Min.), 156 fols., 182 x 128 mm; binder's collection of eight works; six of these, by Yūsofī, copied by the same scribe.
Tadbīr-e maʾkūl va-mashrūb on fols. 105a–109a.

For the description of the MS see **No. 61 : MS 24 I.**

Incipit, fol. 105a, 6, and Explicit, fol. 109a, 3, the same as in **MS 25 IX.**

PL II 238, no. 408 (7); Monzavī I 592b, nos. 5540–50; Panjāb P.L., p. 150, no. 114 XVI; Miklukho-Maklaĭ, p. 276, no. 1971; Tashkent V 274, no. 3924 (49 III); ibid., IX 302–303, nos. 6465–66 (5534 IV and 3334 X, resp.).

No. 49 : MS 26 II

Yūsof b. Moḥammad b. Yūsof "Yūsofī"

Tadbīr-e maʾkūl va-mashrūb تدبیر مأکول ومشروب

MS 26 (ex Coll. Min.), 103 fols., 178 x 120 mm; binder's collection of eleven works.
Tadbīr-e maʾkūl va-mashrūb on fols. 46–51.

For the description of the MS see **No. 62 : MS 26 I.**

Incipit, fol. 46b, and Explicit, fol. 51a, as in **MS 25 IX.**

No. 50 : MS 27 III

Yūsof b. Moḥammad b. Yūsof "Yūsofī"

Tadbīr-e maʾkūl va-mashrūb تدبیر مأکول ومشروب

MS 27 (ex Coll. Min.), 88 fols., 175 x 115 mm; binder's collection of four works; three of these, by Yūsofī, copied by the same scribe.
Tadbīr-e maʾkūl va-mashrūb on fols. 69–72.

For the description of the MS see **No. 63 : MS 27 I.**

Incipit, fol. 69b, as in **MS 25 IX.**

Explicit, fol. 72b, -6

تشنج فرو گیردت استوار   تولد کند رعشه پایان کار
بتاریخ . . .

In this MS, the *khātemä* is missing; cf. **MS 25 IX.**

No. 51 : MS 28 III

Yūsof b. Moḥammad b. Yūsof "Yūsofī"

Tadbīr-e maʾkūl va-mashrūb تدبیر مأکول ومشروب

MS 28 (ex Coll. Min.), 72 fols., 170 x 110 mm; scribe's collection of four works by Yūsofī and excerpts from various sources.
Tadbīr-e maʾkūl va-mashrūb on fols. 63b–66a.

For the description of the MS see **No. 64 : MS 28 I.**

Incipit, fol. 63b, 6

رساله مسمّی بمأکول ومشروب.
ز حکمت اگر هیچ داری خبر   غم خود خورای خواجه و پرمخور

Explicit, fol. 66a, -5

ازاین گونه ابی گر آید بدست   ترا حافظ محرت صحت است

In this MS, the first seven and the last fourteen verses of *Tadbīr-e maʾkūl va-mashrūb* were not copied; cf. **MS 25 IX.**

No. 52 : MS 29 VI

Yūsof b. Moḥammad b. Yūsof "Yūsofī"

Tadbīr-e maʾkūl va-mashrūb تدبير مأكول ومشروب

MS 29 (ex Coll. Min.), 119 fols., 200 x 135 mm; scribe's collection of ten works.
Tadbīr-e maʾkūl va-mashrūb on fols. 104–107.

For the description of the MS see **No. 79 : MS 29 I.**

Incipit, fol. 104a, 6, and Explicit, fol. 107b, as in **MS 25 IX.**

No. 53 : MS Ar. 98 XII

Yūsof b. Moḥammad b. Yūsof "Yūsofī"

Tadbīr-e maʾkūl va-mashrūb تدبير مأكول ومشروب

MS Ar. 98, 135 fols., 193 x 138 mm; fols. 89–135 a scribe's collection of six works by Yūsofī.
Tadbīr-e maʾkūl va-mashrūb on fols. 131b–135a.

For the description of the MS see **No. 85 : MS Ar. 98 IX.**

Incipit, fol. 131b, 4, and Explicit, fol. 135a, -1, as in **MS 25 IX.**

No. 54 : MS 24 IV

Yūsof b. Moḥammad b. Yūsof "Yūsofī"

Favāyed-e akhyār فوايد اخيار

MS 24 (ex Coll. Min.), 156 fols., 182 x 128 mm; binder's collection of eight works; six of these, by Yūsofī, copied by the same scribe.
Favāyed-e akhyār on fols. 88b–105a.

For the description of the MS see **No. 61 : MS 24 I.**

Incipit, fol. 88b, 2, and Explicit, fol. 105a, -7, the same as in **MS 25 VIII.**

PL II 236, no. 408 (4); Monzavī I 575a, nos. 5350-67; Shīrānī II 398, no. 2156; Nūrbakhsh I 157, no. 133 IV; Miklukho-Maklaĭ, p. 409, nos. 3158-59; Osmania Univ., p. 53, no. 40 (see also p. 152); Tashkent V 275-76, nos. 3925-27 (1404 II, 1356 XXI, 1355 V, resp.).

No. 55 : MS 27 II

Yūsof b. Moḥammad b. Yūsof "Yūsofī"

Favāyed-e akhyār فوايد اخيار

MS 27 (ex Coll. Min.), 88 fols., 175 x 115 mm; binder's collection of four works; three of these, by Yūsofī, copied by the same scribe.
Favāyed-e akhyār on fols. 50–68.

For the description of the MS see **No. 63 : MS 27 I.**

Incipit, fol. 50b, and Explicit, fol. 68b, as in **MS 25 VIII.**

No. 56 : MS 28 II

Yūsof b. Moḥammad b. Yūsof "Yūsofī"

Favāyed-e akhyār فوايد اخيار

MS 28 (ex Coll. Min.), 72 fols., 170 x 110 mm; scribe's collection of four works by Yūsofī and excerpts from various sources.
Favāyed-e akhyār on fols. 56b–63.

For the description of the MS see **No. 64 : MS 28 I.**

Incipit, fol. 56b, and Explicit, fol. 63b, 5, as in **MS 25 VIII.**

No. 57 : MS 29 V

Yūsof b. Moḥammad b. Yūsof "Yūsofī"

Favāyed-e akhyār فوايد اخيار

MS 29 (ex Coll. Min.), 119 fols., 200 x 135 mm; scribe's collection of ten works.
Favāyed-e akhyār on fols. 59–65, etc. (see below).

For the description of the MS see **No. 79 : MS 29 I.**

Incipit, fol. 59a, 3, and Explicit, fol. 104a, 6, as in **MS 25 VIII.**

The correct order of fols. in this MS is: 59–65, 96–104.

No. 58 : MS 35

Yūsof b. Moḥammad b. Yūsof "Yūsofī"

Favāyed-e akhyār فوايد اخيار

MS 35 (ex Coll. Min.), 26 fols., 178 x 120 mm

Bound in flexible black leather; simple blind-tooled borders; binding too small for MS. Binding not original. Written on Eastern paper, medium thick, burnished, tan; fols. 1–3, 18–26 substituted later in European paper, medium thin, polished, tan; watermark: part of an emblem and CASA MALL (?) visible. First four fols. affected by moisture, some edges mended.

I. 13–14 lines, 125 x 75 mm; greyish-black with red rubrics; medium-sized, good *nastaʿlīq*. II. substituted fols. 3 and 18: 13–14 lines, 115 x 70 mm, on blind-ruled bicolumnar frame and lines; black; medium-sized, fair *shekastä-āmīz*. Catchwords throughout. Fols. 1–3a, 18b–26 blank.

Anonymous, undated copy (end of original MS missing); eleventh/seventeenth century. Fols. 3 and 18 copied, and dated in the last third of Rajab 1251/11–21 November 1835, by Hādī b. Mahdī Eṣfahānī.

Notes by Hādī b. Mahdī Eṣfahānī.

Incipit, fol. 3b, and Explicit, fol. 18a, as in **MS 25 VIII.**

No. 59 : MS Ar. 98 XI

Yūsof b. Moḥammad b. Yūsof "Yūsofī"

Favāyed-e akhyār فوايد اخيار

MS Ar. 98, 135 fols., 193 x 138 mm; fols. 89–135 a scribe's collection of six works by Yūsofī.
Favāyed-e akhyār on fols. 112b–131b.

For the description of the MS see **No. 85 : MS Ar. 98 IX.**

Incipit, fol. 112b, 3, and Explicit, fol. 131b, 1, as in **MS 25 VIII.**

No. 60 : MS 60 IV

Yūsof b. Moḥammad b. Yūsof "Yūsofī"

ʿElājo l-amrāż علاج الامراض

MS 60 (ex Coll. Min.), 74 fols., 240 x 150 mm; binder's collection in five sections. *ʿElājo l-amrāż* on fols. 61–64.

For the description of the MS see **No. 177 : MS 60 II.**

Incipit, fol. 61a

تفصیل ادویه مفرده از کتاب علاج الامراض .
بسمله. برای دفع صداع وشقیقه مجربست برگ

Explicit, fol. 62b, -1

وبرای سرخی وبثور زبان رسوت[؟] باآب لیمو
سائیده برزبان بمالند مفید است]

This fragment of Yūsofī's[1] (fol. 61a, 1) *ʿElājo l-amrāż*[2] (ibid.) is divided into unnumbered *faṣl* according to diseases *a capite ad calcem.* In this MS, the text breaks off within the section on the treatment of lips, tongue, and gums. The leaves have to be reordered as follows: 61, 63, 64, 62.

1. See **MSS 24, 25,** etc.
2. See PL II 237, no. 408 (5, 6).

PL II 237, no. 408 (5, 6); Monzavī I 569a, nos. 5299-5301; Miklukho-Maklaĭ, p. 383, nos. 2942–43, 2946. Verses from *Favāyed-e akhyār* and *ʿElājo l-amrāż* translated into Turkish and titled *Maghzu ṭ-ṭibb* by Ṭalʿatī: Chester Beatty, p. 122, no. 484 [translator's autograph copy, dated 1067/1656].

No. 61 : MS 24 I

Yūsof b. Moḥammad b. Yūsof "Yūsofī"

Jāmeʿo l-favāyed جامع الفواید

MS 24 (ex Coll. Min.), 156 fols., 182 x 128 mm; binder's collection of eight works; six of these, by Yūsofī, copied by the same scribe. Work VI, *Monājāt dar ṭalab-e ʿeshq va-maḥabbat*, of non-medical contents, not catalogued. (See also **Nos. 40, 48, 54, 77, 80,** and **207**.)
Jāmeʿo l-favāyed on fols. 1-73.

Bound in dark brown leather over stiff cardboard; flap; simple blind-tooled borders and center ornament, also on flap; new endpapers, but inner flap pasted with older marbled paper. Written on Eastern paper of four varieties: 1) fols. 1-74: medium thin to medium thick, burnished, cream-colored; 2) fols. 75-110: thick, layered, burnished, cream-colored; 3) fols. 111-120: medium thick, burnished, cream-colored; 4) fols. 121-156: medium thick, burnished, cream-colored; nos. 3 and 4 later additions to original Yūsofī collection. Water stains, spots, foxing, few leaves show original color of paper; some wormholes.

I. Fols. 1-110: 12-19 lines, 130-45 x 70-80 mm, blind-ruled frame and lines not closely followed; greyish-black with red rubrics; medium-large, uneven, undistinguished *nastaʿlīq*. Fol. 74 blank. II. Fols. 111-120: 18-19 lines, 125-35 x 75 mm, on blind-ruled frame and lines; greyish-black, with red rubrics; medium-small, flowing, fine *nastaʿlīq*. III. Fols. 121-152: 15 lines, 132-40 x 74-78 mm, on blind-ruled frame and lines; border of single red line on fols. 121-128; greyish-black with red rubrics; medium-sized, fair *nastaʿlīq*. Catchwords throughout.

Collations: in works I and III by scribe; in I-VII by a Turkish reader, İbrāhīm, who dated his collations of I-IV between 1098/1687 and 1101/1689 (his hand is a distinguished, copperplate *nastaʿlīq*); IV also collated by another Turkish reader who left glosses in IV and VII (see below).

Anonymous copies, undated except I: Shaʿbān 963/10 June-8 July 1556; II-VI of approximately the same date, since they were copied by the same scribe; VII and VIII possibly also tenth/sixteenth century. A *terminus ad quem* is furnished by the collations (see above).

On fol. 73b a note by İbrāhīm on his collation, partial vocalization, and glosses in I, dated 7 Rajab 1098/19 May 1687; glosses by him on fol. 156a; notes in four more hands in I-VI; among these there are glosses from *Farhang-e Jahāngīrī* in a Turkish hand in IV and VII (see above); recipes by readers on fols. 110, 111, 120a, 153-156.

Incipit, fol. 1b, as in **MS 25 VI.**[1]

Explicit, fol. 73a, -3

باتمام رسید و باختیار [کذا] انجامید تسوید این بیاض
و ترشیح این ریاض بیت بروز هژده ز ماه مبارک رمضان
بسال نهصد و هفده ز هجرت نبوی ببلدهٔ فاخرهٔ هرات
صینت عن تطرق الآفات والحمد لله علی الاتمام
والصلواة [کذا] علی محمد خیر الانام و آله البرة [کذا] الکرام
بتاریخ ...

On this, apparently the author's own epilogue, see **No. 62 : MS 26 I.**

1. Monzavī (I 566b) lists a treatise *Ṭebb-e Nāṣerī* in 47 *faṣl* by Ṭāher b. a. Bakr Ṭabīb, a descendant of Shāh Jalāloddīn Pānīpatī; its Incipit follows Yūsofī's *Jāmeʿ* verbatim. In PL (II 254, no. 434), apparently the same book is titled *Favāyedo l-foʾād* and the fact that its Incipit is identical with that of Yūsofī's treatise is noted.

PL II 237, no. 408 (6); Monzavī I 513b, nos. 4749-70; see note 1 above; cf. PL II 329, no. 584 (172); Tabrīz I 329, 387, nos. 262 (*shomārä-ye daftar* 3430) and 325 (*shomārä-ye daftar* 3414 V), resp.; Shīrānī II 388, nos. 2103-05; Madras III 939, no. 805; Miklukho-Maklaĭ, p. 383, nos. 2944-45, 2947-48; Osmania Med. Coll., p. 112, no. 33; Osmania Univ., p. 53, no. 36; Tashkent VI 151-52, nos. 4347-48 (3767 II and 9211, resp.); ibid., VII 292, no. 5448 (8391); ibid., IX 292-94, nos. 6443-48 (6277, 7689 II, 5538 III, 5534 I, 4936 I, 11259, resp.); *Bayāż-e Yūsofī* (Charminar, p. 238, no. 44) identical with *Jāmeʿ*? Cf. also *Morakkab-e Yūsofī* by Moḥammad Māh b. Valīyollāh b. Moḥammad: Tashkent IX 312-15, nos. 6479-80 (8896 I and 3531, resp.).

No. 62 : MS 26 I

Yūsof b. Moḥammad b. Yūsof "Yūsofī"

Jāmeʿo l-favāyed جامع الفواید

MS 26 (ex Coll. Min.), 103 fols., 178 x 120 mm; binder's collection of eleven works; VIII and IX, of non-medical contents, not catalogued. (See also **Nos. 49, 75, 78, 81, 112, 160, 188,** and **215**.)
Jāmeʿo l-favāyed on fols. 1-46.

Bound in flexible plain brown leather; warped, stained, worn, MS almost totally out of binding. Written on Eastern paper of two varieties: 1) fols. 1-20: thin, slightly transparent, burnished, tan; 2) fols. 21-103: thicker, but much like 1). Some wear and tear. On lacunae see single items.

I. Fols. 1-72, 82b-103: 12-17 lines, 110-50 x 60-85 mm, on blind-ruled frame and lines (on some fols. a bicolumnar frame for the copying of verses); black with red or black rubrics, these sometimes left out; various styles of *naskh* and *nastaʿlīq*, fair to good. II. Fols. 80-81: 18 lines, 150 x 85 mm, on blind-ruled frame and lines; greyish-black; medium-small, ordinary *nastaʿlīq*. Catchwords throughout the MS.

Collations by scribe in work I.

I. Works I-VII, XI: copied by Mīr Māh b. Mīr Qāsem "Monajjem-e Samarqandī"; no. I is signed and dated by him in Shavvāl 999/23 July-20 August 1591. II. Work X is an anonymous copy, dated Ramażān 981/25 December 1573-23 January 1574 (see **No. 188 : MS 26 X**).

Notes by readers throughout.

Incipit, fol. 1a (the first part of the text is missing in this MS)

بعد از قبض طبیعت حادث گردد وچون تخم ریحان
وکنوجه واسبغول ...

Explicit, fol. 46a

واگر غذا أكراء بشیر گاو بخورند نافع بود انشا لله [کذا]
تعالی باتمام رسید وباختتام انجامید تسوید این بیاض
وترشیح این ریاض بروز از هژده ماه مبارك رمضان مصراع
بسال نهصد وهفده زهجرت نبوی صلی الله علیه وسلم به بلده
فاخره هرات صینت عن تطرق الافات والحمد لله علی
الاتمام والصلواه [کذا] علی محمد خیر الانام واله البررة الکرام تمت...

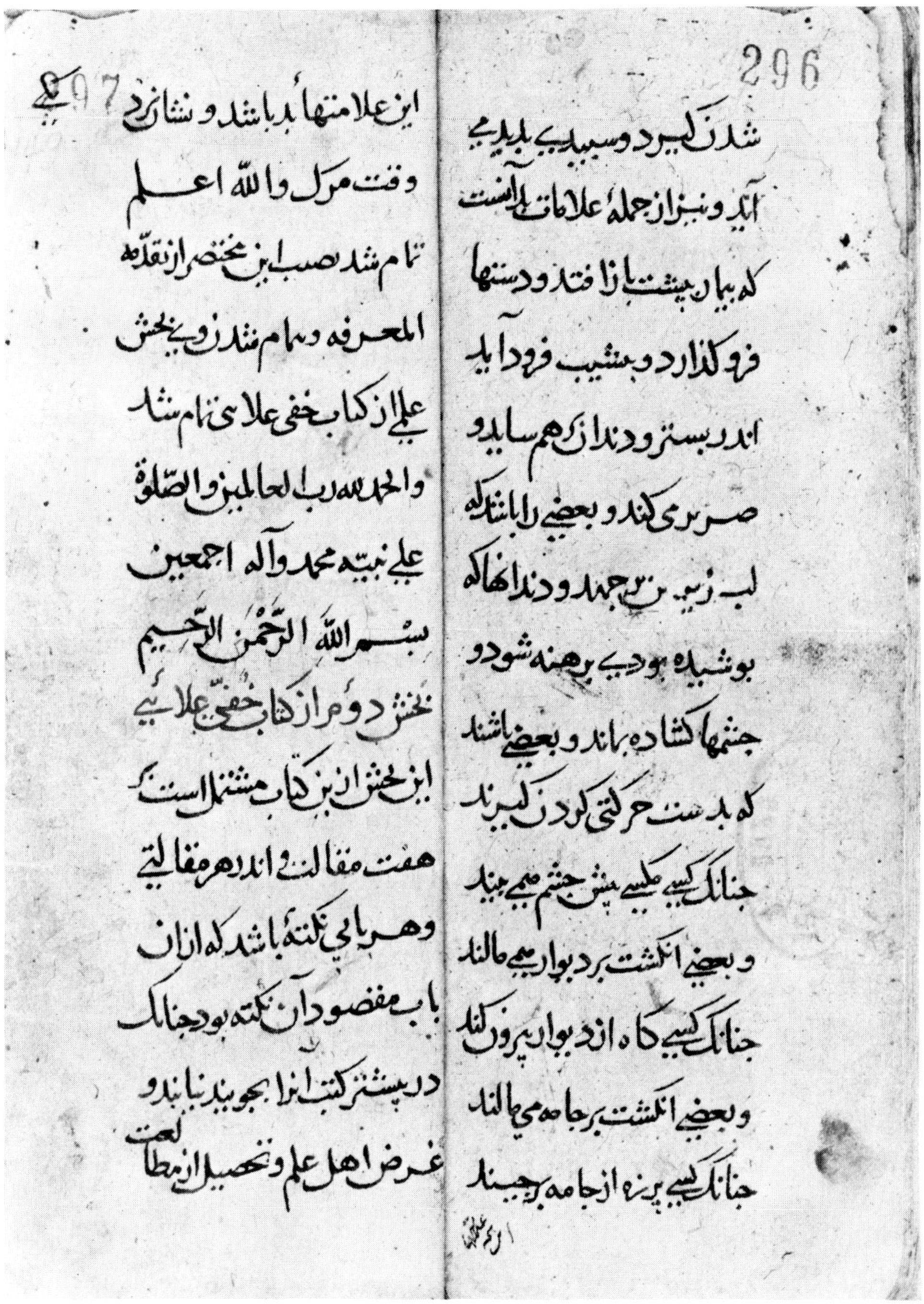

1. MS 8, fols. 148b–149a: Esmāʿīl Jorjānī, *Khoffī-ye ʿAlāʾī* (see page 15)

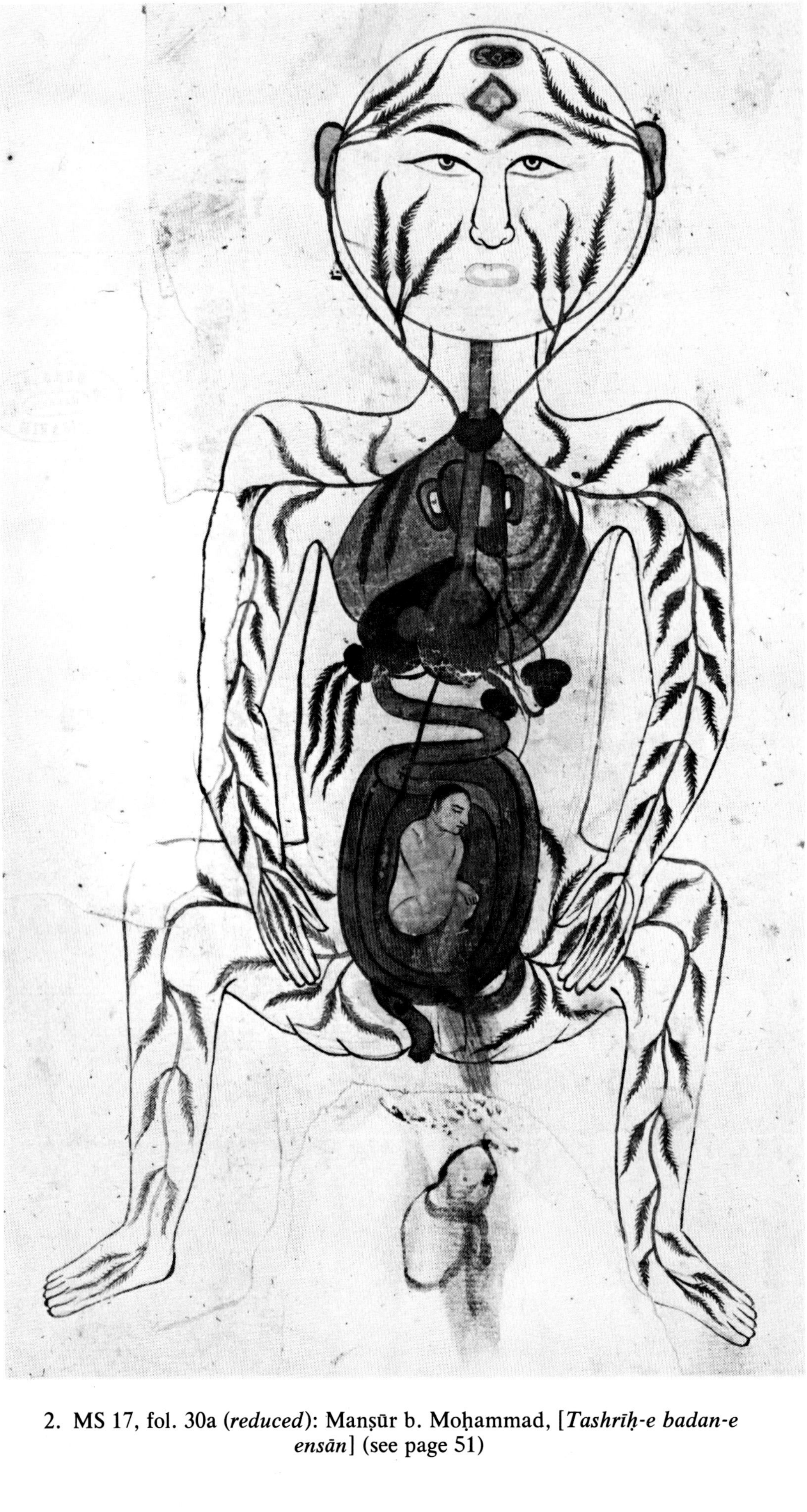

2. MS 17, fol. 30a (*reduced*): Manṣūr b. Moḥammad, [*Tashrīḥ-e badan-e ensān*] (see page 51)

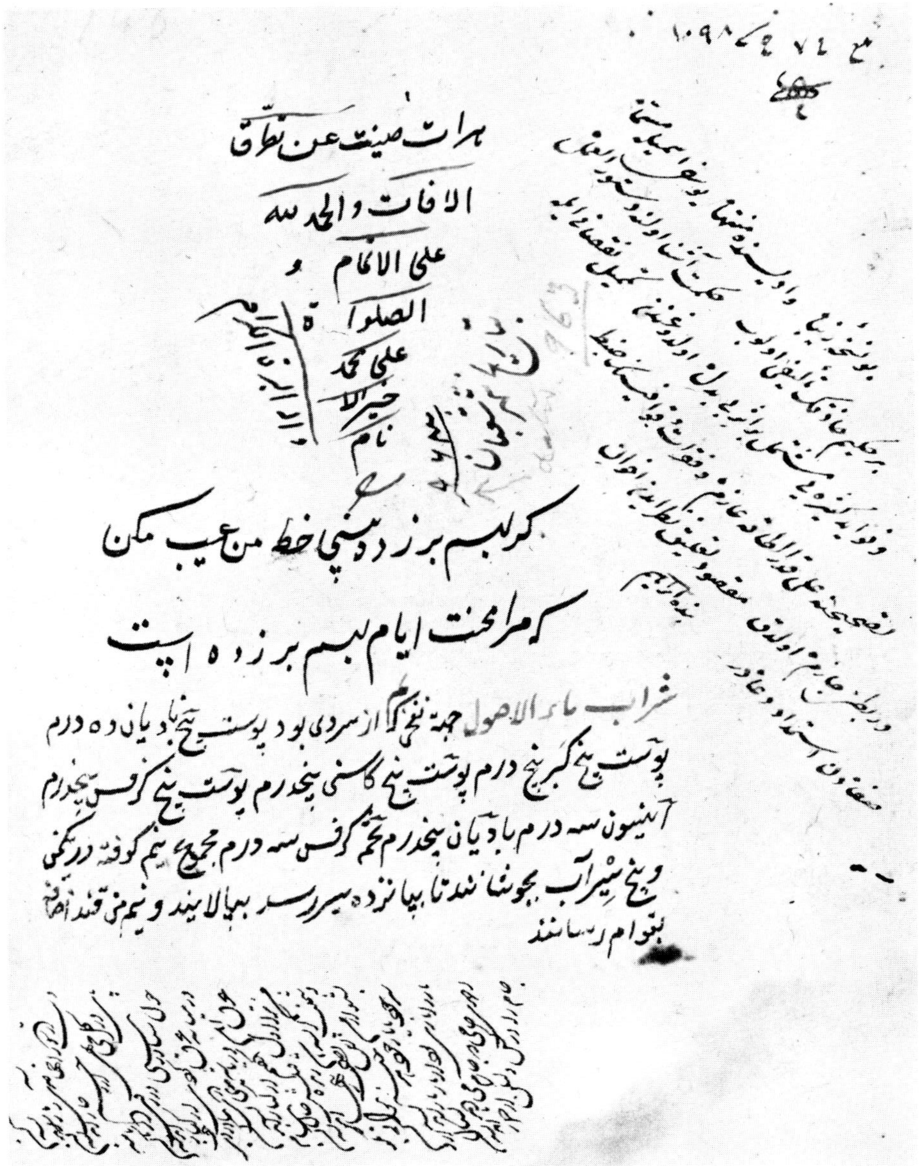

3. MS 24 I, fol. 73b: "Yūsofī," *Jāmeʿo l-favāyed* (see page 77)

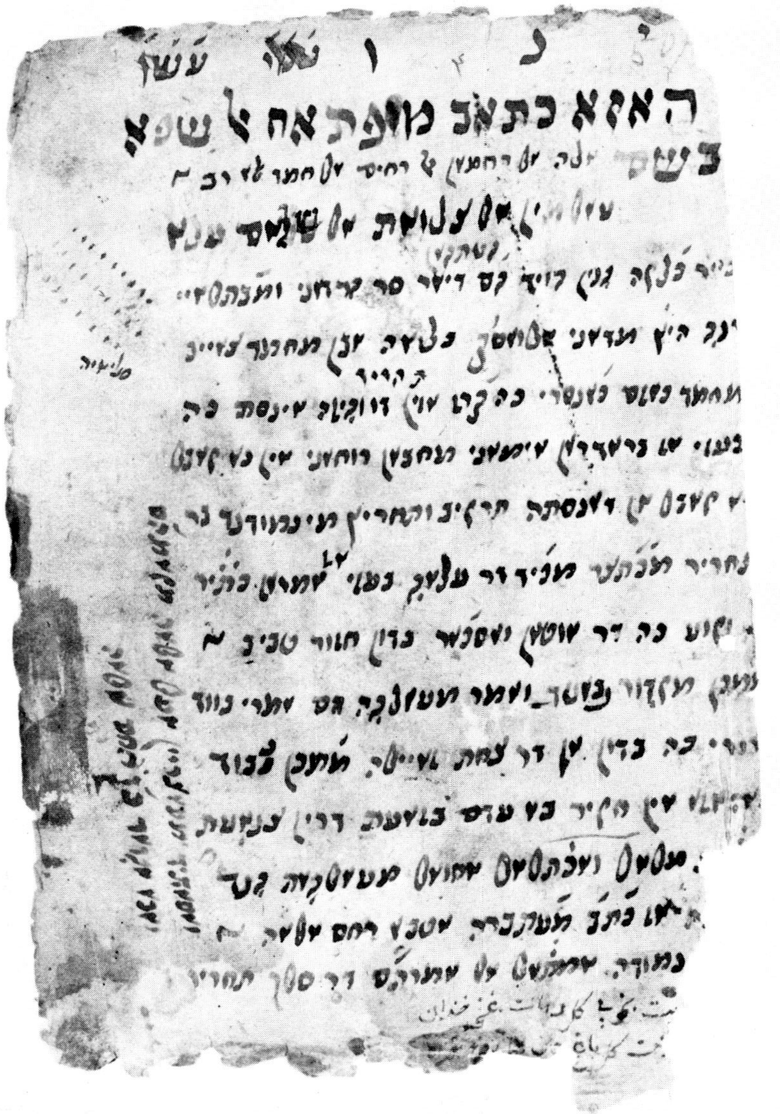

4. MS 59a, recto: Moḥammad Kāẓem b. Moḥammad Ṣāʾeb al-Khwānsārī, *Meftāḥo sh-shefāʾ* (see page 161)

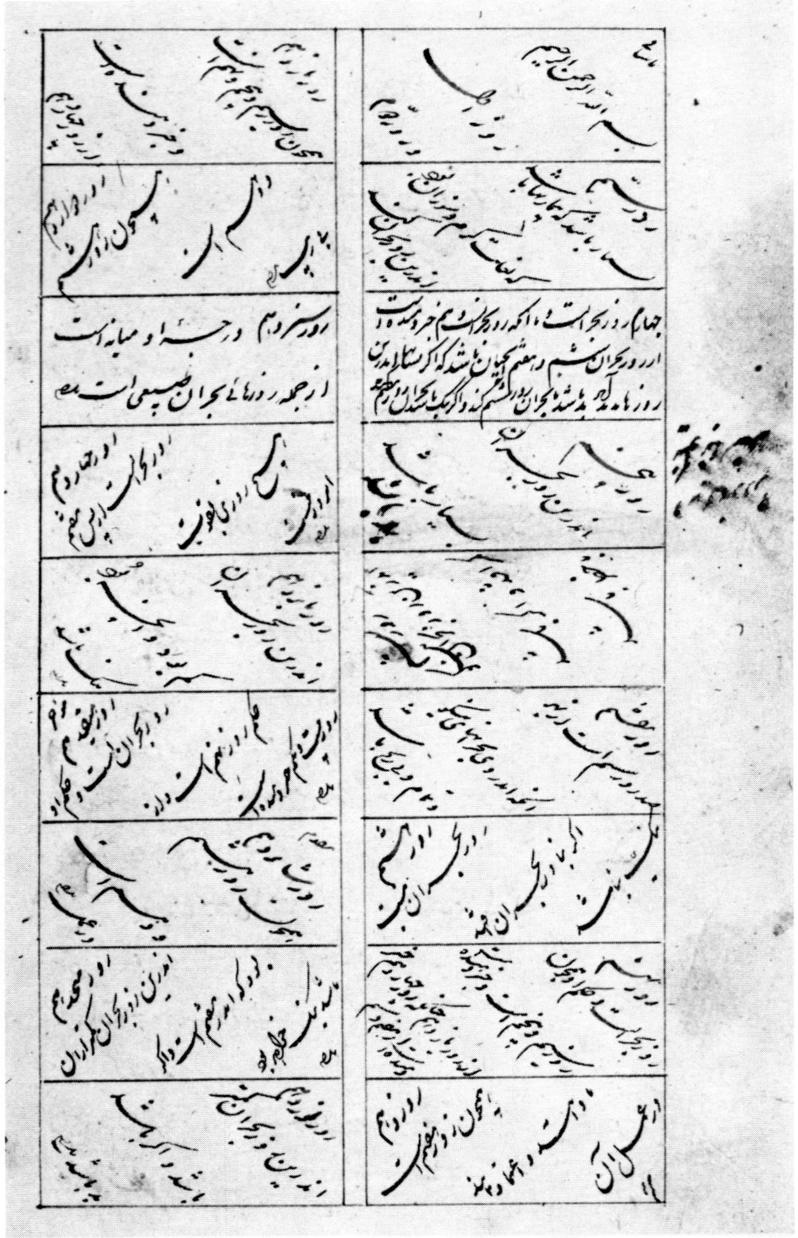

5. MS 120 III, fol. 39b: Anonymous, [*Dar rūzhā-ye boḥrān*] (see pages 136, 185)

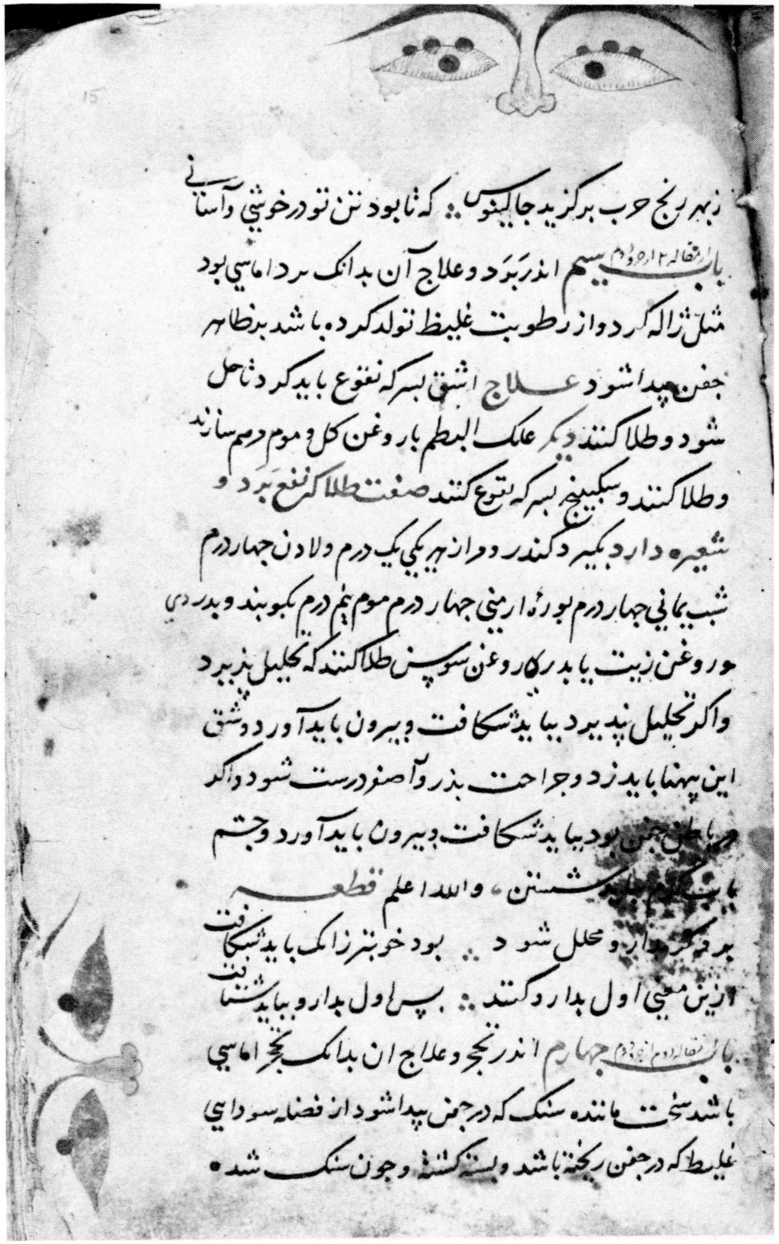

6. MS 75, fol. 15a (*reduced*): Anonymous, [*Kaḥḥālī*] (see page 215)

This epilogue, apparently the author's own conclusion of his work, gives Herāt, 18 Ramażān 917/9 December 1511, as place and date of composition. It is not preserved in all MSS of *Jāmeᶜo l-favāyed* (see, e.g., **Nos. 47** and **63 : MSS 25 VI** and **27 I**).

No. 63 : MS 27 I

Yūsof b. Moḥammad b. Yūsof "Yūsofī"

Jāmeᶜo l-favāyed جامع الفوايد

MS 27 (ex Coll. Min.), 88 fols., 175 x 115 mm; binder's collection of four works; three of these, by Yūsofī, copied by the same scribe. Work IV, *Modkhal-e manẓūm* on astrology, not catalogued. (See also **Nos. 50** and **55 : MSS 27 III** and **27 II**.)
Jāmeᶜo l-favāyed on fols. 2–49.

Bound in brown leather over thick, stiff cardboard; simple blind-tooled borders, blind-stamped three-flower design three times on front and back covers; some wear. Binding not original. Written on Eastern paper, medium thin, burnished, cream-colored; fols. 1, 69, 70, 88 later substituted in European paper, medium thin, burnished, white, no watermarks. Much foxed and water stained, most edges torn; worst damage repaired.

Fols. 1–72: 16 lines, 135 x 80 mm, on blind-ruled frame and lines, works II and III on bicolumnar lines; black with red and green rubrics; medium-small to small, even, fine *shekastä-āmīz*. Catchwords.

Copied by ebn Moḥammad Raḥīm Moḥammad Karīm Torkmān; he dated work I on 19, works II and III on 25, Moḥarram 1136/19 and 25 October 1723, corresponding to *toshqan il*, "the year of the hare," of the Turkish animal-cycle calendar.

Marginal notes by readers.

On fol. 1a a *tamlīk* by Naṣīroddīn Moḥammad Khwājä-ye Naṣīrī, dated 20 Rabīᶜo l-ūlī (*sic*) $\frac{1324}{1366}$/11 February 1947. Another *tamlīk* on fol. 69a by Shams al-afāḍil al-Kashmīrī al-Khalīlābādī al-Khuwāja Naṣīrī (*sic*) al-muqīm bi-Ṭihrān is dated: sanat 1305 *h. sh.*/1926; apparently he was related to the later owner who wrote the *tamlīk* on fol. 1a.

Incipit, fol. 2b, and Explicit, fol. 49a, 5, as in **MS 25 VI.**

No. 64 : MS 28 I

Yūsof b. Moḥammad b. Yūsof "Yūsofī"

Jāmeᶜo l-favāyed جامع الفوايد

MS 28 (ex Coll. Min.), 72 fols., 170 x 110 mm; scribe's collection of four works by Yūsofī and excerpts from various sources. (See also **Nos. 51, 56, 76,** and **208.**)
Jāmeᶜo l-favāyed on fols. 2–56a.

Bound in flexible plain brown leather. Written on Eastern paper, medium thick, burnished, greyish-aquamarine; some wear and tear. For lacunae see below.

13–18 lines, ca. 130 x 65 mm; greyish-black with crimson overlinings; medium-small, uneven, ugly *nastaᶜlīq*. Catchwords.

Anonymous, undated copy; ca. 1200/1800.
Marginal notes by reader.
On fol. 2a a *vaqfīyä* by Moḥammad Esmāʿīl b. Shamsoddīn Moḥammad, dated Rajab 1230/9 June–8 July 1815; below this note his stamp: al-ʿabd Muḥammad Ismāʿīl 1174/1760. On fol. 2a also a stamp of his father: Shams ad-Dīn Muḥammad b. ʿAlī al-Ḥusainī; on fol. 2b one of his and his father's: ʿabduhū ʿAlī Muḥammad al-Ḥusainī.

Incipit, fol. 2b, and Explicit, fol. 56a, as in **MS 25 VI.**

No. 65 : MS 29 III

Yūsof b. Moḥammad b. Yūsof "Yūsofī"

Jāmeʿo l-favāyed جامع الفواید

MS 29 (ex Coll. Min.), 119 fols., 200 x 135 mm; scribe's collection of ten works.
Jāmeʿo l-favāyed on fols. 9–57, etc. (see below).

For the description of the MS see **No. 79 : MS 29 I.**

Incipit, fol. 9b, as in **MS 25 VI.**

Explicit, fol. 83b, -7

و حیوانی چون زراریح [کذا] وزهره افعی وزهره پلنگ
وکژدم وگوزن وحسکل برشیر [آیا یعنی جند بید ستر؟] [

The text breaks off within the section on poisons; cf. **MS 25**, fol. 85b, 2. It appears to be copied here from an incomplete MS. The correct order of fols. is as follows: 9–57, 66–80, 89–95, 81–83, end missing.

No. 66 : MS 30 I

Yūsof b. Moḥammad b. Yūsof "Yūsofī"

Jāmeʿo l-favāyed جامع الفواید

MS 30 (ex Coll. Min.), 85 fols., 185 x 110 mm; scribe's collection of two works. (See also **No. 29 : MS 30 II.**)
Jāmeʿo l-favāyed on fols. 1–8, etc. (see below).

Modern brochure of brown paper; endpapers stiff white paper; spine broken twice, most of MS out of binding. Written on Eastern paper, medium thick, burnished, tan; some ink smears, edges mended. On lacunae see below.

17 lines, 142 x 72 mm, on blind-ruled frame and lines; greyish-black with red rubrics; small, even, deliberate *nastaʿlīq*; simple designs in some margins. Catchwords.

Collations by scribe.

Anonymous copy, work II dated last third of Ṣafar 940/10–19 September 1533.

Many recipes on first and last fols. and in margins. On fol. 1a-b two prescriptions to help overcome an opium addiction; the first of these is incomplete, the second is titled طریق ترك كردن افیون بطریق اهل هند; one recipe on fol. 1a is ascribed to Ghāzī Rūmlū.

On fol. 4a an erased *tamlīk*.

On fols. 4a and 85b an erased stamp; one stamp on fol. 4b reads: ʿabduhū samīʿan 121 (i.e., 1121/1709?).

Incipit, fol. 4b, as in **MS 25 VI.**

Explicit, fol. 14b, -2

چون دست دهد ز شرب سمّت حالی
گر رنج شوی براه غم پامالی
از بهر خلاصیت بنزدیك حکیم [...

The text breaks off in the paragraph on poisons. As far as preserved, this MS is misbound; the correct order of fols. is as follows: 1-8, 28-60, 9-13, lacuna, 14, end missing.

No. 67 : MS 31

Yūsof b. Moḥammad b. Yūsof "Yūsofī"

Jāmeʿo l-favāyed جامع الفواید

MS 31 (ex Coll. Min.), 65 fols., 170 x 115 mm

Bound in plain black leather over cardboard; endpapers yellow. Binding not original. Written on Eastern paper, medium thick, burnished, off-white; most edges repaired in European paper; fols. 1, 2, 65 substituted in the same European paper; watermark partly visible on fol. 65.

15 lines, 132 x 80 mm, on blind-ruled frame and lines; borders added later: red, green, blue, and in outer margins two hair-thin black lines; black with red rubrics; medium-sized, fine *nastaʿlīq*; beginning of text on fol. 2b supplied later in different hand. Catchwords.

Anonymous copy, dated 29 Jomādā II 1053/14 September 1643.

Notes on fol. 64 and in margins throughout.

Tamlīk on fol. 1a by Moḥammad Reżā b. Moḥammad Ṭāher al-Eṣfahānī, dated Rabīʿ II 1131/21 February–21 March 1719.

On fol. 2b a stamp, partly legible: . . . ʿabduhū . . . Mahdī.

Incipit, fol. 2b, as in **MS 25 VI.**

Explicit, fol. 63b, 7

یا روغن گاو اضافه نمایند ونیم گرم بیاشامند نافع باشد
انشاء الله تعالی وتقدس تمام شد...

No. 68 : MS 32

Yūsof b. Moḥammad b. Yūsof "Yūsofī"

Jāmeʿo l-favāyed جامع الفواید

MS 32 (ex Coll. Min.), 26 fols., 180 x 130 mm

Modern brochure, thin flexible light blue cardboard; white endpapers. Written on Eastern paper, medium thin, burnished, tan; fols. 25-26 European paper, thin, white, no watermark; edges torn, waterstained, foxed. For lacunae see below.

13 lines, 120 x 70 mm, on blind-ruled frame and lines; black with red rubrics; medium-sized, flowing, fair *nastaʿlīq*. Catchwords. Fols. 25-26: 13-14 lines, 125 x 70 mm, on blind-ruled frame and lines; black with red rubrics; medium-large, ordinary *nastaʿlīq*.

Anonymous, undated copy (end missing); ca. 1100/1700.

Marginal notes by readers. Fols. 25-26, later bound together with this MS, contain a fragment on therapy with an appendix on fruits and herbs.

Incipit, fol. 1b, as in **MS 25 VI.**

Explicit, fol. 24b, -3

واگر علامت سردی وتری از عدم تشنگی وآب رفتن
دهان وغیرها ظاهر باشد هر صباح آبی که ده عدد انجیر
دران جوشانیده باشند بده مثقال عسل شیرین کرده
نیم گرم]

The text breaks off within the section on the treatment of persons who have swallowed sharp objects.

No. 69 : MS 33

Yūsof b. Moḥammad b. Yūsof "Yūsofī"

Jāmeʿo l-favāyed جامع الفواید

MS 33 (ex Coll. Min.), 81 fols., 153 x 105 mm

Bound in flexible plain crimson leather; some wear, some leaves loose. Written on European paper, medium thin, burnished, white; watermark: coat of arms. First and last fols. foxed, some spots throughout.

12 lines, 105 x 65 mm, on blind-ruled frame and lines; greyish-black with red rubrics and punctuation; medium-small, driving, open, fine *shekastä-āmīz*. Catchwords.

Anonymous copy, dated Sunday, 8 Shaʿbān 1235/21 May 1820.

Notes by readers on fols. 1a and 81b and in margins.

Incipit, fol. 1b, as in **MS 25 VI.**

Explicit, fol. 81a, -3

رباعی چون دست دهد زشرّ سمّت حالی
کز رنج شوی براه غم پامالی
از بهر خلاصیت بنزدیك حکیم
کافی بود از مخلصه منقالی
تمام شد ...

The text ends here with the paragraph on poisons as in **MS 30** (see fol. 14b, -2 there).

No. 70 : MS 34

Yūsof b. Moḥammad b. Yūsof "Yūsofī"

Jāmeʿo l-favāyed جامع الفواید

MS 34 (ex Coll. Min.), 116 fols., 170 x 105 mm

Bound in flexible plain brown leather; worn, one corner torn off. Written on Russian (?) paper, medium thin, glazed, white; some wear and tear.

12 lines, 110 x 62 mm, on blind-ruled frame and lines; black with crimson rubrics and punctuation; small to medium-sized, very even *naskh*. Catchwords. Fols. 1a, 114b–116 blank.

Collations by scribe.

Copied, and dated 7 Zū l-qaʿdä 1274/19 June 1858, by Bāqer b. Jaʿfar.

On fol. 116b a *tamlīk* in European cursive script in purple ink, written by an unpracticed hand: Ce livre appartien (!) à petit persons (!) dr Mohamed Réza Hakim Zadak.

Incipit, fol. 1b, and Explicit, fol. 114a, -4, as in **MS 25 VI.**

No. 71 : MS 59 II

Yūsof b. Moḥammad b. Yūsof "Yūsofī"

Jāmeʿo l-favāyed جامع الفواید

MS 59 (ex Coll. Min.), 142 fols., 208 x 150 mm; scribe's collection of two works. *Jāmeʿo l-favāyed* in the margins of fols. 13a, 15b–45a, 46b–124a.

For the description of the MS see **No. 138 : MS 59 I.**

Incipit, fol. 13a, margin, as in **MS 25 VI.**

Explicit, fol. 124a, margin

دو درم روغن زیت با روغن گاو اضافه نمایند
نیم گرم بیاشامند وغذا اگرا بشیر گاو خورند نافع
باشد انشاء الله تعالی خاتمه باتمام واختتام
انجامید تسوید این بیاض وترشیح این ریاض بروز هژده
زماه مبارک رمضان بسال نهصد وهفده زهجرت نبوی
ببلدهٔ فاخرهٔ هرات صانت عن تطرق الافات
والحمد لله علی الاتمام والصلوة علی محمد خیر الانام واله
البررة الکرام حرره [و] مؤلفه یوسفی جیلانی غفر ذنوبه
وستر عیوبه بمحمد واله حرره...

This MS of Yūsofī's *Jāmeʿo l-favāyed* was obviously transcribed from a copy that faithfully preserved the author's own colophon to his work.[1]

1. Cf. **MS 26 I**, etc.

No. 72 : MS 66 IV

Yūsof b. Moḥammad b. Yūsof "Yūsofī"

Jāmeᶜo l-favāyed جامع الفواید

MS 66 (ex Coll. Min.), 130 fols., 310 x 215 mm; owner's collection of four medical works.
Jāmeᶜo l-favāyed on fols. 75, 81–115, margin.

For the description of the MS see **No. 194 : MS 66 I.**

Incipit, fol. 75a, margin

بسمله . حمد نامحدود حکیمی را که بقانون حکمت
کامل القناعة [کذا] رحمترافع [کذا] انواع امراض ...

Explicit, fol. 115b, margin

و دو درم روغن زیت با روغن گاو اضافه کنند
و نیمگر بیاشامند و غذا اکثر [کذا] بشیر گاو بود
نافع باشد این [کذا] شاء الله تعالی تمام شد ...

Another copy of *Jāmeᶜo l-favāyed* (fol. 75b, right margin) by Yūsofī (*sic*) b. Moḥammad b. Yūsof aṭ-Ṭabīb (fol. 75a, left margin).

No. 73 : MS 78 IV

Yūsof b. Moḥammad b. Yūsof "Yūsofī"

Jāmeᶜo l-favāyed جامع الفواید

MS 78 (ex Coll. Min.), 117 fols., 115 x 230 mm (*jong*); scribe's collection of three medical texts and prayers, etc.
Jāmeᶜo l-favāyed on fols. 95–117.

For the description of the MS see **No. 186 : MS 78 I.**

Incipit, fol. 95a, 4, as in **MS 25 VI.**

In this MS of Yūsofī's *Jāmeᶜo l-favāyed* (fol. 95b, 2) the text is divided into 250 *bāb* (ibid., 5); it breaks off within *bāb* 116 در امراض پستان و ورم الثدی (begins on fol. 115a, 7). Fols. 116 and 117 are small fragments.

No. 74 : MS 93 II

Yūsof b. Moḥammad b. Yūsof "Yūsofī"

Jāmeᶜo l-favāyed جامع الفوايد

MS 93 (ex Coll. Min.), 81 fols., 110 x 210 mm (*jong*); binder's collection in six sections; nos. II (fols. 28b-42b) and IV (fols. 49a to 52b, 9) catalogued (see also **No. 172 : MS 93 IV**); on the others see below. On lacunae see below.
Jāmeᶜo l-favāyed on fols. 28–42.

Bound in dark brown cloth over flexible cardboard; spine greyish-pink cloth; inner covers pasted with white paper; four flyleaves in front and two in back of white Russian (?) paper. Cardboard of binding broken; binding not original. Written on different papers, medium-thick, coarse, grey Eastern, and medium-thick, burnished, white Russian (?).

A. Fols. 1-28: black; different styles of *naskh* and *nastaᶜlīq*. B. Fols. 28-54: 15–16 lines, 85 x 160 mm; black with black overlinings; medium-sized, undistinguished *shekastä-āmīz,* rubrics in *naskh.* Catchwords. C. Fols. 54-81: different hands.

Anonymous, undated copies; thirteenth/nineteenth century.

I. Fols. 1-28a filled with recipes for compound medicines in different hands, incomplete, misbound; scrapbook. III. Fols. 43-48 filled with recipes for amulets, recipes, astrological excerpts, etc., mostly in hand of scribe B, among them a quotation from *Rāḥatᵒ l-ensān* (fol. 45b, 3) on hygiene. V and VI. Fols. 52b, 10 to 81b filled with short sections on omens, etc., in different hands; on fols. 52b-54a (V) a short tract *Naṣīḥatnāmä-ye jamīᶜ-e ḥakīmān* on the regimen of ascesis.

Marginal notes on fols. 28–42.

Incipit, fol. 28b, as in **MS 25 VI.**

The text of Yūsofī's (fol. 28b, 5) *Jāmeᶜo l-favāyed* (no title mentioned, see fol. 28b, 7) breaks off with the rubric *robāᶜī* in the section on *esterkhāᵓo l-lesä,* on fol. 42b.

No. 75 : MS 26 III

Yūsof b. Moḥammad b. Yūsof "Yūsofī"

Qaṣīdä dar ḥefẓ-e ṣeḥḥat قصیده در حفظ صحت

MS 26 (ex Coll. Min.), 103 fols., 178 x 120 mm; binder's collection of eleven works.
Qaṣīdä dar ḥefẓ-e ṣeḥḥat on fols. 51b to 55a, 9.

For the description of the MS see **No. 62 : MS 26 I.**

Incipit, fol. 51b, and Explicit, fol. 55a, as in **MS 25 II.**

PL II 239, no. 408 (12); Monzavī I 523a, nos. 4819–28; Tashkent IX 303–304, nos. 6467–68 (5534 V and 3334 IX, resp.).

No. 76 : MS 28 IV

Yūsof b. Moḥammad b. Yūsof "Yūsofī"

Qaṣīdä dar ḥefẓ-e ṣeḥḥat قصیده در حفظ صحت

MS 28 (ex Coll. Min.), 72 fols., 170 x 110 mm; scribe's collection of four works by Yūsofī and excerpts from various sources.
Qaṣīdä dar ḥefẓ-e ṣeḥḥat on fols. 66–67.

For the description of the MS see **No. 64 : MS 28 I.**

Incipit, fol. 66a, -4

قصیده ایست که انوار حکمتش نام است.
ایکه داری تندرستی از در حکمت درا
تا بعلتهای گوناگون نگردی مبتلا.

Explicit, fol. 67b, 5

خانه ما و شما چلپاسه باشد در مقام
گر نباشد زعفران درخانه ما و شما

In this MS, the prose preface and dedicatory *masnavī* and the conclusion "on various questions" are not copied. In the heading, the text is wrongly called *Anvār-e ḥekmat.*

No. 77 : MS 24 II

Yūsof b. Moḥammad b. Yūsof "Yūsofī"

Dalāyelo n-nabż دلايل النبض

MS 24 (ex Coll. Min.), 156 fols., 182 x 128 mm; binder's collection of eight works; six of these, by Yūsofī, copied by the same scribe.
Dalāyelo n-nabż on fols. 75b-81a.

For the description of the MS see **No. 61 : MS 24 I.**

Incipit, fol. 75b

دلایل نبض. بسمله. الحمد لله النافع الحکیم العلام
والصلواه [کذا] علی زبدة الانبیا ... وبعد پوشیده نماند
که این سطری چندست از صناعت طبّ درادلّهٔ نبض
برحال بدن ... مثنوی وارد امید یوسفی که مدام
فیض گیرند ازین چه خاص و‹چه›عام

Explicit, fol. 81a, -3

زد رقم خامه ام دلایل نبض نظری کن تاملی فرمای
تا شود نبض سال تاریخش ده زصد کم کن وبراو افزای

Yūsofī wrote this treatise on the pulse, *Dalāyelo n-nabż* (fol. 81a, -3), in 942/1535 (for the chronogram see Explicit).

PL II 236, no. 408 (3); Monzavī I 537a, nos. 4967-75; cf. PL II 314, no. 584 (31); Miklukho-Maklaĭ, p. 195, no. 1340; Osmania Univ., p. 53, no. 39; Tashkent IX 299-300, nos. 6457-59 (11665 IV, 5534 VI, 3334 VI, resp.).

No. 78 : MS 26 VI

Yūsof b. Moḥammad b. Yūsof "Yūsofī"

Dalāyelo n-nabż دلایل النبض

MS 26 (ex Coll. Min.), 103 fols., 178 x 120 mm; binder's collection of eleven works. *Dalāyelo n-nabż* on fols. 58–70.

For the description of the MS see **No. 62 : MS 26 I.**

Incipit, fol. 58a, 1

ازین محفوظ [نبض حرکت] اینه ایست از روح
مرکّب از انبساط وانقباض ...

Explicit, fol. 69b, -2

وغیرها نزدیک است بدلایل نبض برحال بدن والله
اعلم زد رقم خامه ام دلایل نبض نظری کن تامل فرما
تا شود نبض سال تاریخش ده زصد کم کن وبراو افزا
تمت ...

There is a lacuna of one fol. between fols. 57 and 58, and the beginning of this text corresponds to **MS 24**, fol. 75b, 8. The concluding verses of the treatise give 942/1535 as the date of composition.

No. 79 : MS 29 I

Yūsof b. Moḥammad b. Yūsof "Yūsofī"

Dalāyelo n-nabż دلایل النبض

MS 29 (ex Coll. Min.), 119 fols., 200 x 135 mm; scribe's collection of ten works; VII, Yūsofī's *Monājāt dar ṭalab-e ᶜeshq va-maḥabbat,* of non-medical contents, not catalogued. (See also **Nos. 52, 57, 65, 82, 84, 151, 173,** and **209.**)
Dalāyelo n-nabż on fol. 1a, 1–7.
Bound in thick but not stiff cardboard, pasted with faded greenish paper; spine of black cloth; modern endpapers and two front flyleaves added when rebound. Written on European paper, medium thick, burnished, cream-colored; heavily foxed; edges trimmed, few tears. For lacunae see below.

15–16 lines, 135–50 x 70–75 mm, on blind-ruled frame and lines; black with red rubrics; on fol. 81a a border of a single green line; various styles of *nastaᶜlīq,* mostly medium sized, undistinguished. Catchwords.

Copied by Mollā Ḥasan Beheshtī; he dated works II and IV Tuesday, 20 Rabīᶜ I 1233/*Wednesday,* 28 January 1818, and work X Sunday, 29 Rabīᶜ II 1233/8 March 1818; on fol. 118b a scribe's verse of his in Turkish.

Marginal notes throughout.

On fol. 1a a stamp of one Majdoddīn, on fol. 13b an illegible stamp.

Incipit, fol. 1a, 1

درمطرقی [؟] جزبی است از انبساطی
که فرعه اولی [؟] اول اوست

Explicit, fol. 1a, 6

تا شود نبض سار[کذا] تاریخش
نبض گیر ونود براو افزای والله اعلم بالصواب

Only the end of *Dalāyelo n-nabż* is preserved in this MS; cf. **No. 77 : MS 24 II.**

No. 80 : MS 24 III

Yūsof b. Moḥammad b. Yūsof "Yūsofī"

Dalāyelo l-bowl دلایل البول

MS 24 (ex Coll. Min.), 156 fols., 182 x 128 mm; binder's collection of eight works; six of these, by Yūsofī, copied by the same scribe.
Dalāyelo l-bowl on fols. 81b–88b.

For the description of the MS see **No. 61 : MS 24 I.**

Incipit, fol. 81b

رساله فی دلائل البَول . بسمله. بعد از سپاس حکیم مطلق
جلّ ذکره وبعد از درود رسول برحق صلی الله علیه واله
واصحابه مخفی نماند که چون رسالهٔ دلایل النبض باختتام
انجامید بخاطر بعضی از مخادیم... که در ادلّهٔ بول نیز کلمهٔ
چند نوشته شود... این مختصر که بدلایل البول موسوم است...

Explicit, fol. 88a, -4

دلایل بُراز[کذا] در صفرت وسواد وبیاض وغیرها نزدیک
است بدلایل بول فتامّل خاتمه حکام بول را زره فکر
یوسفی بهر تو جمع کرد وجمیع برادران
تاریخ سال تاکه شود روشنت بگیر
قاروره وچهارصد وسی فزا دران

Yūsofī wrote this short tract on uroscopy as a companion piece to his *Dalāyelo n-nabż* in the same year 942/1535 (for the chronogram see Explicit) and gave it a corresponding title, *Dalāyelo l-bowl* (fol. 81b, 7).

PL II 236, no. 408 (2); Monzavī I 536b, nos. 4959–66; cf. PL II 314, no. 584 (30); Miklukho-Maklaĭ, p. 195, no. 1339; Tashkent IX 300–301, nos. 6460–61 (11665 V and 3334 VII, resp.).

No. 81 : MS 26 VII

Yūsof b. Moḥammad b. Yūsof "Yūsofī"

Dalāyelo l-bowl دلایل البول

MS 26 (ex Coll. Min.), 103 fols., 178 x 120 mm; binder's collection of eleven works.
Dalāyelo l-bowl on fols. 70–72.

For the description of the MS see **No. 62 : MS 26 I.**

Incipit, fol. 70b, as in **MS 24 III.**

Explicit, fol. 72b, -2

بخلاف ناری که مشابه صبغ زعفرانست
و دلالت کننده است بر حرارت زایده ...

The text breaks off on fol. 72b, corresponding to **MS 24**, fol. 82b, -4.

No. 82 : MS 29 II

Yūsof b. Moḥammad b. Yūsof "Yūsofī"

Dalāyelo l-bowl دلایل البول

MS 29 (ex Coll. Min.), 119 fols., 200 x 135 mm; scribe's collection of ten works. *Dalāyelo l-bowl* on fols. 1a–9a.

For the description of the MS see **No. 79 : MS 29 I.**

Incipit, fol. 1a, -7, and Explicit, fol. 9a, as in **MS 24 III.**

No. 83 : MS Ar. 98 X

Yūsof b. Moḥammad b. Yūsof "Yūsofī"

Dalāyelo l-bowl دلایل البول

MS Ar. 98, 135 fols., 193 x 138 mm; fols. 89–135 a scribe's collection of six works by Yūsofī. *Dalāyelo l-bowl* on fols. 105b–112a.

For the description of the MS see **No. 85 : MS Ar. 98 IX.**

Incipit, fol. 105b, 2, and Explicit, fol. 112a, -3, as in **MS 24 III.**

No. 84 : MS 29 IV

Yūsof b. Moḥammad b. Yūsof "Yūsofī"

Settä-ye żarūrīyä ستّهٔ ضروریّه

MS 29 (ex Coll. Min.), 119 fols., 200 x 135 mm; scribe's collection of ten works. *Settä-ye żarūrīyä* on fols. 83-88, etc. (see below).

For the description of the MS see **No. 79 : MS 29 I.**

Incipit, fol. 83b, -6

بسمله. نسخهٔ دیگر از طبّ که جز دعای او نگوید

روز شب]

جز رضای او نجوید روز شب

Explicit, fol. 58b, -2

خاتمه   این محقّر که باد فایده مند

همه آفاق را چه خاص <و> چه عام

یافت در سال نهصد و چل چار

سمت ختم <و> صورت اتمام تمت ...

The preface and most of the dedicatory *maṣnavī* are not transcribed in this MS (cf. **MS 25**, fol. 86a, -6). The correct order of fols. is: 83-88, 58-59.

PL II 240, no. 408 (15); Monzavī I 550a, nos. 5144-47; Shīrānī II 395, nos. 2138-39; Amritsar, p. 100, no. 246 I (S. H. R. 2270) [?]; Tashkent IX 301, nos. 6462-63 (11665 VI and 3334 V, resp.).

No. 85 : MS Ar. 98 IX

Yūsof b. Moḥammad b. Yūsof "Yūsofī"

Settä-ye żarūrīyä ستّهٔ ضروریّه

MS Ar. 98, 135 fols., 193 x 138 mm; a *majmūʿā* in Arabic (fols. 1-88) and Persian. Fols. 89-135 comprise a scribe's collection of six works by Yūsofī (nos. VIII-XIII of the whole *majmūʿā*); nos. VIII, *Anvār-e ḥekmat* (acephalous), and XIII, *Monājāt dar ṭalab-e ʿeshq va-maḥabbat*, of non-medical contents (incomplete at the end), not catalogued. (See also **Nos. 53, 59,** and **83.**)
Settā-ye żarūrīyā on fols. 99b-105a.

Bound in dark brown leather over thick stiff cardboard; simple blind-tooled borders; three-medallion design and corresponding corner pieces with blind-stamped floral scrolls on front and back; inner covers pasted with blue paper; one flyleaf each in front and back of Eastern paper, thin, transparent, burnished, cream-colored; some wear and tear. Binding not original. Written on European paper, medium thin, burnished, cream-colored.

15 lines, 135 x 85 mm, on blind-ruled frame and lines; verses in hemistichs and verse lines; black with red rubrics and punctuation; medium-large, even, careful *nastaʿlīq*. Catchwords.

Collations by scribe.

Anonymous, undated copy (end missing); ca. 1200/1800.

Marginal notes by readers.

Incipit, fol. 99b, 3, and Explicit, fol. 105a, 5, as in **MS 25 VII.**

No. 86 : MS 57 III

Esmāʿīl b. Moḥammad Yūsof

Favāyed-e Saʿdīyā فواید سعدیه

MS 57 (ex Coll. Min.), 91 fols., 215 x 172 mm; scribe's collection of three medical texts in Persian.
Favāyed-e Saʿdīyā on fols. 61-83.

For the description of the MS see **No. 136 : MS 57 I.**

Incipit, fol. 61b

بسمله. حمد وثنای بی شمار خالق را
که اثار متنوعه او در مخلوقات ظاهر وپیدا است ...

Explicit, fol. 83a, 11

وشاخه [یعنی شاخه] بروانَد وگل کند ومیوه بار اودر [؟]
بارها بتجربه رسیده وازموده است بکنند وبه بینند
والسلام علی من اتبع الهدی

Esmāᶜīl b. Moḥammad Yūsof (fol. 62a, 5) divided his treatise *Favāyed-e Saᶜdīyä* (ibid., 10) into five *maqālä*:

1. (begins on fol. 62a, 14) in five *bāb* — در منافع انسان و یتعلق بها
2. (begins on fol. 64a, -4) in four *bāb* — در منافع حیوانات و بهایم و حشرات،
3. (begins on fol. 67a, 11) in four *bāb* — در منافع اشجار و نباتات و نظایران
4. (begins on fol. 70a, -3) in eight *bāb* — در غرایب و عجایب حکما و اطبا
5. (begins on fol. 72a, 1) in ten *bāb* — در اسرار توالد [کذا] و تناسل و ما یتعلق بها و خواص و منافع متفرقه

The text contains much occult matter, especially in the last two *maqālä*. The author states in the preface that he composed this treatise in Samarqand in 959/1551, *dar jolūs-e ḥażrat-e salṭanatpanāhī,* but he does not mention his name (fol. 62a, 12–13).[1]

It appears probable that Esmāᶜīl b. Moḥammad Yūsof was a younger brother of Yūsof b. Moḥammad b. Yūsof "Yūsofī."[2] Yūsofī's works span a period of more than three decades, from 913/1507–08 to 946/1539–40.[3] Their father, Moḥammad b. Yūsof, had also been a medical author: he wrote *K. jawāhir al-lugha,* a medical dictionary, in 898/1492, and in 924/1518 another medical glossary and dictionary of technical terms in Arabic and Persian, *Baḥr al-jawāhir fī taḥqīq al-muṣṭalaḥāt aṭ-ṭibbīya.*[4] Yūsofī is said to have been born at Khwāf,[5] but his father bears the *nisba* Harawī, and in Herāt Yūsofī wrote his *Jāmeᶜo l-favāyed.*[6]

Two other works by Esmāᶜīl b. Moḥammad Yūsof have been preserved in MSS: *Ḥallo l-asāmī,*[7] a commentary on *K. at-tanwīr fī l-muṣṭalaḥāt aṭ-ṭibbīya* by abū Manṣūr al-Ḥasan b. Nūḥ al-Qumrī,[8] and a short section *dar bāb-e mafāṣel va-neqreṣ,* perhaps taken from a larger work.[9]

1. In 959/1552, the Shaibānid Nowrūz Aḥmad came to the throne; does the title "Auspicious Information" allude to this event?
2. See **MSS 24–35.**
3. See PL II 235–40, no. 408.
4. See Ullmann, pp. 233, 237.
5. See note 3 above.
6. See **MS 25 VI.**
7. Miklukho-Maklaĭ, p. 164, no. 1107; Tashkent VI 159, no. 4363 (6171).
8. Ullmann, pp. 147, 320, and esp. 236.
9. Miklukho-Maklaĭ, p. 373, no. 2852, fols. 281b–286b.

Not in PL or Monzavī; no other MS known.

No. 87 : MS 22 II

Nūrollāh

[*Resālä dar bīkh-e čīnī*] [رساله در بیخ چینی]

MS 22 (ex Coll. Min.), 194 fols., 210 x 135 mm; contains Sharafoddīn Ḥasan's *Resālä-ye yanbūᶜ* and in the margins of fols. 20b–22a Nūrollāh's tract on chinaroot, in a different hand.
[*Resālä dar bīkh-e čīnī*] on fols. 20b–22a, margin.

For the description of the MS see **No. 44 : MS 22 I.**

Incipit, fol. 20b, margin

بسمله. الحمد لله رب العالمین والصلوة والسلام علی خیر خلقه
محمد وآله اجمعین اما بعد محرر این رساله ومقرر این مقاله
خادم الحکما نور الله قریب به بیست سال در هندوستان
روزگار گذرانیدم وبا حکیمان انجا درباب فواید ومنافع
بیخ چینی سخنان میگفتم ...

Explicit, fol. 22a, margin

وبه شیرینی اندکی میل نماید شاید وخورنده بیخ چینی
باید که علی الدوام از یاد حضرت پروردگار غافل نباشد تمت

In this MS of Nūrollāh's (fol. 20b) tract on chinaroot, no title is mentioned. In the introduction, the author speaks of his twenty-year stay in Hendūstān and of a Frankish physician Aresṭū who introduced him to the healing properties of *bīkh-e čīnī* (fol. 20b). This copy does not give a date of composition. In some other MSS, 944/1537-38 or 954/1547 is mentioned as the date of writing.[1] In Sālekoddīn Moḥammad Ḥamavī's collection *Ḥajalato l-ᶜarāyes,* it is said that Aresṭū was the author's original name, that he considered himself a descendant of Aristotle, and had converted to Islam from Christianity.[2] There is no reason to doubt Nūrollāh's authorship of this tract, even though in some MSS ᶜEmādoddīn Maḥmūd is named as its writer.[3] None of the known facts of his biography suggests the possibility that he spent twenty years of his life in India.[4] Confusion between the two authors may have been started by the fact that ᶜEmādoddīn wrote a short tract on chinaroot himself, included by Sālekoddīn Moḥammad in his collection[5] and different from his longer discussion of the same subject.[6]

1. See PL II 240f., no. 410.
2. Nashrīyä III 16b, no. 28.
3. See note 1.
4. See PL II 241, 243 (6); cf. **No. 99 : MS 46 II.**
5. Nashrīyä III 15a, no. 13.
6. See PL II 242–43, no. 411 (2), (5); **No. 104 : MS 87 II**. In a MS in the library of the Royal College of Physicians in London (JRAS [1951], p. 188, no. 41 X), a tract on chinaroot is ascribed to Nūrollāh that according to the catalogue appears to be much longer than the short section in the UCLA manuscript (pp. 353–99 of the London MS). The question requires further study.

PL II 240, no. 410; Monzavī I 400b, nos. 3715-21; cf. PL II 243, no. 411 (6); Tashkent VI 160, no. 4364 (2873 III).

No. 88 : MS 105 II

Moẓaffar b. Moḥammad al-Ḥosainī "Shefāʾī"

[*Qarābāẕīn*] [قرابادین]

MS 105 (ex Coll. Min.), 283 fols., 233 x 145 mm; binder's collection of three works.
[*Qarābāẕīn*] on fols. 128–220.

For the description of the MS see **No. 110 : MS 105 I.**

Incipit, fol. 128b

بسمله . وبه نثقی . نسخه قرابادین شفائی . الحمد لله الحکیم
العلیم والصلوة علی من اوتی الحکمه والکتاب الکریم
وهو یشفی بلطفه السقیم وانه لعلی خلق عظیم وآله
الهادین الی صراط مستقیم وبعد پوشیده نماند که فقیر
حقیر مظفر محمد الحسینی الشفائی درمدتی مدید ترکیبی چند...

Explicit, fol. 219b, -2

عسل صاف بقدر احتیاج بطریق معهود معجون سازند شربتی
یک مثقال بعد از چهل روز تمت هذه النسخه ...

Moẓaffar-e Moḥammad al-Ḥosainī ash-Shefāʾī (fol. 128b, 3) did not title his well-known dispensatory; in the preface he just states his intention to write کتاب جامع ومستغنی از سایر قرابادینات . It is arranged in *bāb* of alphabetical order, listing the compound drugs according to their preparation. Taqī Kāshī records that his fellow townsman Shefāʾī died in 963/1555.[1] Besides poetry and a work on ethics,[2] he composed the following books on medical subjects, in addition to his *Qarābāẕīn:*[3] *Ābestanī va-bāh,*[4] *Bīst bāb fī ṭ-ṭebb,*[5] *Kholāṣato sh-shefāʾ,*[6] and possibly *Dastūr-e gheẕā-ye Shefāʾī.*[7] In *Dharīʿa*[8] it is recorded that he and after him his descendants exploited the cobalt[9] mines of Qamṣar[10] in the vicinity of Kāshān.

1. PL II 245, no. 415.
2. See note 1.
3. PL II 245, no. 415 (3); Monzavī I 580a, nos. 5391–5416; cf. 553a, no. 5165, *Sharḥ-e Qarābāẕīn-e Shefāʾī*, and 587b, no. 5501, *Kollīyāt-e Ḥakīm-e Shefāʾī* (according to the Incipit identical with his *Qarābāẕīn*).

4. Monzavī I 460a, no. 4227.
5. PL II 245, no. 415 (1); Monzavī I 483b, no. 4475; al-Khāliṣī, p. 267, no. 19 III (? Incipit same as that of his *Qarābāẕīn*).
6. PL II 245, no. 415 (2) has this title; Monzavī I 529b, nos. 4898–4903, enters it as *Kholāṣā-ye Shefāʾī*.
7. Monzavī I 536a, no. 4956; according to him, it has to have been written by this Shefāʾī.
8. VII 229, no. 1101.
9. *maʿdin al-lājuward* (see note 8 for reference); on the use of *lājward* to denote cobalt see Hans E. Wulff, *The Traditional Crafts of Persia* (Cambridge, Mass., and London, 1966), pp. 147, 148, 163.
10. See *Farhang-e Joghrāfyāʾī-ye Īrān* III 216b.

PL II 245, no. 415 (3); Monzavī I 580a, nos. 5391-5416; cf. ibid., 583a, no. 5439; Panjāb P.L., p. 350, no. 264; Shīrānī II 398, nos. 2158–59; al-Mauṣil, p. 275, no. 54 II; Nūrbakhsh I 38, no. 29 I; Kekelidze, p. 83, no. 83 (P K 48); Leeds IX 45, no. P. 48; Miklukho-Maklaĭ, p. 373, no. 2854; Naniana II 243, nos. CXI–CXII; Osmania Med. Coll., p. 110, no. 4; Rampur, p. 130, no. 322; Tashkent IX 354-56, nos. 6528-32 (3885, 4724 II, 3496 II, 6651 I, 3334 I, resp.).

Kholāṣā-ye Shefāʾī: Panjāb P.L., p. 325, no. 250; al-Mauṣil, p. 107, no. 104; Miklukho-Maklaĭ, p. 173, no. 1177.

No. 89 : MS 106

Moẓaffar b. Moḥammad al-Ḥosainī "Shefāʾī"

[*Qarābāẕīn*] [قرابادين]

MS 106 (ex Coll. Min.), 231 fols., 200 x 113 mm

Bound in dark brown leather over stiff cardboard; flap; simple blind-tooled borders and three-medallion design with blind-stamped floral scrolls on covers and flap; inner covers pasted with dark beige leather; one flyleaf each in front and back, of thin, burnished, yellowish paper (modern?). Some wear and tear. Binding not original. Written on Eastern paper, medium thin, slightly transparent, burnished, tan.

12 lines, 120 x 65 mm, on blind-ruled frame and lines; black with red rubrics; medium-sized *naskh* leaning to *nastaʿlīq*, deliberate and clear, but undistinguished. Catchwords.

Collations by scribe.

Copied, and dated 4 Rabīʿ II 1074/5 November 1663, by Maḥmūd Ṭabasī.

Numerous marginal notes in different hands; fols. 228b–231a filled with several short recipes, written by scribe (?), twelve lines of plain neat *naskh*; among these is a quotation from Esmāʿīl Jorjānī on a *barshaʿṣā*, and a *qeṭʿā*, giving the recipe for an aphrodisiac, by one Neẓāmoddīn.[1]

On fol. 231a an owner's stamp reading Muḥammad Ṣāliḥ al-Ḥusainī.

Incipit, fol. 1b

بسمله. الحمد لله الحكيم العليم والصلوة على من اوتى الحكمة
والكتاب الكريم وهو يشفى بلطفه السقيم ... وبعد پوشيده
نماند كه فقير حقير مظفر بن محمد الحسينى الشفايى درمدتى
مديد ...

Explicit, fol. 228a, 7

بقدر احتیاج بطریق معهود معجون سازند شربتی یکمثقال
بعد از چهل روز تمام توان خورد تم الکتاب ...

1. See **No. 112 : MS 26 IV.**

No. 90 : MS 107

Moẓaffar b. Moḥammad al-Ḥosainī "Shefāʾī"

[*Qarābāẕīn*] [قرابادین]

MS 107 (ex Coll. Min.), 117 fols., 220 x 123 mm

Bound in flexible dark brown leather; simple blind-tooled borders; inner covers pasted with white paper; warped; spine repaired, separated from MS; last four fols. loose. Written on European paper, medium thick, burnished, white; watermark obscure; fols. 1-3, 115-117 added later of different European paper; some wear and tear. For lacunae see below.

15 lines, 165 x 75 mm, on blind-ruled frame and lines; black with red rubrics; medium-sized, uneven, mostly fair *nastaʿlīq*. Catchwords.

Collations by scribe.

Anonymous, undated copy; fol. 115 with the end of the text substituted later; twelfth/eighteenth century.

Notes in different hands in margins and on fols. 1-4a, 115-117; in a recipe on fol. 3b, Moḥammad Bāqer b. ʿEmādoddīn Maḥmūd Šīrāzī[1] is quoted as authority.

On fol. 4b a *tamlīk* by Ṣadroddīn Moḥammad b. Moḥammad Masīḥ Ṭabīb; his stamp on fols. 4b and 11a (date illegible); on fol. 2a a note by Ḥājj Mortażā Ḥasanpūr, son of the late ʿAbbās, presenting this volume to C. M. and dated 4 Ābānmāh 1339 *h. sh.*/26 October 1960.

Incipit, fol. 4b, 1

بسمله. وبه نستعین. الحمد لله ربّ العالمین انوش دارو
که اعضای رئیسه را قوت دهد ...

Explicit, fol. 115a, 2, as in **MS 105 II.**

The preface of Shefāʾī's work is not copied in this MS; cf. **MS 105**, fol. 128b, -6.

No. 91 : MS 108

Mozaffar b. Moḥammad al-Ḥosainī "Shefāʾī"

[*Qarābāzīn*] [قرابادين]

MS 108 (ex Coll. Min.), 130 fols., 230 x 160 mm

Bound in black leather over stiff cardboard; simple blind-tooled borders; inner covers pasted with yellowish-green paper; half the MS out of binding, spine broken; worm-eaten. Written on Eastern paper, medium thick, burnished, off-white; stains, spots, edges torn, especially of first fols., repaired. For lacunae see below.

15 lines, 145 x 90 mm, on blind-ruled frame and lines; black with red rubrics; medium-large, bold *nastaʿlīq*. Catchwords. Collations by scribe.

Anonymous, undated copy. A note on fol. 1b, above the text, is dated 1088/1677 (by the scribe?).

On fols. 125a, -4 to 130b, -1 some short paragraphs, copied by scribe, on the calcination (*koshtan*) of metals, on *nushdārū-ye loʾloʾī*, on good and bad symptoms of diseases, etc.; they break off with fol. 130b.

On fol. 1a a *tamlīk* by one Moḥammad ʿAlī.

Incipit, fol. 1b, and Explicit, fol. 125a, 10, as in **MS 105 II.**

In this MS, there is a lacuna between fols. 77 and 78.

No. 92 : MS 109

Mozaffar b. Moḥammad al-Ḥosainī "Shefāʾī"

[*Qarābāzīn*] [قرابادين]

MS 109 (ex Coll. Qāʾenī), 160 fols., 245 x 130 mm

Bound in brownish paper over stiff cardboard; spine of dark brown leather; inner covers pasted with white paper, dotted with a pattern of light green and yellow inkspots; binding stained, worn and torn. Original (?) binding. Written on European paper, medium thin, transparent, burnished, white; watermark obscure; fols. 1 and 160 pasted on Russian paper, medium thin, yellowish; some margins repaired with the same paper (blind stamp on fol. 159 reads: bumaga no 6); fol. 160 out of binding; MS stained and spotted.

15 lines, 180 x 83 mm, on blind-ruled frame and lines; borders of one thin red line; black with red rubrics; medium-large, energetic, good *nastaʿlīq*; qurʾānic and other quotations in large, good *naskh*. Catchwords.

Collations by scribe and readers.

Anonymous copy (part of fol. 160 with colophon torn off), dated Ṣafar 1126/16 February–16 March 1714.

Many marginal notes by readers; recipes by Moḥammad Hāshem Tehrānī[1] (fol. 132b), Moḥammad Saʿīd Qommī Ḥakīmbāshī-ye Ṣāḥebqerān (fol. 135b), Mīrzā Qāżī (fol. 153b); on fol. 53a, a note dated Thursday, 19 Żū l-ḥejjā 1179/ 29 May 1766; another note, commemorating a successful treatment by Mīrzā Gholāmrezā, son of Čaparbāshī (?), dated 1274/1857.

Incipit, fol. 1b, and Explicit, fol. 160a, as in **MS 105 II.**

1. See **Nos. 123–24 : MSS 48–49.**

No. 93 : MS 110

Moẓaffar b. Moḥammad al-Ḥosainī "Shefāʾī"

[*Qarābāẕīn*] [قراباذین]

MS 110 (ex Coll. Min.), 200 fols., 210 x 155 mm

Bound in black leather over stiff cardboard; simple blind-tooled borders, three-medallion design, supplemented by two more medallions and corresponding corners, all blind-stamped with floral scrolls; inner covers pasted with European pink-dyed paper. Binding somewhat worn; one quire loose. Written on European paper, medium thin, slightly transparent, burnished, white; watermark: a shield with a crenellated tower; two names in capitals illegible, because bound in (Italian?). Ink sometimes blotted through; stained, worn.

12–15 lines, 140–60 x 75–100 mm, on blind-ruled frame and lines; black with crimson and orange rubrics; medium-large, fair to good, undistinguished *naskh* of different styles, one scribe (?). Catchwords. Fols. 197b, 198a, 200b blank.

Anonymous, undated copy; thirteenth/nineteenth century.

On fols. 1a, 194b–200a, and in margins medical notes; on fols. 195b–196a recipes by Moḥammad al-Ḥosainī Ṭabīb-e Eṣfahānī.

On fol. 1b owner's stamp: Muḥammad al-Ḥusainī, dated 1214/1799 (?). Is this owner identical with the author of the recipes on fols. 195b–196a?

Incipit, fol. 1b

بسمله. وبه نستعين. الحمد لله الحكيم العليم والصّلوة على
من اوتى الحكمته [كذا] والكتاب الكريم ... [ا ب، ٤] اما بعد
پوشیده نماند که فقیر حقیر مظفر بن محمّد الحسینی الشفائی ...

Explicit, fol. 194a, -6

عسل مصفى بقدر احتیاج بطریق معهود معجون سازند
شربتی یکمثقال بعد از چهل روز تمام توان خورد والله اعلم
تمت الکتاب [کذا] ...

No. 94 : MS 111

Moẓaffar b. Moḥammad al-Ḥosainī "Shefāʾī"

[*Qarābāẕīn*] [قرابادين]

MS 111 (ex Coll. Min.), 66 fols., 183 x 115 mm

Bound in flexible dark brown leather; simple blind-tooled borders; spine torn, back cover missing, front cover worn and warped. Binding too small for MS, not original (thirteenth/nineteenth century). Written on Eastern paper of two varieties: 1) fols. 1-6: medium thin, burnished, cream-colored; 2) fols. 7-66: medium thick, burnished, beige. Surface of paper partly worn, stained; inkblots; edges torn off. On lacunae see below.

On fols. 1-6 see below. Fols. 7-66: 13 lines, 120 x 65 mm, on blind-ruled frame and lines; black with red rubrics; medium-sized, fine, energetic *nastaʿlīq*. Catchwords.

Fragmentary copy, anonymous, undated; eleventh/seventeenth century.

Fols. 1-6 filled with recipes, short fragments of texts, etc., in different hands; several dates from the year 1257/1841 in the same hand; another note dated Jomādā II 1253/2-30 September 1837. Many marginal notes throughout the MS, among them a recipe by Ḥakīm Kūček, on fol. 12a.

Fols. 7-66 of this MS contain fragments of Shefāʾī's *Qarābāẕīn*. The order of fols. is disrupted; the correct order is: lacuna, 9 (*īāraj*, etc.), lacuna, 11 (*govāresh*), lacuna, 13-16 (*ḥabb*), lacuna, 48-49, 44-46 (*ḥabb*), lacuna, 50-53 (*davā* to *ẕarūr*), lacuna, 30-43 (*rowghan* to *safūf*), lacuna, 20-28 (*safūf* to *sharāb*), lacuna, 54-57 (*sharāb*), lacuna, 62, 10 (*shīāf*), lacuna, 58-61 (*żemād*), lacuna, 64 (*ṭelā*), lacuna, 19 (*ṭelā*), lacuna, 47 (*ṭelā*), lacuna, 17-18 (*ghargharä* to *fīrūznūsh*), 12 (*fandārīqūn* to *farzajä*), lacuna, 63 (*kalkalānäj* to *koḥl*), 8 (*koḥl*), lacuna, 66 (*lazūq* to *laʿūq*), lacuna, 7 (*maʿjūn*), lacuna, 65 (*maʿjūn*), lacuna, 29 (*morabbā*), end missing.

No. 95 : MS 112

Moẓaffar b. Moḥammad al-Ḥosainī "Shefāʾī"

[*Qarābāẕīn*] [قرابادين]

MS 112 (ex Coll. Min.), 87 fols., 80 x 180 mm

Bound in white paper, a large sheet folded and pasted together (heading: *pāknevīs-e dīktä*); warped. Written on Eastern paper, medium thin, surface of uneven smoothness, yellow, pinkish-grey, mustard-colored; first and last fols. badly damaged; stained, blotted, mouse-eaten; fol. 1 torn out and pasted on cover. On lacunae see below.

17-21 lines, 60 x 150 mm; black with red overlinings; medium-small, undistinguished *shekastä-āmīz* of varying styles, but probably by one hand. Catchwords.

Collations by scribe.

Anonymous, undated copy (end missing); twelfth/eighteenth century.

Marginal notes, partly Persian in Hebrew characters.

On fol. 1 stamp of a former owner: Muḥammad Mahdī, dated 119 (1190/1776?).

In this copy of Shefāʾī's *Qarābāẕīn*, beginning and end are missing; fol. 1 begins with *īāraj-e lūghādīā*; the lower part of fol. 87 is torn away; on fol. 87a a *marham*, on fol. 87b a *naṭūl*, are discussed.

No. 96 : MS 113

Moẓaffar b. Moḥammad al-Ḥosainī "Shefāʾī"

[*Qarābāẕīn*] [قرابادين]

MS 113 (ex Coll. Min.), 28 fols., 240 x 120 mm

Modern brochure of thin, coarse, yellowish paper; torn. Written on Eastern paper, medium thin; heavily soiled, soaked, stained; original surface and color cannot be determined; ink not blotted out. On lacunae see below.

27–29 lines, 170 x 75 mm; black with red rubrics; medium-sized good *naskh*. Catchwords.

Collations by scribe.

Fragmentary copy, anonymous, undated; twelfth/eighteenth century.

Marginal notes by readers.

On fol. 1a owner's stamp; only part of the date is legible: twelfth/eighteenth century.

The text of this MS is transcribed from a misbound copy; this MS is itself misbound. The correct order of fols. is the following: beginning missing, 17a, 1–13 (*ḥabb*), 17b, -11 (from *ṣefat-e ān*) to 18a, -7 (*ḥabb sāzand*), 17a, 14–15 (in collation on margin *ad* 18a, -8), 17a, -13 to 17b, -12, 18a, -7 (*ḥabb-e moql*) to 19b, -1, 27-28, 20-26 (*ḥabb* to *rowghan*), lacuna, 1-12 (*rowghan* to *sharāb*), lacuna of one fol., 13-16 (*sharāb* to *shīāf*), rest missing.

No. 97 : MS 114

Moẓaffar b. Moḥammad al-Ḥosainī "Shefāʾī"

[*Qarābāẕīn*] [قرابادين]

MS 114 (ex Coll. Min.), 30 fols., 280 x 150 mm

Unbound, but sewn together in a makeshift way. Written on Eastern paper, medium thin, slightly transparent, burnished, cream-colored; margins torn or cut off, one corner clipped; stained. For lacunae see below.

15–17 lines, 185 x 90 mm, on blind-ruled frame and lines; black with black overlinings; large fair *nastaʿlīq*. Catchwords.

Fragmentary copy, anonymous, undated; twelfth/eighteenth century.

The MS is misbound; the correct order of fols. is the following: beginning missing, 1–3, 7 (*żemād* to *fīrūznūsh*), lacuna, 8–12, 4, 25–28, 13–22 (*farzajā* to *maʿjūn*), lacuna, 23–24 (*maʿjūn*), lacuna, 29–30 (*maʿjūn*), lacuna, 5-6 (*mofarreḥ* to *morabbā*), end missing.

No. 98 : MS 85 II

Moẓaffar b. Moḥammad al-Ḥosainī "Shefāʾī"

[*Qarābāzīn*] [قرابادين]

MS 85 (ex Coll. Min.), 51 fols., 190 x 110 mm; scribe's collection of two works on medicine. [*Qarābāzīn*] on fols. 41, etc. (see below).

For the description of the MS see **No. 169 : MS 85 I.**

Incipit, fol. 41a

زهردارا دفع کند ودافع همه زهرهای کشنده
است وجذام وفالج وصرع وسکته ولقوه ورعشه
ومالیخولیا وضیق النفس وخناق سوداوی وبلغمی ...

This *qarābāzīn* was obviously excerpted from Shefāʾī's work.[1] It is divided into *bāb* of alphabetical order. The order of fols. is disrupted; it can be corrected as follows: beginning missing, fol. 41, 4-11, 50 (within *bāb tāʾ, teryāq,* to within *bāb sīn, sekangobīn*), lacuna, 34-36 (*shorbat* to *shīāf*), lacuna, 51, 49, 46 (*bāb ṭāʾ, ṭelā,* to within *bāb mīm, meṣrūzīṭūs*), lacuna, 44, 39-40, 45 (*maʿjūn* to *marham*), end missing.

1. See **MSS 105–114.**

No. 99 : MS 46 II

ʿEmādoddīn Maḥmūd b. Serājoddīn Masʿūd Shīrāzī

[***Resālä-ye āteshak***] [رسالهٔ آتشک]

MS 46 (ex Coll. Min.), 149 fols., 210 x 120 mm; owner's collection of two Arabic texts (I, IV), two groups of short Arabic excerpts (VI, VIII), and four Persian texts (II, III, V, VII), all on medical subjects. (See also **Nos. 102, 103,** and **113.**) [***Resālä-ye āteshak***] on fols. 37-56.

Bound in polished burgundy-colored leather over thick, stiff cardboard; three-medallion design on front and back, inset with thin leather, blind-stamped floral scrolls of light grey against a background of dark grey; spine of rust-colored leather; inner covers pasted with cream-colored paper; corners worn or broken off; wormholes, worn and torn; some leaves loose. Written on Eastern paper, medium thick, transparent, brittle, burnished, white; spots and stains; in parts foxed; torn, wormholes; three fols. torn out after fol. 149, and two after fol. 92.

A. Works I, IV–VI, VIII, fols. 1–36, 75b, -2 to 78, 79–92, 142–146: 18 lines, 160 x 80 mm, on blind-ruled frame and lines; black with black and crimson overlinings; medium-sized, very hasty, undistinguished *shekastä-āmīz.* Catchwords. B. Works II, III, VII, fols. 37 to 75b, -2, 93–141: 12 lines, 145 x 65 mm, on blind-ruled frame and lines; black with rubrics occasionally in red; ink sometimes blotted through paper; beginnings of texts in medium-large, fine *nastaʿlīq,* then changing to medium-large, dense, spidery, undistinguished *shekastä-āmīz.* Catchwords. Fols. 50a (lower half), 50b, 142a, 143b, 144a blank.

Collations by Moḥammad Kāẓem Lāhejānī; the collation of VII is dated first third of Ṣafar 1081/20–30 June 1670.

A. Copied by Moḥammad Kāẓem Lāhejānī; no. I he dated Monday, 18 Moḥarram 1082/*Wednesday,* 27 May 1671, and no. V Ūjjain, second third of Shaʿbān 1081/23 December 1670–2 January 1671; nos. IV, VI, and VIII are undated and unsigned. B. Copied by Mollā Rażīyoddīn Moḥammad Astarābādī, named in the colophon of II on fol. 56a, written by Moḥammad Kāẓem; in the colophon of VII, fol. 141b, Rażīyoddīn calls himself only فراست وزیرخانی [؟]. He signed and dated no. VII Dāro l-fatḥ-e Ojjain, 25 Moḥarram 1081/14 June 1670; nos. II and III are undated and unsigned (but see above). Rażīyoddīn writes in the colophon of VII that he transcribed it

لاجل جالینوس الزمانی حکیم محمد کاظم
المتوطن بگیلان صانها الله عن بلیات الاوان

It appears that Moḥammad Kāẓem was the owner of this *majmūʿä* who copied some of the collected texts himself and had the others copied for him; afterwards all of them were bound together.

Medical notes on inner covers, fols. 92b, 147–149a, from *Kāmil aṣ-ṣinaʿa* by al-Majūsī,[1] *Irshād aṭ-ṭibb* by ibn Jumaiʿ (?),[2] from works by ʿEmādoddin Maḥmūd, Ḥakīm Masīḥo z-zamān (?),[3] etc.

On fols. 1a, 37a, 79a, 93a (attempted erasure on fols. 37a and 79a) an anonymous *vaqfīyä,* dated 1211/1796, forbidding the sale of the book and reserving its use for the students of religious sciences who live in the village of ʿAqdā.[4] *Waqf* written on many fols. verso.

Incipit, fol. 37b

بسمله. باید دانست که مرض آتشك را اقسام متباینه
هست چنانچه متعذر است که انرا در حد واحد
ارتباط دهند اما بحسب الامکان در تعریف او
کلامی که موافق قوانین این فن است بیاوریم
والتوفیق من الله وحده وارباب جدری گفته اند...

Explicit, fol. 56a, 5

سفوف مقوی دارچینی رازیانه مصطکی بالسّویه کوفته
و بخته نگاه دارند اینست تمام کلام سید بهاء
الدّین مؤلفها الحقیر الفقیر علی الله الحبیب ابن مسعود بن
محمود الطبیب والحمد لله اولا وآخرا وظاهر[کذا]
وباطنا والصلوه علی نبیّنا محمد وآله اجمعین

Toward the end of this untitled treatise on *āteshak*, the author quotes extensively from Sayyed Bahā᾽oddīn[5] on the treatment of the disease and gives his formula for a *ma῾jūn-e sīmāb*; the *safūf* copied here in the Explicit is part of it. The author concludes his quotation by saying این است تمام کلام سیّد بهاء الدین, then names himself as ebn Mas῾ūd b. Maḥmūd aṭ-Ṭabīb.[6] In another version, not represented in the collection at UCLA,[7] the quotation from Bahā᾽oddīn is followed by a longer discussion by the author himself. At the end his name is given as ebn Mas῾ūd b. Maḥmūd Maḥmūd aṭ-Ṭabīb.[8] He did not title his treatise, but in the introduction, missing in this MS, he immediately announces his subject after short opening eulogies (see **MS Ar. 41**, fols. 42b to 43a, 9; **MS Ar. 96**, fol. 144a, -5 to 144b). In this MS, on fol. 37a, Moḥammad Kāẓem Lāhejānī gives author's name and subject as follows:

رسالة تحقیق مرض نار فارسی که مشهور بآتشک
است از حکیم نحریر فاضل حکیم عماد الدین
محمود شیرازی رحمه الله

The author of this text is ῾Emādoddīn Maḥmūd b. Serājoddīn Mas῾ūd b. ῾Emādoddīn Maḥmūd Shīrāzī.[9] His grandfather Maḥmūd was physician to Shāh Esmā῾īl.[10] In the years 902–04/1496–98, at Shīrāz, he taught medicine to Maḥmūd b. Moḥammad ῾Abdollāh, the author of *Toḥfä-ye Khānī.*[11] Of his works on medicine, a treatise *dar taḥqīq-e mofarreḥāt-e yāqūtī* is preserved.[12] At present it cannot be determined whether or not more of the writings transmitted under ῾Emādoddīn Maḥmūd's name belong to him rather than to his grandson of the same name.[13] In his treatise on *āteshak,* ῾Emādoddīn Maḥmūd the younger quotes his grandfather with a prescription.[14]

῾Emādoddīn Maḥmūd the younger[15] was first in the service of ῾Abdollāh Khān Ostājlū, governor of Shīrvān, but for some reason incurred his wrath. As a punishment he had to spend one night out in the cold and snow, during which ordeal he resorted to opium. Although he recovered, he had a tremor, *ra῾shä,* for the rest of his life. Since he was an *afyūnī* himself, he held the therapeutic virtues of opium in high esteem.[16] After a time in direct service to Shāh Ṭahmāsp, he was appointed physician-in-residence at the hospital in Mashhad, where he spent the later part of his life. It was probably there that in or after 979/1571–72, Nūrollāh Shūshtarī read with him the *Shāfīä,* the abridgment of *Ma῾ālemo sh-shefā᾽*, by Ghīāṣoddīn Manṣūr Shīrāzī. The sources are silent about the date of his death. In the preface to his *al-Murakkabāt ash-shāhīya,*[17] ῾Emādoddīn Maḥmūd says that he first studied the standard works of medicine with his father and other men in the field and then practiced for nearly twenty years before coming to the court of Shāh Ṭahmāsp and presenting this work to him. Unfortunately, there is no indication as to when this was, and Eskandar Monshī also remains silent about Maḥmūd's period at the court. The only date that can be fixed is 977/1569, when at Mashhad he wrote his tract on *āteshak.*[18]

Maḥmūd's writings on medical subjects[19] and his formulas for compound medicines earned him a reputation as a skilled physician, but he was especially known for his treatment of chronic diseases and of those of a "hot nature," such as "the small and big scab," *jarab-e ṣaghīr va-kabīr,* popularly known as "syphilis," *āteshak.* His work on this subject is indeed the first monographic treatment in Persian of this "new" disease.

In the introduction the author explains why none of his predecessors had discussed it fully: the ancients could not have observed it, and modern authors had not paid much attention to it. They had either dealt with it in an abridged form, without offering any clues as to its treatment, as had Mīr Bahā᾽o d-dowlä Nūrbakhshī,[20] or did not find an opportunity to include it in their writings because they were addicted to intoxicants and hallucinogens,[21] as was Mollā Sharafoddīn Ḥasan Shīrāzī, who spent all his time with hemp and wine.[22] Still others were too occupied with their duties in the service of princes. He himself had for a long time been unable to carry out his plans to write about the subject because he was in attendance at the court, but now, in Mashhad, he had the leisure to put his ideas on paper, even though he was without the standard textbooks.[23]

The judgments passed here by the author on his predecessors Bahāʾo d-dowlä and Sharafoddīn Ḥasan should not be taken literally: Maḥmūd himself says that he will quote from Bahāʾ,[24] and Sharaf was at least enough master of his senses to write an extensive treatise on therapy and simple and compound drugs, the *Resālä-ye yanbūʿ*.[25] One writer not mentioned here by Maḥmūd is Yūsofī, who in his *Jāmeʿo l-favāyed* and *Favāyed-e akhyār*[26] gives prescriptions for syphilis.

1. See Ullmann, p. 140.
2. See Ullmann, p. 164.
3. A Ḥakīm Masīḥo z-zamān dedicated a treatise *Ḥefẓo ṣ-ṣeḥḥä* to the Mughal emperor Owrangzēb (reigned 1069-1119/1659-1707); see PL II 267, no. 460.
4. A village district to the south of Nāʾīn and east of Ardakān, part of the province (*shahrestān*) of Yazd (*Farhang-e joghrāfyāʾī-ye Īrān*, X 135b-136a).
5. See note 24 below.
6. In the MS of Teheran Med. Fac., the name is given more fully as ibn Masʿūd b. Maḥmūd Maḥmūd aṭ-Ṭabīb (Nashrīyä III 361a, no. 2). Blochet misunderstood the author's name as Bahāʾoddīn b. Masʿūd b. Maḥmūd (II no. 890 V).
7. Cf. **MS Ar. 96**, fol. 158b (in **MS Ar. 41**, the end is missing).
8. This is a MS in the Royal College of Physicians, copied by a nephew of the author, ʿAlī b. Ḥasan b. Masʿūd (see below, note 19), in 1037/1627-28 (JRAS [1951], p. 191, no. 56 II; this MS was formerly in the collection of C. Elgood, who also translated it: *Annals of Medical History*, 3 [September 1931, no. 57], pp. 465-86).
9. Maḥmūd's name is given in this form by Sālekoddīn Moḥammad Ḥamavī in his collection *Ḥajalato l-ʿarāyes*, copied by himself in 1006/1597 (see, e.g., Nashrīyä III 15a, no. 9). Maḥmūd's nephew ʿAlī b. Ḥasan, who transcribed Maḥmūd's treatise on phlebotomy, etc. (see **No. 103 : MS 46 V**), added the following names of his forebears: Maḥmūd [the elder] b. Moḥammad b. Aḥmad b. Ḥosain b. ʿAlāʾ (see Monzavī I 574a, no. 5345).
10. See previous note for reference. Other relatives of ʿEmādoddīn Maḥmūd the younger who were active in medicine include his son Moḥammad Bāqer (PL II 251, no. 428; Nashrīyä III 16b, -2, no. 33; *Ẕail-e Tārīkh-e ʿĀlamārā-ye ʿAbbāsī*, p. 275, -8 to -4; a Moḥammad Bāqer b. Maḥmūd is mentioned as the author of *Resālä-ye akmal dar maqālä-ye ajmal* in Charminar, p. 240, no. 116), Ḥakīm abū Naṣr Gīlānī, and Mīrzā Moḥammad Shīrāzī (Eskandar Monshī I 123). The latter is also mentioned, along with his brothers Mīrzā Moḥammad Ḥosain and Mīrzā Moḥammad Saʿīd, as *ketābdār-e khāṣṣä-ye sharīfä* of Shāh Ṣafī in *Ẕail-e . . . ʿĀlamārā* (p. 275, -8 to end).
11. See Nashrīyä III 304a, s.v. They read together Aqsarāʾī's commentary on the *Qānūn* (see Dietrich, p. 91, no. 34), the Kullīyāt of the *Qānūn* itself (see Ullmann, p. 152), Nafīs b. ʿIwaḍ al-Kirmānī's *Sharḥ* of ibn an-Nafīs's *Mūjiz al-Qānūn* (see Dietrich, p. 86, no. 32, and p. 92, no. 35; Ullmann, p. 173), *Īḍāḥ maḥajjat al-ʿilāj* by Ṭāhir b. Muḥammad as-Sijzī (see Dietrich, p. 236, no. 121; cf. Ullmann, p. 28), and Galen's anatomy (*Tashrīḥ-e Jālīnūs*; see Ullmann, pp. 40-41, nos. 13-14; pp. 53-55, nos. 74-80). This was the medical curriculum of the author of *Toḥfä* according to his own testimony. Compare the same passage in the printed text of *Toḥfä* (Madras Gov't Or. Ser. No. CLII, 1959, p. 2, 10-14); see also PL II 232, no. 40.
12. Besides **MS 46 III**, two MSS in Teheran University, dated 996/1587 and 1101/1689, are preserved of this text (Monzavī I 602b, s.v. *Mofarreḥ-e yāqūtī*, nos. 5623-24; the latter is catalogued in Meshkāt III (2) 808, s.v. *Mofarreḥ-e yāqūtī*). It is not known whether the two Teheran MSS are consecutive links in one line of transmission, but both give as the date of composition 902/1496. The author's grandfather, Fakhroddīn Shīrāzī, and Sharafoddīn Ḥasan are quoted as the authors of a recipe for Solṭān Yaʿqūb (see **No. 102 : MS 46 III**). If this is Yaʿqūb Aq Qoyunlu, who reigned 883-96/1478-90, the time between Yaʿqūb's reign and 902/1496 would appear rather short to accommodate two generations. Moreover the text begins exactly like some treatises by ʿEmādoddīn Maḥmūd the younger: *Resālä-ye āteshak* (see **Nos. 100-101: MSS Ar. 41 II** and **Ar. 96 VII**) and *Resālä-ye afyūn* (Rahāvard, p. 189, no. 287 I). Did the younger Maḥmūd imitate his grandfather's eulogies, or did he revise the elder's tract on *mofarreḥāt*? The MS of 996/1587, copied by Moḥammad Bāqer, a son of the younger Maḥmūd, is a collection of works by the latter on *pādzahr, āteshak, čūb-e čīnī, qalʿ-e āṣār*, etc. (Monzavī I 602b, no. 5623). Here, the question has to be left undecided.
13. See **No. 103 : MS 46 V** and note 19 below.
14. **MS Ar. 41**, fol. 47b, -4.
15. The following short biographical note is taken from Eskandar Monshī I 123-24; see also PL II 241, no. 411; Elgood, p. 381; Rieu II 474.
16. Cf. his tract on *afyūn*, Rahāvard, p. 189, no. 287 I; PL II 242, no. 411 (1).
17. Rieu II 474b, *ad* Add. 23560 II; the MS was copied in 1099/1687.
18. The MS transcribed by Maḥmūd's nephew ʿAlī (see note 8 above) gives the second Thursday of Rabīʿ I (II?) 977/25 August (22 September?) 1569 as the date of completion.

19. See **Nos. 102–103 : MSS 46 III** and **46 V; No. 104 : MS 87 II**; PL II 241–44, no. 411; Nashrīyä III 10b–15b, s.v. *Ḥajalato l-ʿarāyes*; in addition to these a *Resālä-ye amrāż-e aṭfāl*, or *Resālä dar amrāż-e ṣebyān* (identical?), is preserved in one MS each in the Inst. Hist. Med., New Delhi (*Cat.* I 35, no. 11965) and Punjab University (Shīrānī II 392, no. 2123).
The Majles Library, Teheran, contains a MS of a treatise by ʿEmādoddīn Maḥmūd b. Masʿūd, titled (?) *Advīä* (Majles, no. 2475 III; Monzavī I 469a, no. 4340); it cannot now be determined whether or not this is a version of his Arabic work *al-Murakkabāt ash-shāhīya*.
On fols. 1-36 in **MS 46**, Moḥammad Kāẓem Lāhejānī copied a *Risālat al-mushil*, without title or author's name, that he ascribed to "Hakīm ʿEmādoddīn Maḥmūd Shīrāzī" (fol. 1a). It cannot now be decided whether this ascription is correct and to which of the two physicians of this name it would belong. An Arabic *Risāla fī l-mushil* by "Muḥammad Bāqir b. Maḥmūd aṭ-Ṭabīb" is preserved in a Bankipore MS (*Cat.* IV 127, no. 81 [nineteenth century], the cataloguer of which identifies its author with ʿEmādoddīn Maḥmūd the younger's son of this name. In a Kābol MS, a Persian *resālä dar ṭarīq-e moshel kardan* is preserved, the author of which is supposed to be ʿEmādoddīn Maḥmūd. The MS is dated 949/1542; its

Incipit reads هرچند فکر کردم که معنی که معلوم آن مخدوم نباشد نیافتم (Monzavī I 597a, no. 5583)

The relationship of this Persian text to the Arabic tract in the UCLA manuscript remains subject to further study.
In *Haft eqlīm* (Ethé I 396, no. 233; ed. *Bibl. Ind.* I 284), four works by ʿEmādoddīn are mentioned by title: 1) a treatise on chinaroot; 2) a treatise on the properties of opium; 3) a tract on anatomy, *tashrīḥ*; and 4) *Sharḥ dar baʿżī mabāḥeṣ-e Qānūn*. No MSS are known as yet of nos. 3 and 4. Again it is not clear to which of the two ʿEmādoddīn the name refers.
20. See **No. 46 : MS 23.**
21. *moskerāt va-moghayyerāt-e ʿaql.*
22. **MS Ar. 41**, fol. 42b, -3, has *bang va-khamr*, and **MS Ar. 96**, fol. 144b, 5, has *bang va-afyūn*; the former reading appears to be preferable, giving one inhaled and one liquid drug; cf. also the title *bang va-bādä.*
23. For this introduction see **Nos. 100–101 : MSS Ar. 41 II** and **Ar. 96 VII.**
24. Cf. also Elgood, pp. 379-81. In **MSS 46 II** and **Ar. 96 VII**, the recipes quoted toward the end of the treatise are attributed to Sayyed Bahāʾoddīn, however. This is very likely to be a scribal error, though, Maḥmūd's nephew having the name Bahāʾo d-dowlä (see Elgood's translation, p. 484b; see note 8 above for references).
25. See **No. 44 : MS 22 I.** ʿEmādoddīn Maḥmūd the younger quotes him in his *Mofarreḥ-e yāqūtī* (**No. 102 : MS 46 III**).
26. See **No. 47 : MS 25 VI, VIII**; Elgood, p. 379.

PL II 242, no. 411 (4); Monzavī I 461b, nos. 4235–39; cf. Monzavī I 460b, nos. 4229–31, s.v. *Ābelä*; Shīrānī II 392, no. 2120.

ʿEmādoddīn Maḥmūd Shīrāzī is quoted with prescriptions in a collection of medicines: Miklukho-Maklaĭ, p. 587, no. 4430.

ʿEmād's *Afyūnīyä*: Shīrānī II 391, no. 2118.

No. 100 : MS Ar. 41 II

ʿEmādoddīn Maḥmūd b. Serājoddīn Masʿūd Shīrāzī

[***Resālä-ye āteshak***] [رسالهٔ آتشک]

MS Ar. 41, 49 fols., 170 x 95 mm; scribe's (?) collection of one Arabic and one Persian work on medicine; work I, fols. 1-37, an incomplete copy of Jaghmīnī's *Qānūnja*.
[*Resālä-ye āteshak*] on fols. 42b-49b.

Bound in flexible, plain, pale crimson leather; inner covers bare; one flyleaf each in front and back, waterstained, foxed; binding worn and torn. Binding not original. Written on Eastern paper, medium thin, burnished, light brownish; fol. 38 European paper. For lacunae see below.

Fols. 42b-49b: 14-22 lines, 120 x 55-60 mm, 140 x 70 mm, and whole page, on blind-ruled frame and lines of 120 x 55 mm; black; small, hasty, uneven *shekastä-āmīz*, not fully punctuated; same hand as no. I? Catchwords. Fols. 38, 39a, 40a, 41a, 42a blank.

Collations by scribe.

Anonymous, undated copy (end missing); no later than 1042/1632 (see below on notes).

Recipes in Persian on fols. 39b, 40b, 41b; date on fol. 39b: Sunday, 5 Jomādā II 1042/*Saturday*, 18 December 1632; verses on fol. 40b, copied by Moḥammad Saʿīd on 1 Rabīʿ I 1043/5 September 1633; another note on fol. 40b dated in the *madrasa*, in the teaching room (*dar ḥojrä-ye āmūzī*) of Mollā Moḥammad Reżā Gīlānī, 1044/1634.

Incipit, fol. 42b

بسمله . الحمد لله المحمود ى كل وعاله والصلوه على سىدىا
محمدًا محمودًا احمدا [كذا] وآله حون مرضى كه
معروفست ىاتسك در رمان ساىق نبود ...

Explicit, fol. 49b, -3 (cf. **MS Ar. 96,** fol. 154b, 1)[1]

المحمود رىىں [؟] معل كىرا صمع عرىى رىوىد ترىد
عارىعوں ابرروب ىكه سه [؟] نشاسته رعفران ىكه اىاں
ترك حىاىكه كاىور مصطكى پسته معر بادام محموده ىكه
حعىر گوىد كه در اصل اىں ىسحه]

The MS contains an untitled treatise on *āteshak* (fol. 42b, 3); the author's name does not appear here since the end is missing (probably three fols. are lost). A comparison with **MS 46 II** and **MS Ar. 96 VII** shows that the text is ʿEmādoddīn Maḥmūd Shīrāzī's treatise on *āteshak* (syphilis).

1. Fully punctuated, the text reads as follows:

المحمود زيبق [؟] مقل كثيرا صمغ عربى ريوند تربد غاريقون
انزروت يكه سه [؟] نشاسته زعفران يكه انبان ترك چنانكه
كافور مصطكى پسته مغز بادام محموده يكه حقير گويد
كه در اصل اين نسخه]

No. 101 : MS Ar. 96 VII

ʿEmādoddīn Maḥmūd b. Serājoddīn Masʿūd Shīrāzī

[*Resālä-ye āteshak*] [رسالهٔ آتشك]

MS Ar. 96 (ex Coll. Min.), 159 fols., 212 x 150 mm; binder's collection of eight Arabic and Persian works.
[*Resālā-ye āteshak*] on fols. 144–158.

For the description of the MS see **No. 144 : MS Ar. 96 I.**

Incipit, fol. 144a, -6

بسمله. رساله در امراض سودا.
الحمد لله المحمود فى كلّ فعاله والصّلوة على سيده [كذا]
محمّد محمود احمد وآله چون مرض كه معروف باتشك
است در زمان سابق نبود...

Explicit, fol. 158b, 1

سفوف مقوى دارچينى رازيانه مصطكى بالسّويه كوفته
وبختته [كذا] نگاهدارند اين است تمام كلام سيد بهاء
الدين مؤلف الحقير الحلقفير [كذا] ملا بحسب [كذا] الدّين
ابن مسعود محمود الطبيب والحمد لله اولا د [كذا] واخرا
وظاهرا وباطنا والصّلوه على نبيّنا محمد واله اجمعين

As is shown in the Explicit, the author's name is incorrectly given here as Mollā Najīboddīn b. Masʿūd-e Maḥmūd aṭ-Ṭabīb; for the correct wording of the Explicit see **MS 46 II.**

No. 102 : MS 46 III

ʿEmādoddīn Maḥmūd b. Serājoddīn Masʿūd Shīrāzī

[*Dar taḥqīq-e mofarreḥāt-e yāqūtī*] [در تحقيق مفرّحات ياقوتى]

MS 46 (ex Coll. Min.), 149 fols., 210 x 120 mm; owner's collection of Arabic and Persian medical texts.
[*Dar taḥqīq-e mofarreḥāt-e yāqūtī*] on fols. 56–78.

For the description of the MS see **No. 99 : MS 46 II.**

Incipit, fol. 56b

بسمله. الحمد لله المحمود فی کل فعاله والصلوة والسلام
علی نبینا محمد وآله وبعد بدانکه از کمال مردم
فاضل در این زمان که ما در اینیم چنان شده که
آدمی را از رو وریش می شناسند وطبیبی چند
پیدا شده اند که...

Explicit, fol. 78b, -6

وخاصیتی که بآن ممتاز است انست که تولید عقل کند
ومغز دماغ می افزاید هذا ذلك ما[؟] هذا المحافظه علیه
والرکون الیه والطلب المانع [کذا] الدیه کلها لدیه والله
سبحانه تعالی تمت الرساله الموسومه بتالیف ارسطو الحکیم
لاسکندر حس طلب[؟] علی[؟] الخدار والشیب والله اعلم

The author of this untitled treatise on *mofarreḥ-e yāqūtī* (fol. 57a, 3) does not name himself in the text. His grandfather Fakhroddīn[1] and Sharafoddīn Ḥasan[2] are quoted with several recipes; they together prescribed a medicament for Solṭān Yaᶜqūb (*scil.* Aq Qoyunlu).[3] The introductory eulogies to Allah and Mohammed (see Incipit) are nearly verbatim the same as those in ᶜEmādoddīn Maḥmūd's treatise on *āteshak* in **MS Ar. 41 II.** On fol. 56b, Moḥammad Kāẓem wrote above the text

رسالة حکیم فاضل حکیم عماد الدین محمود شیرازی در تحقیق
مفرحات یاقوتی از ترکیب وغیره

It appears reasonably safe to hold this ascription to be correct.[4]

The *khātemä* of this tract is formed by an extract from the Pseudo-Aristotelian *Sirr al-asrār* (fols. 75b, -2 to 78b) in Arabic.[5] Beginning of *khātemä*, fol. 75b, -4:

حقیر گوید که بیدارم که مشک نیم مثقال عنبر نیم مثقال
الحاق کردن مناسبست خاتمه مسك مرکبات
السیاسة فی تدبیر الریاسة المعروف بسر الاسرار این کتابیست
که ارسطو در وقتی نوشته که اسکندر اورا طلب کرده از یونان

بواسطة پیری و دور مسافة استعفا جسته درین کتاب چنین
آورده که آن من میدانم که بآن رجوع است درین کتاب
و در تدبیر حفظ صحة آدمی می آورد باین عبارت
انی لما اعتقدت افشاء کل ما علمته الیك لمرار ان اکتمك [؟]
الدواء الذی یعرف بالعصمة وهو کنز الحکما المکنون...

1. E.g., fol. 75b, 2.
2. See **No. 44 : MS 22 I.**
3. Reigned 883–96/1478–90.
4. Another copy of this text, Meshkāt III (2) 808, no. 1035, also gives ʿEmādoddīn Maḥmūd as its author, but apparently not on the authority of the text itself either.
5. Cf. PL II 194, no. 346 (2).

Not in PL; Monzavī I 602b, nos. 5623–24. Cf. note 5 above.

No. 103 : MS 46 V

ʿEmādoddīn Maḥmūd b. Serājoddīn Masʿūd Shīrāzī

[*Resālä-ye ḥejāmä*] [رسالهٔ حجامه]

MS 46 (ex Coll. Min.), 149 fols., 210 x 120 mm; owner's collection of Persian and Arabic medical texts. [*Resālä-ye ḥejāmä*] on fols. 79–91.

For the description of the MS see **No. 99 : MS 46 II.**

Incipit, fol. 79b

بسمله. و به ثقتی واعتمادی.
حمد لك والصلوة علی رسولك بعد از توفیق فراغ از بیان
معالجة بفصد شروع در معالجه بحجامه میکنم و درو از
قلیل و کثیر و قطمیر و نقیر چیزی فروگذار نمیکنم
والتوفیق من الله المتعالی فی کل حال بدانکه حجامة
عبارتست از لزوم محجمه ظاهر عضوی را...

Explicit, fol. 91a, 6

فان الدم يقل سيلا فيها فلا بد من انتظار الاجتماع *
قد وقع الفراغ من تسويد هذه الرساله الموسومة
برساله الحجامة للفاضل النحرير حكيم عماد الدين محمود ...

The subject of this treatise on cupping is mentioned after a few short introductory eulogies (fol. 79b, 3; see Incipit), but not in the form of a title. The author does not name himself, but the copyist ascribes the tract to ʿEmādoddīn Maḥmūd in a short note on fol. 79b as well as in the colophon (see Explicit). From the first sentence of this treatise, it can be gathered that Maḥmūd wrote a parallel essay on bleeding, *faṣd*, before he began to compose this. In a MS of Majles library, Teheran, these two parts, on *faṣd* and *ḥejāmä*, form one treatise together with a third section on ʿ*alaq* (Majles, no. 8085 II). The MS was copied by the author's nephew ʿAlī Reżā b. Ḥasan in 990/1582 (see Monzavī I 574a, no. 5345).

Not in PL; Monzavī I 574a, no. 5345.

No. 104 : MS 87 II

ʿEmādoddīn Maḥmūd b. Serājoddīn Masʿūd Shīrāzī

[*Resālä-ye bīkh-e čīnī*] [رسالهٔ بیخ چینی]

MS 87 (ex Coll. Min.), 134 fols., 210 x 115 mm; scribe's collection of three works.
[*Resālä-ye bīkh-e čīnī*] on fols. 35–57.

For the description of the MS see **No. 114 : MS 87 I.**

Incipit, fol. 35b

بسمله . پوشیده نماند که این بیخ درین تاریخ مردم بران اطلاع
واز استعمال این [کذا] انتفاع یافته اند چنین مسموع شد
که بعضی اوقات دران بلاد که بیخ ازانجا می اورند قحطی دران
شهر پیدا شده بود ...

Explicit, fol. 57a, 3

امّا ان دو بزرگوار که بر تسدید رفته بودند این معنی را مذکور ساختند
اما بحد ومصر نبودند بلکه درانحال ازاین قول رجوع نمودند با
وجود قوت احتمال تمت الرساله

The MS contains an anonymous, untitled treatise on *bīkh-e čīnī* in an unnumbered sequence of *faṣl*. Its identification as ʿEmādoddīn's work rests on a comparison with Rieu II 844b (on MS Add. 19619 V). In both copies there is no preface, whereas the Paris version is, according to Blochet, dedicated *à un prince séfévi* and divided into an introduction and nine chapters.[1] The MS of Teheran Medical Faculty[2] is divided into a *moqaddemä* and six *faṣl*. It cannot now be determined whether that version is the same as in the UCLA manuscript.[3]

1. Blochet II, no. 890 II.
2. Rahāvard, p. 194, no. 287 III.
3. Cf. PL II 242–43, no. 411 (2, 5).

PL II 242–43, no. 411 (2, 5); Monzavī I 415b, nos. 3848–53; Shīrānī II 391, no. 2119.

No. 105 : MS 88

Kamāloddīn Ḥosain Shīrāzī

[*Resālä dar teryāq-e kabīr*] [رساله در ترياق كبير]

MS 88 (ex Coll. Min.), 191 fols., 190 x 120 mm

Bound in black leather over thick stiff cardboard; simple blind-tooled borders, three-medallion design with blind-stamped floral scrolls; inner covers pasted with pink-dyed European paper. Binding not original. Written on two randomly used varieties of Eastern paper: 1) medium thick, slightly transparent, burnished, cream colored; 2) medium thin, transparent, burnished, beige; on first and last fols. some spots, occasional waterstains, inkspots; edges trimmed when MS was restored; mouse-eaten in one small part. Very clean overall.

9 lines, 115 x 65 mm, on blind-ruled frame and lines; greyish-black with red rubrics and punctuation; medium-large, distinguished, copperplate *nastaʿlīq*. Catchwords cut off when MS was rebound?

Copied, and dated Dāro s-salṭanä-ye Aḥmadnagar 992/1584, by al-Matīn b. Shāh Aḥmad Qoṭboddīn.

Recipes by readers in margins.

On fol. 2a owner's stamp, effaced by water; only legible word (name?): Maḥmūd.

Incipit, fol. 1b

بسمله . حمد وسپاس سزاوار حکیمیست که ترکیب
بدن انسانرا از اجزاء لطیفه وجواهر شریفه ترتیب نمود
واز عطاخانهٔ جود مادة الحیوة وجودرا عطا فرمود ...

Explicit, fol. 191b, 2

اما در امراض معده و مانند آن اگر حل نسازند بلکه همچنان
بدهند که فرو برد در معده بیشتر درنگ کند و اثرش بهتر
ظاهر شود والله اعلم بالصواب تمت هذه الرسالة...

Kamāloddīn Ḥosain Shīrāzī (fol. 3a, 3) did not title this treatise on the composition of the famous great antidote; he described his subject as follows (fol. 5a, 2-5):

رسالهٔ جامع کامل در بیان اصول ترکیب حاوی بر قانون
ترتیب شامل بر زبدهٔ اغراض حکما در اختیارات اجزاء
و وجوه تاثیر تریاق کبیر که اجلّ تریاقات واشرف
مرکّباتست...

The text is divided into a *moqaddemä* in two *maṭlab* (begins on fol. 6a, 5); three *rokn*, the first in two *jozv* (begins on fol. 17a, 9), the second also in two *jozv* (begins on fol. 58a, 8), and the third in three *jozv* (begins on fol. 156b, 6); and into a *khātemä* in four *jomlä* (begins on fol. 178a, 6). Among the authorities quoted indirectly or directly are Andromachus,[1] Dioscorides,[2] Galen,[3] ibn Māsawaih,[4] Ḥunain b. Isḥāq,[5] Isḥāq b. Ḥunain,[6] ar-Rāzī,[7] ibn Sīnā,[8] al-Bīrūnī,[9] ibn abī Ṣādiq,[10] Esmāʿīl Jorjānī,[11] and Ṣāḥeb-e *Jāmeʿ*.[12]

Kamāloddīn Ḥosain b. Nūroddīn Moḥammad b. Kamāloddīn Ḥosain Shīrāzī[13] was at first physician to Shāh Nūroddīn Neʿmatollāh Yazdī.[14] This patron is very likely to be Shāh Nūroddīn Neʿmatollāh Bāqī, who was married to a sister of Shāh Ṭahmāsp, Khānesh Bēgom.[15] Kamāl dedicated his treatise on *teryāq* to him (fol. 4a, 1).[16] After Nūroddīn's death, Kamāl came to the court of Shāh Ṭahmāsp,[17] and in 974/1566 inscribed his treatise on hygiene, *ḥefẓ-e ṣeḥḥat*, to him.[18] Since Kamāl's habit of wine-drinking became too well known in public, he incurred Shāh Ṭahmāsp's disfavor, and during the reign of Moḥammad Khodābandä (985-95/1577-87), he went to the court of Khān Aḥmad Gīlānī. Khān Aḥmad held him in high esteem and engaged in discussions of medical subjects with him. At his court Kamāl died.[19]

In *Haft eqlīm* a Ḥakīm Kamāloddīn is mentioned as the author of a commentary on a medical treatise by Ghīāṣoddīn Manṣūr.[20] It is not clear whether the two physicians are identical, especially since Kamāl's grandfather bore the same name.[21] In *Toḥfä-ye Sāmī*, it is reported that Kamāloddīn Ḥosain b. Roknoddīn Shīrāzī died in 953/1546.[22] It is tempting to take this to mean the elder Kamāl's death, but the date somewhat conflicts with Sālekoddīn Moḥammad Ḥamavī's statement that he lived during the reign of Shāh Esmāʿīl I.[23]

1. Ullmann, pp. 91, 304, 310f., 323, 328; cf. Cataloguer, *Theriaca*, pp. 116-17.
2. Ullmann, pp. 257-63 and index.
3. On his writings on *materia medica* and pharmacy see Ullmann, pp. 47-50, nos. 49-55; pp. 60-61, nos. 102-106.
4. Ullmann, pp. 112-15, 326.
5. Ullmann, pp. 115-19; on his work on theriaca see ibid., p. 327.
6. Ullmann, pp. 119, 228.
7. Ullmann, pp. 128-36.

8. Ullmann, pp. 152–55, 304. The section on theriaca is *Qānūn* III 310–15.
9. His *Kitāb aṣ-ṣaidana fī ṭ-ṭibb* is here quoted as *Ketāb-e ṣaidīyä*; cf. **MS 87 I.**
10. Ullmann, p. 160; GAL I 484, Supp. I 886. He wrote commentaries on Hippocrates' *Aphorisms*, Galen's *De usu partium*, Ḥunain's *Masāʾil ṭibbīya*, and a *Risālat al-adwiya wa-l-aṭʿima al-muqtabasa min al-aḥādīth al-mukarrama*; are the quotations here taken from this last work?
11. Simple and compound drugs are discussed in *ketāb* 10 of *Zakhīrä-ye Khwārezmshāhī*; see **MS 1**, etc.
12. The most famous medical book titled *al-Jāmiʿ* was ibn al-Baiṭār's *K. al-jāmiʿ li-mufradāt al-adwiya wa-l-aghdhiya*; see Ullmann, p. 281.
13. This form of his name appears in Sālekoddīn Moḥammad's *Ḥajalato l-ʿarāyes* (Nashrīyä III 16a, no. 22); its correctness is also attested by MSS of Kamāl's works: see Nashrīyä III 309b, s.v. *Ḥefẓ-e ṣeḥḥat*.
14. Eskandar Monshī I 168, 2.
15. *Jāmeʿ-e Mofīdī* III, ed. Afshār (Tehrān [Asadī] 1340), p. 686, 10. This brother-in-law of Shāh Ṭahmāsp is called Shāh Naʿīmoddīn Neʿmatollāh Bāqī by Afshār in *Yādgārhā-ye Yazd* I, *Sels. Entesh. Anjom. Āṣār-e Mellī* 68 (Tehrān 1348), p. 413. Sālekoddīn Moḥammad writes that Kamāl was in the service of Shāh Neʿmatollāh II (see note 13 above for reference), but there is a conflict of chronology here, since Shāh Nūroddīn Neʿmatollāh II was one of the notables of Ardabīl at the time of the Timurid abū Saʿīd's campaign in Āzarbayjān, in 872/1467 (Khworshāh b. Qobād, *Tārīkh-e Qoṭbī* V, ed. Mojāhed Ḥosain Zaidī [New Delhi 1965], pp. 397, 3, etc., esp. 7; Khworshāh relates the event on the authority of Jalāloddīn Moḥammad Dawānī. See EI² I 148a bottom, s.v. abū Saʿīd [Aubin].).
16. Kamāl calls him Shāh Nūroddīn Neʿmatollāh al-Bāqī al-Ḥosainī.
17. Eskandar Monshī I 168, 2.
18. Nashrīyä III 309b, s.v. *Ḥefẓ-e ṣeḥḥat*. It is not clear whether the two MSS in the Majles library represent one and the same text. See Nashrīyä III 16a, no. 23; PL II 247, no. 418. Storey doubtfully discusses Kamāloddīn Ḥosain, the author of *resālä-ye teryāq*, and Kamāloddīn b. Nūroddīn, the author of *ḥefẓ-e ṣeḥḥat*, as two different authors, but there is no reason to assume that they are not identical (cf. Sālekoddīn Moḥammad, Nashrīyä III 16a, nos. 22–23).
19. See note 17 above for reference. According to Sālekoddīn Moḥammad (see note 13 above), Kamāl became Aḥmad's vizier: *ṣadr*.
20. Ethé I 396, no. 234; ed. *Bibl. Ind.* I 284.
21. In a late work on sexual medicine, *Toḥfato l-ʿāsheqīn*, a Kamāloddīn Ḥosain b. Ḥakīm Aḥmad Shīrāzī is quoted; if "Aḥmad" is correct here, it cannot be Kamāl the younger (see Nashrīyä III 305b, 4).
22. Rieu Supp., p. 113a, *ad* Or. 4691.
23. Reigned 907–30/1501–23; see note 13 above for reference.

PL II 246, no. 417; cf. ibid., 247, no. 418; Monzavī I 506b, no. 4682.

No. 106 : MS 82

Fakhroddīn b. Mortażā Mahābādī

Toḥfä-ye Khānīyä تحفهٔ خانیه

MS 82 (ex Coll. Min.), 5 fols., 220 x 140 mm; **MSS 62, 80–83** are obviously parts of a scribe's collection of medical treatises that was only recently taken apart and bound separately.

For the description of the MS see **No. 150 : MS 62.**

Incipit, fol. 1a

بسمله. حمد بیحد وسپاس بیعد مرحکیمی را که دقایق
حکمت او بی پایان است وصلوة مرطبیبی [؟] که

طبیب داروخانه گناه مومنان است و بر آل و اصحاب
او که راه نمایان دین اند رضوان الله علیهم اجمعین
اما بعد این مختصری است در بیان شناختن پادزهر
وکیفیت خوردن آن بنابر اشارت عالیحضرت گردون
اقتداری ...

Explicit, fol. 5b, 7

وچون بر موضع زخم نهند بر سر زخم بچسپد
رباعی این نسخه که از کتم عدم روی نمود ∴
در نهصد و هفتاد و شش آمد بوجود ∴
امید که بر احباب مبارک باشد ∴ از پرتو لطف کردگار معبود ∴
جامعه العبد الفقیر الی الله الهادی فخرالدین بن مرتضی مهابادی
فی سنه ۹۷۷ ط ط تمت ...

Fakhroddīn b. Mortażā Mahābādī (fol. 5b, -4) wrote his treatise *Toḥfä-ye Khānīyä*[1] (fol. 1b, 1) in twelve short *bāb* on the bezoar stone (see Incipit) at the suggestion of Eʿtemādo d-dowlä Moghīṣoddīn Moẓaffar Khān (fol. 1a, -4) in 977/1569 (fol. 5b, -3). Since Fakhroddīn's treatise on chinaroot (see **No. 107 : MS 83**) was written at Agra, it appears probable that this tract was also composed in India. Besides the two short treatises preserved in UCLA manuscripts, he left a note

در بیان امتحان وتجربه بعض ادویه مرکبه و مفرده

in a MS in Teheran.[2]

1. The other MSS of this tract do not bear this title (Monzavī I 485b, nos. 4486–87).
2. Nashrīyä III 360b, no. 286 XII (cf. Rahāvard, p. 434, no. 286 X [!]).

Not in PL; Monzavī I 485b, nos. 4486–87.

No. 107 : MS 83

Fakhroddīn b. Mortażā Mahābādī

[*Resālä-ye čūb-e čīnī*] [رسالهٔ چوب چینی]

MS 83 (ex Coll. Min.), 7 fols., 220 x 140 mm; **MSS 62, 80–83** are obviously parts of a scribe's collection of medical treatises that was only recently taken apart and bound separately.

Fols. 1a and 7b blank; for further description of the MS see **No. 150 : MS 62.**

Incipit, fol. 1b

بسمله. الحمد لله الکریم الجلیل الذی یشفی بکمال حکمته
ولطفه السقیم والعلیل والصلوة علی محمد وآله المرشدین
الی سواء السبیل اما بعد چنین گوید بندهٔ کمین
فخر الدین که این رساله ایست در بیان شناختن چوب
چینی وکیفیت خوردن ان بنا براشاره عالی جناب
فضایلماب...

Explicit, fol. 6a, 6

واگر کسی معرفت نداشته باشد مقدار دویست استار
زیر دیك بسوزانند که کافیست والله اعلم تم
التالیف فی سنه ۹۷۹ فی بلدة اکره ط تمام شد...

The close resemblance of the preface in this tract to that of **MS 82** appears to warrant identifying their respective authors as the same person. Here, the author's name is given only as Fakhroddīn (see Incipit). He did not title his work on chinaroot in eight short *bāb* (see Incipit for reference to his subject). It was written at the suggestion of a physician of high rank, Ḥakīm Esḥāq, who practiced at Agra and Lahore and was called by Fakhroddīn *Boqrāṭ-e zamān-e mā* in a *robāʿī* (fol. 1b, 6). This tract was composed at Agra in 979/1571 (see Explicit).

On fols. 6a–7a a short section titled *ṭarīq-e ertekāb-e čūb-e čīnī* is written in the scribe's hand.

Not in PL or Monzavī.

No. 108 : MS 86 V

Moḥammad Maʿṣūm b. Sayyed Ṣafāʾī Bhakkarī "Nāmī"

Mofradāt-e ṣaḥīḥ مفردات صحیح

MS 86, 140 fols., 260 x 150 mm; scribe's collection in five sections.
Mofradāt-e ṣaḥīḥ on fols. 109–140.

For the description of the MS see **No. 187 : MS 86 II.**

Incipit, fol. 109b

رب یسر تمم بالخیر. بسمله. حمد خداوندی را کش بدر کبریا
هست برابر بهم حشمت شاه گدا
هرکه بتحقیق دید جانب را زین کران
نایدش در نظر هیچکس در دو جهان
[س ۷] امّا از برای عاقبت آرای ارباب نظر ضمیر حشمت افزای
اصحاب معروض میدارد که محمّد معصوم بن سید صفهانی
الحسینی الترمذی اصلاً < البهکری > مسکناً والنامی تخلصاً
که چون اختیارات بدیعی بعضی...

Explicit, fol. 140a, 3

این حب برای سگ دیوانه باشغال دیوانه گزیده باشد
به شود حب که اوّل گفته شد همین است

These leaves contain a copy of *Mofradāt-e ṣaḥīḥ* (fol. 110a) by Moḥammad Maᶜṣūm b. Sayyed Ṣefahānī al-Ḥosainī at-Termeẕī *aṣlan* [al-Bhakkarī] *maskinan* va-n-Nāmī *takhalluṣan* (fol. 109b, 7; instead of "Ṣefahānī" read "Ṣafāʾī").[1] In the preface the author says that he excerpted simple and handy preparations from books like ***Ekhtīārāt-e Badīᶜī***[2] and collected them in his own work (fol. 109b, -4, etc.). In this MS, there are lacunae between fols. 114 and 115, 121 and 122, and 124 and 125. Moreover, the text appears incomplete on fol. 139, 3, where the treatment of snakebites follows immediately after that of expectoration of blood, *nafs-e dam*.

1. See PL I 651–53 for his biography; Moḥammad Maᶜṣūm's main work is *Tārīkh-e Send*; he died soon after 1015/1606–07.
2. See **MS 36**, etc.

PL II 250, no. 426; Monzavī I 602b, nos. 5625–26; Eilers-Heinz, p. 157, no. 194; Katrak, p. 103, no. 410 [?]; Tashkent IX 378, no. 6555 (8126).

No. 109 : MS 105 III

Amānollāh Fīrūz-Jang Khān-Zamān Amānī (?)

Dastūro l-Honūd دستور الهنود

MS 105 (ex Coll. Min.), 283 fols., 233 x 145 mm; binder's collection of three works. *Dastūro l-Honūd* on fols. 221–280.

For the description of the MS see **No. 110 : MS 105 I.**

Incipit, fol. 221b

بسمله. کتاب دستور الهنود منقسم ساخته بمقدمه ودو
باب وخاتمه مقدمه در بیان بعضی جزئیات علمی وتدابیر
اسباب ضروری که مصطلح ومختار این طایفه است

Explicit, fol. 280b

از هر کدام چهار دام در آب سائیده داخل تیل [؟] مذکور
کرده چندان بجوشانند که یکی شود تمام شد نسخه
دستور الهنود ...

In a note on fol. 221a, the scribe gives Nūroddīn Moḥammad[1] as the author of this comprehensive account of Indian medicine, *Dastūro l-Honūd.* In the text itself, no author is mentioned, and the title appears only in the first, introductory sentence and in the colophon (see above). The treatise is divided into a *moqaddemä,* two *bāb,* and a *khātemä.* A work of the same title is preserved in three other MSS,[2] naming Amānollāh Fīrūz-Jang Khān-Zamān Amānī[3] as the author. Further study will have to determine the identity of texts and authors.

1. See **No. 110 : MS 105 I.**
2. *Lindesiana,* pp. xx and 113, no. 721; Fonahn, no. 185; PL II 254, no. 435 (1); Inst. Hist. Med., New Delhi, I 26, no. 9864; Shīrānī II 390, no. 2114.
3. PL I 812, note 1. He is supposedly also the author of a work on medicine, talismans, and alchemy, *Ganj-e bād āvardä-ye ṣāḥebqerānī,* based on Arabic, Persian, and Indian sources (see Monzavī I 590a, nos. 5524–26), and of *Ommo l-ʿelāj,* on purgatives (PL II 254, no. 435 (3)).

PL II 254, no. 435 (1); not in Monzavī; see above, note 2.

Ommo l-ʿelāj: Tashkent IX 357–59, no. 6534 (5534 II).

Ganj-e bādāvard: Inst. Hist. Med., New Delhi, I 31, nos. MMS 7816–17.

No. 110 : MS 105 I

Nūroddīn Moḥammad b. ᶜAbdollāh b. Ḥakīm ᶜAino l-molk Qoraishī Shīrāzī

Alfāẓ-e advīä الفاظ ادویه

MS 105 (ex Coll. Min.), 283 fols., 233 x 145 mm; binder's collection of three works. (See also **Nos. 88** and **109 : MSS 105 II** and **105 III**.)
Alfāẓ-e advīä on fols. 1–127.

Bound in plain black leather over stiff cardboard; inner covers pasted with thin pink paper. Binding somewhat worn, MS partly loose. Written on Eastern paper of two varieties: 1) fols. 1–127, 221–283: thin, burnished, light grey; 2) fols. 128–220: thin to medium thin, burnished, greenish-grey; stained along edges, worm-eaten, edges repaired. On lacunae see below.

I. Fols. 1–127: 17 lines, 185 x 105 mm, on blind-ruled frame and lines; black with red rubrics and overlinings, on fols. 60b–64a rubrics in green; small (fols. 1 to 26a, 2) and medium-large (fols. 26a, 3 to 127), neat *nastaᶜlīq*. II. Fols. 221–280: 16–18, 22 lines, 185 x 98 mm, on blind-ruled frame and lines; black with red rubrics and overlinings; fols. 221–226a, large, aggressive *shekastä*; fols. 226b–280, medium-small, neat *nastaᶜlīq*, leaning to *naskh*. Same scribe as I (?). III. Fols. 128–220: 17 lines, 143 x 83 mm, on blind-ruled frame and lines; black with red rubrics; small, fine, neat *nastaᶜlīq*. Catchwords throughout, in III mostly cut away by trimming.

Collations by scribes throughout.

Works I and III anonymous copies, I dated Morshedābād, 17 Rajab 7 "Farrokhshāhī" (i.e., A.H. 1130)/16 June 1718, and III dated Friday, 13 Jomādā I 7 (doubtless of the same era as no. I)/*Thursday*, 14 April 1718. This era refers to the Mughal emperor Farrokhsīār, who reigned 1124–31/1712–19. Work II was copied, and dated 1069/1658, by Aḥmad b. Moḥammad al-Mūsavī.

Readers' notes on fols. 1a, 128a, 220b–221a, 281–283, and in margins.

On fol. 1a a note on a gift of *čīnī* by ᶜAlī Moḥammad Khān to ᶜAbdo ṣ-Ṣabūr; on fol. 128a several *tamlīk* and stamps: a purchase note by ebn Loṭfollāh Moḥammad Jaᶜfar al-Madanī (?) al-ᶜĀmelī, his stamp reading "Jaᶜfar b. Luṭf Allāh al-ᶜĀmilī" and dated 1074/1663; purchase note by Moḥammad ᶜAlī b. Shaikh Moḥammad Ṣāleḥ, dated 1116/1704; purchase note by ebn Moḥammad . . . (trimmed away) Moḥammad Khān, dated 1180/1766, his stamp reading "Muḥammad Khān" and dated 1181/1767 (? see also his note on fol. 220a); *tamlīk* by the son of Moḥammad Khān, ebn Moḥammad Khān Moḥammad Reżā. On fol. 281b purchase note by Zaino l-ᶜābedīn, dated 1 Ẕū l-ḥejjä 1237/19 August 1822.

Incipit, fol. 1b

بسمله . هو الله أحد الله الصمد که پایهٔ حقیقت بیچونیش
از دایرهٔ دریافت واحاط شناخت برتراست ...

Explicit, fol. 127a

یوج ف مر جانور شکاری یوز ف مر جانور چرنده
یوزك و یوزه ف مر سگ توله یون مر بنفشه
لله الحمد تمام شد ...

Due to a lacuna of at least one fol. between fols. 2 and 3, the author's name is not preserved in this MS of *Alfāẓ-e advīä* by Nūroddīn Moḥammad b. ʿAbdollāh b. Ḥakīm ʿAino l-molk Qoraishī Shīrāzī.[1] He wrote it in 1038/1628–29 (the title serves as a chronogram, fol. 3a, 4) and dedicated it to the Mughal emperor Shāhjahān (1038-68/1628-58).[2] The text is divided into: 1) a *moqaddemä* in four *fāyedä* (begins on fol. 3a, -7):

1. دربیان علامات تصحیح اعراب
2. دربیان علامات زبان هر دیار
3. درتحقیق طبایع ودرجات دوا وعلاماتی که منسوبست بان وذکر مجملی از دوا بطبع ودرجه وقوت
4. دربیان مختار وشربت ومصلح وبدل دوا وعلامات ان

2) a *natījä* in 28 *bāb* according to the *abtath* alphabet, listing the names of simple drugs in Arabic, Persian, "Hendī," and other tongues; and 3) a *khātemä* on six powerful drugs not discussed in the books of the ancients: *pādzahr, mūmīāʾī, čūb-e čīnī, čāʾī* (sic), *qahvä,* and *tabnākū* (sic). The *khātemä* is missing in this MS. In *fāyedä* 1 of the *moqaddemä, Ṣeḥāḥo l-advīä* by "the son of the author of *Ekhtīārāt-e Badīʿī*"[3] is cited as authority, and in *fāyedä* 4, Mīr Moḥammad Moʾmen Astarābādī is quoted on weights and measures; he wrote a *resālä* on the subject for Moḥammad Qoṭbshāh of Golconda (1020–35/1611–25).[4]

1. PL II 255, no. 439 (1).
2. See preceding note.
3. See **MSS 36** and **45.**
4. PL II 31, no. 61. Apparently this treatise was not given a title by its author.

PL II 255, no. 439 (1); Monzavī I 475b, nos. 4403-07; cf. ibid., 513a, no. 4745 (identical?); Shīrānī II 385, no. 2087; Charminar, p. 237, no. 6; Luzac, p. 22, no. 169; Miklukho-Maklaĭ, p. 53, no. 174; ibid., p. 372, no. 2844 [*khātemä*?]; Osmania Med. Coll., pp. 111-12, nos. 27, 36, resp.; Tashkent V 289, no. 3957 (3085); ibid., IX 359-60, nos. 6535-36 (3494 I and 4614, resp.); Versailles, p. 334, no. 928 (72) [??].

No. 111 : MS Ar. 110

ebn Rashīdoddīn Moḥammad ʿArab

Persian introduction to *Ṭibb al-aʾimma,* by abū ʿItāb ʿAbdallāh wa-l-Ḥusain ibnā Bisṭām

MS Ar. 110 (ex Coll. Min.), 76 fols., 245 x 175 mm; the Arabic text on fols. 3b–75a.

Bound in flexible plain moss-green leather; inner covers pasted with marbled paper; stained and worn. Written on Eastern paper, thin, burnished, off-white.

14 lines, 165 x 95 mm, on blind-ruled frame and lines; black with red rubrics; large, distinguished *naskh*. Catchwords. Copied, and dated 1130/1717, by Yār Moḥammad.

Many marginal notes in Persian throughout MS, in small, elegant *nastaʿlīq* (by scribe?).

On fol. 1a, a *waqfīya* by Muḥammad Jaʿfar b. Muḥammad Ṣafī al-Fārisī, accompanied by his stamp and dated 22 Rajab 1278/23 January 1862.[1] Muḥammad Jaʿfar calls himself *khādim al-madhhab al-jaʿfarī* and donates this book to the students of religious sciences; the *tauliya* of the *waqf* is assigned to his male descendants in the male line, and after them to his male descendants in the female line.

Incipit, fol. 1b

كتاب طب الائمة عليهم السلام
بسمله. حمد وسپاس حكيمي را سزاست كه بحكمت
كامله كيفيت مزاج را از التيام عناصر متضاده مختلف
الاثر ساخته وبروفق ان صورت بسيار بدايع غريب
صنايع انسانرا با حسن صور برداخته

Explicit, fol. 3a, -3

وچون بناى اين كتاب بر احاديث منقوله از حضرات ائمه
معصومين صلوات الله عليهم اجمعين است لهذا اشعار
بذكر معنى حديث وذكر احوال بعض از رواة انها خالى
از مناسبتى نيست

The author of this preface to the Arabic text of *Ṭibb al-aʾimma*,[2] ebn Rashīdoddīn Moḥammad ʿArab (fol. 2b, 4), says that Mīrzā ʿĀdel Khān b. Mīrzā Ḥātem Bēgā,[3] the vizier, ordered him to translate *Ṭibb al-aʾimma* from Arabic into Persian to make it accessible to everyone (fol. 2a, -3). However, the text that follows (from fol. 3b) is in Arabic.

1. Another *vaqfīyä* of his in **No. 42 : MS 21.**
2. Cf. Ullmann, p. 189.
3. If this Ḥātem Bēg is identical with Shāh ʿAbbās I's vizier, Ḥātem Bēg b. Malek Bahrām Ordūbādī Naṣīrī (Eskandar Monshī II 722–23 and index), the date of this edition of *Ṭibb al-aʾimma* would fall into the first half of the eleventh/seventeenth century.

Not in PL or Monzavī.

No. 112 : MS 26 IV

Neẓāmoddīn Aḥmad Gīlānī (?)

[*Ṭalab-e qovvat-e bāh*] [طلب قوت باه]

MS 26 (ex Coll. Min.), 103 fols., 178 x 120 mm; binder's collection of eleven works.
[*Ṭalab-e qovvat-e bāh*] on fols. 55a, 9 to 56b, 1.

For the description of the MS see **No. 62 : MS 26 I.**

Incipit, fol. 55a, 9

طلب قوت باه . حکیم حاذق کامل نظام دولت و دین
که با تو چرخ ستیزه نمای نستیزد
توان حکیم مسیحادمی دراین ایام
که از دوای تو زحمت زخلق بگریزد

Explicit, fol. 56a, -1

هران نگار پری روی که ضرب بند او
چنان مطیع بکرد که هیچ نستیزد

This *qeṭᶜä* in seventeen verses is written in question and answer form. It seems possible that the Neẓāmoddīn mentioned in the scribe's heading is actually its author. Neẓāmoddīn Aḥmad Gīlānī lived at Eṣfahān during the reigns of Shāh ᶜAbbās I and Shāh Ṣafī and went later to the court of Abdollāh Qoṭbshāh of Golconda; he died in 1059/1649.[1] Among the treatises on medical subjects he left is *Bāhīyä,* on drugs influencing sexual powers.[2] It appears probable that the Neẓāmoddīn mentioned in the *qeṭᶜä* is identical with Aḥmad Gīlānī.[3]

1. See PL II 260, no. 447; Monzavī I 472a, s.v. *Asrāro l-aṭebbā*; 595a, s.v. *Majmūᶜä-ye Ḥakīmo l-Molk*; 673b, s.v. *Shajarä-ye dānesh*; 716a (index), s.v. Neẓāmoddīn Aḥmad Gīlānī (all of the works listed under this name by the same author?).
2. See Monzavī I 480b, s.v.
3. In a MS in Teheran Med. Fac., this dialogue is wrongly attributed to Solṭān Sanjar and Avicenna (!); see Monzavī I 480a, no. 4442, s.v. *Bāh-nāmä-ye manẓūm.*

Not in PL; for reference to Monzavī see note 3 above.

No. 113 : MS 46 VII

Mīrzā Qāżī b. Kāshefā

[*Resālä dar čūb-e čīnī va-qahvä va-čāy*] [رساله در چوب چینی وقهوه وچای]

MS 46 (ex Coll. Min.), 149 fols., 210 x 120 mm; binder's collection of eight Arabic and Persian texts. [*Resālä dar čūb-e čīnī*] on fols. 93b–141.

For the description of the MS see **No. 99 : MS 46 II.**

Incipit, fol. 93b

بسمله . الحمد لله ربّ العالمین والصلوة والسّلم علی محمد
خاتم المرسلین وخیر البشر علی ابن [کذا] ابیطالب امیر
المؤمنین ... [س-۲] چون بتوجه خاطر افتاب مآثر
اشرف اقدس مروج مذهب حق ایمّه اثنا عشر کلب
آستان خیر البشر علی ابن [کذا] ابیطالب علیه السلام
شاه عباس صفوی حسینی بهادر خوان [کذا] ...

Explicit, fol. 141a, -3

وبعضی حکایات نقل کرده که هیچ مناسبتی باین چای
خطائی ندارد والله اعلم والعلم عند الله انشا الله لی منافع
ومضار باقی ادویه که از تجربه قیاس برین فقیر ظا شد [کذا.
یعنی ظاهر شد] در کتاب علیحده بیان خواهم کرد تا
شیعیان امیر المومنین علیه السّلام ازین منتفع شوند وثواب
آن بروزگار فیض اثار نواب همایون عاید شود . [بتاریخ ...

Qāżī b. Kāshefā b. Moḥammad Rashīd (fol. 94a, -1) wrote his untitled treatise *dar čūb-e čīnī va-qahvä va-čāy* (fol. 94b, 5) for Shāh ᶜAbbās Ṣafavī (fol. 94a, 2). He divided it into three *bāb*, and the first of these into *faṣl* (fol. 95a, 1).

Mīrzā Qāżī died at Ardabīl in 1075/1664-65, after having been Shaikho l-Eslām at Eṣfahān.[1] His father, "Ḥakīm Kāshefā-ye Yazdī,"[2] was physician to Shāh Ṣafī and served as *ḥakīmbāshī-ye Īrān*; he wrote a Persian treatise *ar-Robᶜo l-mojayyab*.[3] Among Mīrzā Qāżī's works are theological tracts,[4] two treatises on astronomy, *Toḥfä-ye ᶜAbbāsīyä*[5] and *at-Toḥfä al-Moḥammadīyä*;[6] a metrological tract, *Resālä fī l-owzāno sh-sharᶜīyä*;[7] and two books on medical subjects, *Jām-e jahān-nomāy-e ᶜAbbāsī*, on the legitimate uses of wine, and this discussion of chinaroot and other modern drugs.[8] His tract *Jām* was written on command of Shāh ᶜAbbās I in 1037/1627,[9] but it cannot be determined to which shāh of this name the astronomical treatise[10] and the work on chinaroot are dedicated.[11]

1. See *Jāmeᶜ-e Mofīdī*, p. 503, 13, and index; Rieu II 844a, *ad* Add. 19619 I (quotation from *Qeṣaṣo l-khāqānī*).
2. *Zail-e Tārīkh-e ᶜālamārā-ye ᶜAbbāsī*, p. 276, 1.
3. *Dharīᶜa* V 309, 25 (no. 1476).
4. Ibid.
5. PL II 90, no. 136 (1).
6. Ibid. (2), dedicated to Eᶜtemādo d-dowlä Moḥammad Bēg *vazīr-e aᶜẓam*, one of the viziers under Shāh ᶜAbbās II (Vaḥīd Qazvīnī, *ᶜAbbāsnāmä*, pp. 171-72, 298-99, index).
7. PL II 90, no. 136; no MSS are known as yet.
8. On these two see Rieu II 844a, *ad* Add. 19619 I-II.
9. Ibid.; in *Dharīᶜa* (note 3 above) a MS is mentioned that was dated 1026/1617. If that is correct, *Jām* was composed about eleven years earlier at least.
10. Rehatsek, p. 38, no. 72, does not have any details.
11. Rieu II 844a, *ad* Add. 19619 II, states, without giving reasons, that it too was composed under Shāh ᶜAbbās I.

PL II 255, no. 438 (2); Monzavī I 414b, nos. 3837-47; Tashkent VI 162, no. 4366 (2873 II).

Jām-e jahān-nomāy-e ᶜAbbāsī: Miklukho-Maklaĭ, p. 135, no. 889; Tashkent VI 161, no. 4365 (2873 I); ibid., VIII 111, no. 5689 (9269 I).

No. 114 : MS 87 I

Mīrzā Qāżī b. Kashefā

[*Resālä dar čūb-e čīnī va-qahvä va-čāy-e khaṭāʾī*]

[رساله درچوب چینی وقهوه وچای خطائی]

MS 87 (ex Coll. Min.), 134 fols., 210 x 115 mm; scribe's (?) collection of three works; no. III (fols. 59b-127a), *Shajarä-ye elāhīyä*, by Moḥammad b. Ḥaidar *al-madᶜūv be*-Rafīᶜoddīn al-Ḥosainī aṭ-Ṭabāṭabāʾī, non-medical, not catalogued. (See also **No. 104 : MS 87 II**.)
[*Resālä dar čūb-e čīnī*] on fols. 1-34.

Bound in flexible plain black leather; inner covers bare; one flyleaf each in front and back of Eastern paper, thick, burnished, beige; spine torn, part of MS loose, warped. Written on Eastern paper, medium thin, burnished, cream-colored; especially first fols. spotted, stained. Lacuna between fols. 57 and 58.

A. Works I and III, fols. 1-34, 58-127: 12 lines, 130 x 65 mm, on blind-ruled frame and lines; greyish-black with red rubrics, on fols. 1-34 left out, on fols. 58-127 mostly filled in; medium-small neat *naskh*, leaning to *nastaᶜlīq*. Catchwords. B. Fols. 35-57: 12 lines, 130 x 65 mm, on blind-ruled frame and lines; greyish-black with red rubrics, partly left out; medium-small to medium-large neat *naskh*; written with narrower pen than A, but by the same scribe (?). Catchwords. Fols. 34b, 35a, 57b, 127b blank.

Collations by scribe.
I and II anonymous, undated copies; III ends as follows (fol. 127a, 6):

وبتاریخ نهم شهر ربیع الآخر سنه ۱۰۴۸ ز تالیف وتنمیق
این رساله فراغ افتاد بحمد علی متعال وصلوة بر نبی وآل
ختم نمود تم

A comparison with Rieu I 31b shows that this is the author's own colophon to his work, but not the scribe's;[1] III is therefore also an anonymous, undated copy. Since the paper is identical throughout the whole MS, I-III can be attributed to approximately the same period, ca. 1100/1700, even if not transcribed by the same hand.

Fols. 128-134 filled with recipes.

On fol. 1a a *tamlīk* by ʿAbdo l-Ghaffār is dated 1264/1847. On fols. 1b, 2a, 35b, 36a, 58a, etc., the scribe wrote *waqf* in bold letters.

Incipit, fol. 1b

دوائی چند که در کتب حکماء سابق نبوده مثل چوب چینی
وقهوه وچای خطائی این رساله مشتمل است بر سه
باب ...

Explicit, fol. 34a, 4

ودر بعضی حکایات نقل کرده که هیچ مناسبتی باین چا خطائی
ندارد والعلم عند الله انشاء الله تعالی منافع ومضار باقی
ادویه که از تجربه وقیاس برین فقیر ظاهر شده در کتاب علاحده
بیان خواهم کرد خواص وعوام ازین منتفع شوند تم

The MS contains an untitled, anonymous treatise on *čūb-e čīnī, qahvä,* and *čāy-e khaṭāʾī* (Incipit) in three *bāb,* subdivided into *faṣl.* Perhaps it was transcribed from a defective MS lacking the preface, or the copyist of the MS took exception to the very marked Shīʿite tendency in the introductory remarks; this copy at least is not damaged in the beginning. The identification of this tract as that by Qāżī b. Kāshefā rests on its comparison with **No. 113 : MS 46 VII.**

Among the earlier authors quoted are ʿEmādoddīn Maḥmūd Shīrāzī,[2] Kamāloddīn Ḥosain Shīrāzī,[3] the author's own father,[4] and al-Bīrūnī with his *K. aṣ-ṣaidana.*[5]

1. In the British Museum MS the date of composition is given as Rabīʿ II 1047/23 August-20 September 1637, however (see Rieu I 31b); this may well be a copyist's error.
2. See **No. 99 : MS 46 II,** with references.
3. See **No. 105 : MS 88.**
4. All three are quoted on the nature of *čūb-e čīnī,* fol. 1b, -5 to end.
5. Here misspelled *Ketāb-e ṣaidīyä,* fol. 34a, 1; see also PL II 202, no. 356.

No. 115 : MS 115

Moḥammad Moʾmen b. Moḥammad Zamān Tonakābonī

Toḥfato l-moʾmenīn تحفة المؤمنين

MS 115 (ex Coll. Min.), 307 fols., 310 x 210 mm

Bound in lacquered cardboard; outer covers: red borders with floral design in green and blue framed in narrow black and gold borders; dark blue panel with three-medallion design, floral scrolls of green and different shades of pink and rose; inner covers: narrow black and gold borders, red panel with a green and yellow lily; spine of dark brown leather. One flyleaf each in front and back of thin, flexible cardboard; in the back, one more leaf of thick white paper. The corners and edges of the binding, and the front cover, much battered. Written on Italian (?) paper, medium thin, slightly transparent, glazed, white; watermarks, heraldic devices and names written in capital letters, unclear.

23 lines, 215 x 110 mm, on blind-ruled frame and lines; black with crimson overlinings; medium-sized dense, even, but undistinguished *shekastä-āmīz*; some rubrics in *naskh*. Catchwords.

Collations by scribe.

Anonymous copy, dated (fol. 265b, -1) 1273/1856.

Recipes on fol. 1a and in margins.

On fol. 1b a *tamlīk* and two stamps of Moḥammad Bāqer b. Moḥammad Reżā ʿAṭṭār, dated 19 Ṣafar 1290/18 April 1873; on the back flyleaf a *tamlīk* in modern blue ink by Āqā Mīrzā Naṣrollāh Khān, dated "the night of 11-27-1313 (*h.sh.*?)/16 February 1935."

Incipit, fol. 1b

بسمله. وبه نستعين. سبحانك اللهم يا قدوس ويا طبيب
النفوس اتمم لنا انوار معرفتك وارزقنا سعودت مغفرتك ...

Explicit, fol. 307b, 9

از خوردن ان طیور بیهوش گردند وچون دبق را با عسل
ودوشاب طبخ بلیغ داده مانند ریسمان براشجار وغیر ان
گذارند طیوریکه بران نشینند پای بست گردند
قد فرغت ...

Najīboddīn Moḥammad Moʾmen b. Moḥammad Zamān Tonakābonī Dailamī (fol. 1b, -8 to -6) divided his pharmacopoeia and dispensatory *Toḥfato l-moʾmenīn* (fol. 2a, -10)[1] into two main parts: A) (five) *tashkhīṣāt*, and B) *dastūrāt* in three *qesm*. None of the known manuscripts that are described in detail contains the last of these *qesm*.[2] The layout of the work is as follows:

A. *tashkhīṣāt*

1. (begins on fol. 2b, 2)

دربيان سبب اختلاف اقوال در ماهيات وقوة وقدر شربت ادويه وشروط اخذ هر دوا وذكر درجات وانقسام قوتها باقسامه

2. (begins on fol. 4a, 9)

در ذكر صفات احول ادويه وبيان افعال كليه وتغير اسامى ومعانى لغاتى كه در طى انشا اين مجموعه مذكور ميشود ودر كتب ادويه مفرده مدار عليهاست

3. (begins on fol. 7b, -2) دربيان ماهيه وخواص وكيفيت ادويه مفرده واغذيه مفرده ومركبه وذكر مصلح وبدل وقدر شربت وانچه بدان مناسب است

4. (begins on fol. 248a, 7) در مداواى سموم

5. (begins on fol. 253b, 3) دربيان اوزان وانچه بان متعلق است

B. *dastūrāt*, in three *qesm*

1. (begins on fol. 255a, 1) in five *ṭarīq*[3]

دربيان اعمالى كه متعلق است بادويه مفرده مثل شستن وسوختن ادويه وتحميص وتسويه وامثال ان وطريق اشاميدن عشبه وچوب چينى وماء الجبن ومانندان واعمال غريبه

2. (begins on fol. 276a, 1) in 24 *bāb*

دربيان اعمالى كه متعلق است بادويه مركبه وذكر معاجين وحبوب وساير مركبات

3. (mentioned in table of contents on fol. 2b, 1)

در معالجات با رعایت اختصار

Moḥammad Moʾmen wrote this work as a collection of prescriptions well tested by his father and himself in long practice, and also as a corrective to the most widely used work on *materia medica* in his time, *Ekhtīārāt-e Badīʿī.*[4] As his major source he took *Mā lā yasaʿu ṭ-ṭabība jahluhū,* known as *Jāmeʿ-e* Baghdādī,[5] but he also gleaned material from ibn al-Baiṭār's *Jāmiʿ*,[6] Dāvūd Anṭākī's *Tadhkirat ulī l-albāb,*[7] ibn at-Tilmīdh,[8] "moʾallef-e *Moghnī*",[9] "moṣannef-e *Shāmel*"[10] and others, and perused the following standard works of medicine: the *Qānūn, Moʿālajāt-e Boqrāṭī,*[11] *Ekhtīārāt-e* bn-e Hobal,[12] *Ḥāvī-ye kabīr va-ṣaghīr,*[13] *Shefāʾo l-asqām,*[14] *Moʿālajāt-e* Īlāqī,[15] *Konnāsh-e fākher,*[16] Bokhtīshūʿ,[17] Galen's *Munqidh as-sumūm,*[18] *Kāmil aṣ-ṣināʿa,*[19] *Moṣannafāt-e* Moḥammad-e bn-e Zakarīyā,[20] and *Manqūlāt-e* Ḥonain-e bn-e Esḥāq;[21] at the end of this long list, the author enumerates some works by Indian physicians which he studied: *Tarjamä-ye* Bāhar,[22] *Ketāb-e* Čarak,[23] استجوك,[24] and Bhōjdēv-e Fīrūzshāhī.[25] For the sake of brevity, the author adds, he will not quote his sources' names in the places of his book where he cites them. It is remarkable that none of these books, whether Moḥammad Moʾmen actually used them or not,[26] were composed by a Persian author in Persian.[27] He even appears to blame Ḥājjī Zaino l-ʿAṭṭār for his use of this language, saying مولف اختیارات بدیعی بلغت فارسی نوشته ومساهله درتحقیق ادویه نموده (fol. 1b, -5).

At the end of the *tashkhīṣāt, Toḥfato l-moʾmenīn* is dated "in the months of" 1090/1679.[28] The author dedicated it to Shāh Solaimān Ṣafavī, the service at court being a tradition passed on to him from his father and his grandfather (fols. 1b, -9 to 2b, 1 comprise the preface and table of contents).

1. The wording of the preface does not suggest interpreting مؤمنين as a dual. It is rather a *genitivus obiectivus,* and the title is to be translated as "Gift to the Believers." The author introduces the title only *en passant,* and not as referring to his father and himself (cf. Elgood, p. 368).

   Another work by Moḥammad Moʾmen, on theology, shows the same pattern in its title: *Tabṣerato l-moʾmenīn*; it was completed in 1086/1675, according to a MS in Mashhad (*Cat.* I, *faṣl* 1, MS no. 62; *Dharīʿa* III 325, no. 1188; PL II 261, no. 448). Cf. note 28 below.
2. See PL II 261, no. 448; Pertsch, p. 585, note 7.
3. The fifth *ṭarīq* of this *qesm* is not transcribed in all MSS (see **MSS 117** and **120 IV**); its subjects are alchemical processes, implements, and codes.
4. See **No. 20 : MS 36**, etc.
5. Composed in 711/1311 by Yūsuf b. Ismāʿīl b. Ilyās al-Kutubī al-Baghdādī as a practical abridgment of ibn al-Baiṭār's *Jāmiʿ*; see Ullmann, pp. 281, 285.
6. See Ullmann, p. 281.
7. See Ullmann, pp. 181, 287.
8. Ibn at-Tilmīdh wrote an *Aqrābādhīn* that won wide fame; see Ullmann, pp. 163, 306.
9. The text seems to be corrupt in this passage; it reads (fol. 2a, 2):

هرچه ابن تلمیذ مولف مغنی ومصنف شامل
کامل الادویه امین الدوله وغیره ایراد نموده

Ibn at-Tilmīdh was also known under his *laqab* Amīn ad-Daula (see Ullmann, p. 163), but he was not the author of a *Mughnī.* His teacher, abū l-Ḥasan Saʿīd b. Hibatallāh, wrote a *K. al-mughnī fī tadbīr al-amrāḍ wa-maʿrifat al-ʿilal wa-l-aʿrāḍ* (see Ullmann, p. 160), but since in this passage works on pharmacopoeia are listed, probably ibn al-Baiṭār's *K. al-mughnī fī l-adwiya al-mufrada* is meant (Ullmann, p. 281). Abū l-Munā al-Kūhīn al-ʿAṭṭār abridged his dispensatory *K. minhāj ad-dukkān* in *al-Mughnī wa-l-bayān fī l-ḥawānīt wa-l-bīmāristānāt* (Ullmann, p. 309; GAL Supp. I 897), but this work does not appear to have been widely known. A Persian medical text titled *Moghnī ṭ-ṭabīb,* by abū Ṭāleb Sharīf Ḥosainī, cannot be meant here because it is later than *Toḥfä* (see Monzavī I 598b, no. 5593; Dāneshgāh XV, 4216, no. 5359; cf. Monzavī I 513a, no. 4746, s.v. *Jāmeʿo t-tajāreb*). The next title in Moḥammad Moʾmen's list might be understood as *K. ash-shāmil fī l-adwiya al-mufrada,* by Ghiyāth ad-Dīn a. Saʿīd ash-Shīrāzī (Ullmann, p. 285; Dietrich, p. 158, no. 66), again presuming that here books on pharmacopoeia are listed (for medical books in general of this title cf. ibn a. Uṣaibi῾a, index, s.v. abū l-Khaṭṭāb Muḥammad b. Muḥammad; Ullmann and GAS III, resp. indices, s.v. *aš-Šāmil*).

10. See preceding note.
11. By abū l-Ḥasan Aḥmad b. Muḥammad aṭ-Ṭabarī at-Turunjī; see Ullmann, p. 140.
12. *K. al-mukhtārāt fī ṭ-ṭibb*, by Muhadhdhab ad-Dīn ῾Alī b. Hubal; see Ullmann, pp. 161–62.
13. Abū Bakr Muḥammad b. Zakarīyā᾽ ar-Rāzī's famous medical encyclopedia (Ullmann, p. 130) and *K. al-ḥāwī fī ῾ilm at-tadāwī*, by Najmoddīn Maḥmūd Shīrāzī (Ullmann, p. 178; see **No. 17 : MS 20**).
14. By Ḥājjī Bāshā Khiḍr b. ῾Alī al-Āyidīnī; see Ullmann, p. 180.
15. Muḥammad b. ῾Alī al-Īlāqī wrote, around 460/1068, a commentary on ibn Sīnā's *Kullīyāt* (GAL I 485, Supp. I 826c, 887).
16. Ascribed to ar-Rāzī, but in all likelihood not by him; see Ullmann, pp. 132f., 136.
17. It cannot be decided which member of the famous family of physicians is meant here. In a series of medical compendia it is plausible to expect a mention of Jurjīs b. Jibrīl b. Bukhtīshū῾'s *Kunnāsh*, or of Jibrīl b. ῾Ubaidallāh b. Bukhtīshū῾'s *al-Kāfī* (see Ullmann, pp. 108–11; Dietrich, p. 64, no. 21; GAS III 210, 314). (On the name B*u*khtīshū῾, a Syro-Persian hybrid meaning "Jesus saved," see Justi, *Iranisches Namenbuch*, p. 72, s.v. *Buχtyešū῾*.)
18. This could mean Galen's *K. al-adwiya al-muqābila li-l-adwā᾽* or the Pseudo-Galenian *K. as-sumūm* (Ullmann, p. 49, no. 53, and p. 61, no. 106, resp.).
19. By ῾Alī b. al-῾Abbās al-Majūsī; see Ullmann, p. 140.
20. The author adds after this title (fol. 2a, 5):

وسایر کتب که فهرست اسامی ان در خارج
کتاب مرقوم است

He appears to be talking about a collection of shorter works by ar-Rāzī in one volume; see Ullmann, pp. 132–36.

21. Given the number of translations of Greek medical texts done by Ḥunain b. Isḥāq, this formulation does not make much sense; on Ḥunain's adaptations from Greek, and his own writings, see Ullmann, pp. 117–19; GAS III 247–56.
22. According to Dr. Claus Vogel (letter of 4 May 1974), Bāhar represents Bāhaḍa here, a vernacular form of the well-known physician Vāgbhaṭa's name; cf. Claus Vogel, *Vāgbhaṭa's Aṣṭāṅgahṛdayasaṃhitā. The First Five Chapters of Its Tibetan Version*, Abhandlungen für die Kunde des Morgenlandes, 37 II (Wiesbaden 1965), p. 45.
23. On Caraka see Julius Jolly, "Medicin," *Grundriß der Indo-Arischen Philologie* . . . III 10 (Straßburg 1901), § 9; cf. Ullmann, p. 122.
24. Probably *Siddhayoga* by Vṛnda; see Jolly (note 23 above), § 5.
25. This Bhōjdēv is conceivably identical with Rāy Bhōjdēv, the translator into Persian of a (Sanskrit?) book of therapy *a capite ad calcem* in 48 *faṣl* preserved in a seventeenth-century copy from India at Tashkent (*Cat.* X 119, no. 6865 [10032 IV]). However, it cannot at present be determined at the court of which of the Delhi or Bengal sultans of the name Fīrūzshāh this Bhōjdēv was in service (see Bosworth, *Dynasties*, Index, s.v. Fīrūz).
26. In *bāb* 24 of *qesm* 2 of the *dastūrāt*, on the treatment of hunting-birds, Moḥammad Mo᾽men quotes the names of great veterinarians and falconers of the past: Qosṭūn-e Rūmī, ebno l-῾Avvām, Adham, Qeṭrif (!), Sūmāros, and ebn-e Jānes (probably an error for Arkhījānes, Archigenes). See Ullmann, *Naturwissenschaften*, pp. 44–50, esp. p. 50 on Dāwūd b. ῾Umar al-Anṭākī, obviously quoted here by Moḥammad Mo᾽men.
27. In *qesm* 2 of the *dastūrāt*, a physician Moḥammad Bāqer is often mentioned as the author of compound prescriptions. His name is followed by the eulogy *ṭāba tharāhu*, which might point to the fact that he had only recently died when *Toḥfä* was composed. This Moḥammad Bāqer could be the son of ῾Emādoddīn Maḥmūd; see PL II 251, no. 428.
28. Presumably on the authority of the MS, Īraj Afshār dates *Toḥfä* in the year 1080/1669; see "Fehrest-e noskhähā-ye khaṭṭī-ye Ketābkhānä-ye Vezārat-e Omūr-e Khārejä" in Nashrīyä I 2, s.v. *Toḥfato l-mo᾽menīn*. If that is correct, the date given in the UCLA manuscript would refer to a copy somewhere in its chain of transmission (cf. Elgood, p. 368).

PL II 261, no. 448; Monzavī I 491a, nos. 4528–88; ibid., 584b, no. 5457; ibid., 604b, no. 5640; Panjāb P.L., p. 347, no. 262, p. 316, no. 243 (*Entekhāb* titled *Farhang-e advīä*); Täbrīz I 222–24, nos. 165–66 (*shomārä-ye daftar* 2569 and 2593, resp.); al-Khāliṣī, p. 257, no. 1; Nūrbakhsh I 194, no. 197; Charminar, p. 241, nos. 147–50; ibid., p. 238, no. 57 [*Entekhāb az Toḥfä*]; Eilers-Heinz, p. 284, no. 264; Luzac, p. 45, nos. 322–23; Meredith-Owens, p. 29, no. Or. 12419; Miklukho-Maklaĭ, p. 106, nos. 653–54; Osmania Med. Coll., p. 111, no. 24; Osmania Univ., p. 52, no. 24; Rampur, p. 132, nos. 327–29; Tashkent V 276–78, nos. 3929–35 (4224 I and III, 2717, 3502, 3653, 2116 VI, 2479 IV, 3760 I, resp.); ibid., VIII 102, no. 5685 (3516); ibid., IX 315–19, nos. 6481–84 (5031, 2266, 4660, 5842, resp.).

Turkish version of *Toḥfä*, *Ghunyetü l-muḥaṣṣilīn fī terjemet Tuḥfetü l-mu᾽minīn*, by Aḥmed b. Ḥüseyin b. Ḥasan . . . (1164/1750): al-Mauṣil, pp. 44, 61, nos. 57 and 148, resp.

Qarābāẕīn-e jong [?]: Tashkent IX 363–65, no. 6539 (479).

No. 116 : MS 116

Moḥammad Moʾmen b. Moḥammad Zamān Tonakābonī

Toḥfato l-moʾmenīn تحفة المؤمنين

MS 116 (ex Coll. Min.), 115 fols., 250 x 157 mm

Modern brochure of thin, flexible, fading green cardboard; one flyleaf each in front and back of medium-thin, white paper, modern. Written on European paper, medium thin, transparent, burnished, white; watermarks obscure. Stained, spotted, many margins repaired; most of fol. 1 torn out, lost; remaining fragment pasted on European (?) paper, thin, transparent, burnished, greyish. For lacunae see below.

22 lines, 170 x 90 mm, on blind-ruled frame and lines; black with red rubrics; medium-sized even, neat, but undistinguished *naskh*. Catchwords.

Collations by scribe and by a reader marked at regular intervals, as they were proceeding; they were done from a copy written mostly in the author's own hand (fol. 41b, margin) and completed on 2 Shaʿbān 1105/29 March 1694 (fol. 116b, margin); the MS was collated again with a copy transcribed from the author's (note on fol. 116b).

Copied, and dated the last [30] Rajab 1105/27 March 1694, by Mīr Mahdī al-Ḥosainī.

Numerous recipes in margins, quoted from ṣāḥeb-e *Ḥāvī*,[1] ṣāḥeb-e *Kāmelo ṣ-ṣenāʿā*,[2] ebn Sīnā, *Zakhīrā*,[3] *Aghrāżo ṭ-ṭebb*,[4] Najīb ad-Dīn as-Samarqandī's *Qarābāzīn-e khamsā*,[5] *Sadīdī*,[6] Dāvūd Anṭākī,[7] Shefāʾī,[8] ʿEmādoddīn Maḥmūd Shīrāzī,[9] Sālekoddīn Moḥammad Ḥamavī,[10] Moḥammad Hāshem Ṭehrānī,[11] and Emām Reżā;[12] notes by Moḥammad Bāqer Ḥosainī Ṭabīb[13] on fols. 20b and 116b.

Owner's stamp on fol. 106b, illegible but for: Muḥammad; a library stamp (modern) on fol. 2a, giving the name of Majdoddīn.

Incipit, fol. 2a

با دیگری وبعضی درمنافع متفرد وبعضی مضعف
قوة ادویه نافعه اند پس در تراکیب شرط
است که از کثیر المنفعه وشریف واز ضعیف القوه
المنفعة قدر زیاده داخل کنند ...

Explicit, fol. 116b, 1

وچون دبقرا باعسل ودوشاب طبیخ [کذا] بلیغ داده
مانند ریسمان براشجار وغیرآن گذارند طیوری که
بران نشینند [کذا] پای بسته گردند والسلام علی من اتبع
الهدی قد فرغت ...

This MS contains *qesm* 2 of the *dastūrāt* of Moḥammad Moʾmen's *Toḥfato l-moʾmenīn.* Of the first fol. only a small fragment is preserved, and the text begins on fol. 2a within the introduction; cf. **MS 120 IV**, fol. 42a, 3.

1. Abū Bakr Muḥammad b. Zakarīyāʾ ar-Rāzī; see Ullmann, p. 128, etc.
2. ʿAlī b. al-ʿAbbās al-Majūsī; see Ullmann, p. 140, etc.
3. This is either the well-known *K. adh-dhakhīra* by Pseudo-Thābit b. Qurra, or Esmāʿīl Jorjānī's equally famous *Zakhīrä-ye Khwārezmshāhī*; see Ullmann, p. 136, and **No. 2 : MS 1,** etc.
4. By Esmāʿīl Jorjānī; see **No. 13 : MS 6.**
5. A collection of works on *materia medica* and pharmacy by as-Samarqandī; there are four treatises on these subjects and dietetics: *K. aṭʿimat al-marḍā*, *K. uṣūl tarkīb al-adwiya*, *K. al-aghdhiya wa-l-ashriba*, and *Qarābādhīn ʿalā tartīb al-ʿilal*; one MS of this collection contains in addition the author's *K. al-asbāb wa-l-ʿalāmāt* and *K. al-adwiya al-mufrada*; see Ullmann, pp. 170, 201, 278, 308.
6. Sadīd ad-Dīn al-Kāzarūnī's commentary on the *Mūjiz* by ibn an-Nafīs, titled *al-Mughnī*, but often known as *Sadīdī*; see Dietrich, p. 89, no. 33.
7. Dāwūd b. ʿUmar al-Anṭākī composed *Tadhkirat ulī l-albāb wa-l-jāmiʿ li-l-ʿajab al-ʿujāb* and *K. an-nuzha al-mubhija fī tashḥīdh al-adhhān wa-taʿdīl al-amzija*; see Ullmann, pp. 181, 287.
8. See **No. 88 : MS 105 II**, etc.
9. See **No. 99 : MS 46 II**, etc.
10. This is probably Sālekoddīn Moḥammad b. Mālekoddīn Moʾayyad Ḥamavī Yazdī, who lived during the reign of Shāh ʿAbbās I and was more than seventy (lunar) years old in 1032/1622 (Nashrīyä III 12a, 7). According to *Jāmeʿ-e Mofīdī*, he died toward the end of ʿAbbās I's reign. His father's and grandfather's names are given there as Moʾayyadoddīn Moḥammad b. Saʿdoddīn Moḥammad (*Jāmeʿ-e Mofīdī*, pp. 406, 14 to 407, 7). In his treatise on coffee, tea, bezoar, and chinaroot he calls himself a pupil of ʿEmādoddīn Maḥmūd Shīrāzī (Leipzig *Cat.*, p. 512b, no. CCLVII 6). He also wrote *Haikal-e fīl* (Monzavī I 609a, with reference to Rahāvard, pp. 15, 196, 433; cf. *Jāmeʿ-e Mofīdī*, p. 407, 1) and gathered and transcribed in his own hand two collections of medical works, one in Arabic, called *Majmaʿ an-nafāʾis*, and the other in Persian, called *Ḥajalato l-ʿarāyes* (Nashrīyä III 10b, s.v. *Ḥajalato l-ʿarāyes*). See PL II 255, no. 437.
11. See **Nos. 123–124 : MSS 48–49.**
12. This refers either to *ar-Risāla adh-dhahabīya*, an Arabic work on hygiene, etc., ascribed to the eighth imām ʿAlī b. Mūsā ar-Riḍā, or to one of its Persian versions; on these see PL II 196, no. 350; Meshkāt III (2) 735; **Nos. 222** and **218 : MSS 69–70.**
13. A Sayyed Moḥammad Bāqer Mūsavī (thus quoted in PL II 264, no. 452) was court physician to Shāh Solaimān (1077–1105/1666–94) and Shāh Solṭān Ḥosain (1105–35/1693–1722). It is therefore possible that this MS was at one time in his possession.

No. 117 : MS 117

Moḥammad Moʾmen b. Moḥammad Zamān Tonakābonī

Toḥfato l-moʾmenīn تحفة المؤمنين

MS 117, 185 fols., 280 x 180 mm; scribe's collection of several poetical works and the *dastūrāt* of *Toḥfato l-moʾmenīn*. *Toḥfato l-moʾmenīn* on fols. 65–169.

Bound in flexible burgundy-colored leather; three-medallion design with blind-stamped floral scrolls; inner covers thick greyish-green leather; warped, worn, MS out of binding, spine torn and broken; sewing of MS mostly undone, quires and single leaves unattached. Written on European paper, medium thick, burnished, white; watermarks obscure. The MS is incomplete in front and back; for other lacunae see below.

19 lines, 200 x 115 mm, on blind-ruled frame and lines; black with red rubrics, these repeated in margins; medium-sized even, fine *nastaʿlīq*. Catchwords.

Collations by scribe.

Anonymous copy (after fol. 169 one fol., the end of *Toḥfä*, is missing); ca. 1200/1800.

Illegible *tamlīk* on fol. 169b; on fol. 181a several owner's stamps, most of them reading: Moḥammad Ḥosain . . . Ṭabāṭabā'ī and dated 127·/1853–62; on fol. 101b an owner's stamp reading: adīb al-mamālik and dated 13·4 (third digit illegible)/between 1886 and 1915; thus, in all likelihood, Mīrzā Ṣādeq Khān Farāhānī "Adību l-Mamālek" (1277–1336/1860–1917)[1] was at one time the owner of this manuscript.

Incipit, fol. 65a

بسمله. در بیان اعمالی که متعلق است بادویه مفرده
وان مشتمل است طریق دویم در بیان دستور
استعمال بعضی ادویه مثل چوب چینی وماند آن...
[س ۵] ... طریق اوّل در تدابیر ادویه مفرده وان مشتمل
است بر پنج فصل...

Explicit, fol. 169b, -1

واب دهن دافع قمل دوی جمیع حیوان است وحقیر
نیز مجرب یافته است وبتعدیل است]

The MS contains the *dastūrāt* of Moḥammad Mo'men's *Toḥfato l-mo'menīn.* After fol. 169 one fol. is missing; the text breaks off on fol. 169b within *bāb* 24 of *qesm* 2 of the *dastūrāt.* In *qesm* 1 the last, fifth, *ṭarīq* is not copied in this MS; on fol. 78a, 6 the scribe wrote وطریق پنجم مخصوص نسخهٔ اصل است (see **MS 115**, fols. 266–275).

1. See Rypka, p. 348, no. 8, and esp. pp. 375–76.

No. 118 : MS 118

Moḥammad Mo'men b. Moḥammad Zamān Tonakābonī

Toḥfato l-mo'menīn تحفة المؤمنين

MS 118 (ex Coll. Min.), 65 fols., 295 x 200 mm

Bound in thin flexible brown leather; simple blind tooling; stained, worn; spine torn. Binding too small for the size of leaves, not original. Written on Eastern paper, medium thin, burnished, beige; stained, most margins torn, repaired, some more than once; first and last fols. badly torn. For lacunae see below.

25 lines, 235 x 160 mm, on blind-ruled frame and lines; black with red rubrics; medium-sized good *nastaʿlīq*; fols. 64–65 written in slightly smaller, more open *nastaʿlīq*, by the same scribe (?). Catchwords, often torn off or pasted over by repairs.
Anonymous, undated copy (fragment); twelfth/eighteenth century.
Medical notes by readers on fol. 1a and in margins.

This MS is an incomplete copy of the *dastūrāt* of *Toḥfato l-moʾmenīn*; the beginning and end are missing and there are several lacunae in between. The copy is misbound; the order of fols. has to be corrected as follows: beginning missing, 8–17 (*qesm* 1, within *ṭarīq* 1 to within *ṭarīq* 5), lacuna (six fols.?), 19–27, 18, 28–63, 6, 2–4, lacuna of one fol., 5, 64–65 (*qesm* 2, within preface to within *bāb* 23), lacuna (one fol.?), 7 (part of *bāb* 24); fol. 1b contains a long supplement to fol. 20a (cf. the sign over *meṣrūzīṭūn* on fols. 1b and 20a, resp., and see **MS 120**, fol. 48b).

No. 119 : MS 119

Moḥammad Moʾmen b. Moḥammad Zamān Tonakābonī

Toḥfato l-moʾmenīn تحفة المؤمنين

MS 119 (ex Coll. Min.), 191 fols., 168 x 110 mm

Bound in slightly flexible, plain rust-colored leather; inner covers pasted with European paper; one front flyleaf of Italian paper; of the watermark only part of a name in a cartouche legible: ...NANI E. F. Binding worn, warped, brittle; too small for MS, not original. Written on Eastern paper, thin, burnished, beige; stains, holes, margins frayed and repaired; torn. Blank leaves inserted for lacunae; on these see below.
17 lines, 130 x 85 mm, on blind-ruled frame and lines; black with red rubrics; small, good *shekastä-āmīz*. Catchwords. Collations by scribe.
Anonymous, undated copy (end missing); ca. 1200/1800.
Notes in margins.
On fol. 1a an owner's stamp: ʿAlī Ibrāhīm, dated 1221/1806.

Incipit, fol. 1a

از اسا بسریانی و بفارسی مورد نامند

Explicit, fol. 191b, -1

وضماد خشك او با حنا كه در حمام استعمال نمایند
جهة جرب وحكه]

The MS contains *tashkhīṣ* 3 of Moḥammad Moʾmen's *Toḥfato l-moʾmenīn*; beginning and end are missing; in this MS the text starts within the section on *ās*, and ends within the section on *shāhtaraj*. Fols. 6, 7, 21 are blank; they mark the position of lacunae.

No. 120 : MS 120 I

Moḥammad Moʾmen b. Moḥammad Zamān Tonakābonī

Toḥfato l-moʾmenīn تحفة المؤمنين

MS 120 (ex Coll. Min.), 187 fols., 222 x 120 mm; binder's collection of four works, nos. I-III copied by the same scribe. Nos. I and IV are parts of *Toḥfä,* nos. II and III two other medical texts in Persian. (See also **Nos. 121, 158,** and **204.**) *Toḥfato l-moʾmenīn, tashkhīṣ* 4-5 and *qesm* 1 of *dastūrāt* on fols. 1-35.

Bound in rust-colored leather over thick, stiff cardboard; flap; simple blind-tooled borders around covers and flap; inner covers and flap pasted with violet-colored paper; five flyleaves in front, one in back; the first two front flyleaves of medium-thin, burnished, cream-colored Eastern paper, the other flyleaves of white European paper, watermarks obscure. Binding stained, somewhat worn; not original. Written on two varieties of Eastern paper: A. fols. 1-40: thin, transparent, burnished, beige; B. fols. 41-187: thin to medium thick, of varying transparency, burnished, beige; some spots and stains.

A. Fols. 1-40. I. Fols. 1-35a: 21 lines, 150 x 60 mm, on blind-ruled frame and lines; black with crimson rubrics; medium-sized copperplate *naskh.* II. Fols. 35b-39a: medium-small, impeccable *nastaʿlīq* by the same scribe. III. Fols. 39b-40a: tables of 9 x 2 fields, 155 x 77 mm; alternating diagonal lines; medium-small, distinguished *shekastä-āmīz* by the same scribe. Catchwords throughout. B. Fols. 41-187: 21 lines, 150 x 60 mm, on blind-ruled frame and lines; black with red rubrics; three styles of medium-sized *naskh,* probably by one scribe: 1) fols. 41b-97b, nearly copperplate; 2) fols. 98a-106b, less disciplined than 1); 3) fols. 107a-186a, slightly smaller, but finer than 2). Catchwords.

A. Collations by scribe. B. Collations by ebn-e Mowlānā ʿOwnoddīn ʿAlī Shaikh Moḥammad for ash-Shaikh al-jalīl ash-shaikh Zain ad-Dīn al-ʿĀmilī, dated by him in the last third of Jomādā II 1130/21-30 May 1718 (fol. 186b).

A. Anonymous copy (on fol. 40a the names of the scribe and his patron erased); on fol. 40a a date in 1233/1817 is still legible; no. I was dated by the scribe on Saturday, 27 Shavvāl 1233/*Sunday,* 30 August 1818 (fol. 35a). B. Anonymous copy, the collations dated in the last third of Jomādā II 1130 (see above).

Flyleaves, fols. 1a, 40b-41a. and margins filled with medical notes, most of them in the same hand.

A. Copied for a high-ranking physician whose name has been erased on fol. 40a; only part of his honorific titles remain legible: ...عالیجای مقدس القاب جالینوس الزمانی On the collations of B, see above.

On fol. 41a-b illegible stamps; on fols. 1b and 187b owner's stamp reading: Hāshim al-Ḥusainī.

Incipit, fol. 1b

بسمله. وبه نستعين. تشخيص چهارم در مداواى سموم
ومشتمل است بر پنج فصل اول در تاثير [كذا. يعنى
تدابير] منع سموم واحتراز ازان دوم در تدابير مشتركه
سموم سيوم در تدابير مشتركه سموم مشروب
چهارم در تدبير سموم ملدوغه پنجم در بيان انچه
حشرات ازان گريزند فصل اول...

Explicit, fol. 35a, 7

گل سرخ پوست ترنج صندل سفید عود هندی حسن
لبان بالسّویه نبات دو وزن مجموعرا به نبات بقوان
اورده ادویه را با قلیلی از مشك اضافه نموده قرصها
سازند والسلم تمت الرسالة...

This MS contains *tashkhīṣ* 4–5 and *qesm* 1 (fol. 15a) of the *dastūrāt* of Moḥammad Mo᾿men's *Toḥfato l-mo᾿menīn*; *ṭarīq* 5, on *kīmīā*, is not transcribed in this MS of *qesm* 1 of the *dastūrāt* (cf. **No. 117 : MS 117**).

No. 121 : MS 120 IV

Moḥammad Mo᾿men b. Moḥammad Zamān Tonakābonī

Toḥfato l-mo᾿menīn تحفة المؤمنين

MS 120 (ex Coll. Min.), 187 fols., 222 x 120 mm; binder's collection of four works, nos. I-III copied by the same scribe.
Toḥfato l-mo᾿menīn, dastūrāt, qesm 2, on fols. 41–186.

For the description of the MS see **No. 120 : MS 120 I.**

Incipit, fol. 41b

بسمله. قسم ثانی از دستورات جامع موسوم
بتحفة المؤمنین که آن مشتملست بر تشخیصات
و دستورات در بیان اعمالی که متعلق است بادویه
مرکبه و ذکر هریك از مرکبات چون هرعلت و مرضی را
بدوائی مفرد مداوا نمیتوان نمود بنابرین موافق هر
یك باید ترکیب از مفردات کرد...

Explicit, fol. 186a, 12

وچون دبق را باعسل ودوشاب طبخ بلیغ [کذا] نموده
مانند ریسمان بر روی اشجار وغیران گذارند طیوری
که بران نشیند پای بست گردند وچون ورق عنب
الثعلب را باخون ارنب کری بسازند وبریسمانی بسته
دراب اندازند جمیع ماهیان بران گرد جمع گردند والسلم
علی من اتبع الهدی تمت بالخیر والعاقبه

A comparison of this Explicit with the other MSS of *qesm* 2 of the *dastūrāt* shows that it represents a longer version of the text. There appear to be two different chains of transmission since both **MS 116** and **MS 120 IV** are fully collated. On fol. 187a-b, the scribe explains the abbreviations and signs occurring in the text, under the heading: رموز هذه النسخه .

No. 122 : MS 121

Moḥammad Moʾmen b. Moḥammad Zamān Tonakābonī

Toḥfato l-moʾmenīn تحفة المؤمنین

MS 121 (ex Coll. Min.), 277 fols., 210 x 147 mm

Bound in black leather over stiff thick cardboard; simple blind-tooled borders, three-medallion design with blind-stamped floral scrolls; inner covers pasted with yellowish-green paper; binding somewhat worn. Written on Italian paper, medium thin, glazed, white; watermark: a capital *P* in italic script between crossed palm fronds, in a medallion crested with a coronet, dated 1828; first and last fol. each a little soiled, otherwise few stains; MS looks little used.

15 lines, 135 x 75 mm, on blind-ruled frame and lines; black with red rubrics; medium-large, very neat, mannered *naskh*. Catchwords. Fols. 1-2a, 276-277 blank.

Copied by Moḥammad ʿAlī; he dated the *tashkhīṣāt* on 20 Zū l-qaʿdä 1247/21 April 1832 (fol. 25b, 8) and the *dastūrāt* on Wednesday, 6 Moḥarram 1248/*Tuesday*, 5 June 1832.

On fol. 1a one erased *tamlīk*; another *tamlīk* is dated Thursday, 14 Jomādā I 1250/18 September 1834.

Incipit, fol. 2b, 1

تشخیص رابع در مداوای سموم ومشتمل است
بر پنج فصل ...

Explicit, fol. 275b, 2

طیوری که بران نشینند پای بسته گردند والسلام
علی من اتّبع الهدی قد فرغ...

This MS contains *tashkhīṣ* 4–5 and the *dastūrāt* of Moḥammad Moʾmen's *Toḥfato l-moʾmenīn*, including *ṭarīq* 5 of *qesm* 1 of the *dastūrāt* (fols. 68b, 5 to 85b, 4).

No. 123 : MS 48

Moḥammad Hāshem b. Moḥammad Ṭāher Ṭehrānī

Toḥfä-ye Solaimānī تحفهٔ سلیمانی

MS 48 (ex Coll. Min.), 36 fols., 185 x 105 mm

Bound in plain dark brown leather; inner covers bare; one flyleaf each in front and back. Binding somewhat worn, water-soaked, warped; not original. Written on European paper, thin, slightly transparent, burnished, white; watermark obscure. Fols. 1 and 36 soiled, elsewhere water stains along edges. On lacunae see below.

14 lines, 135 x 65 mm, on blind-ruled frame and lines; black with red rubrics and overlinings, these occasionally left out; medium-sized, good, bold *naskh*. Catchwords, mostly cut off by trimming.

Anonymous, undated copy; first half of twelfth century/ca. 1690–1740.

On front flyleaf erased stamps; on fol. 11b a stamp reads: al-ʿabd al-mudhnib Muḥammad Walī, 1164/1750.

Incipit, fol. 1a

علی کریم افضاله ما عُلِّقَ عِلْقٌ فی الشّفاء والتداوی وعُلِّقَ
عَلَقٌ علی الممنوّ المتداوی * ونفایس صلوات طیّبات
نثار روضهٔ مقدّسهٔ منوّرهٔ طبیبی که موخری را معالجاتش
بیماران جهالت را بقانون الشفا ومنهاج دوا راه نمود...

Explicit, fol. 36a, 5

وبدل مومیائی دووزن او قفر الیهود است وبعضی
گفته اند که بدل او یکوزن موم ومثل موم روغن

زيتون است ونختم على هذا القدر من الاطناب
في هذا الباب والله اعلم بالصواب ...

There follow more eulogies after this and then what appears to be the author's original colophon (fol. 36a, 9):[1]

رساله موسومه بتحفهٔ سليمانى در روز هشتم ماه اول
از ماههاى سال نهم عشر نهم بعد الالف من الهجرة
على مهاجرها الف الف الثنا والتحيه سمت اختتام
وصورت اتمام پذيرفت ...

(Pious invocations end fol. 36b, 9)

This MS contains *Toḥfä-ye Solaimānī* (fol. 3a, 13) by Moḥammad Hāshem b. Moḥammad Ṭāher Ṭehrānī Ṭabīb (fol. 1b, 7). There is one leaf missing before fol. 1, including the initial doxologies on Allah. The treatise is divided into three *bāb*:

1. (begins on fol. 4b, 1) in ten *faṣl,* on zedoary (*jadvār*)
2. (begins on fol. 21b, 9) in four *faṣl,* on bezoar (*pādzahr*)
3. (begins on fol. 30a, 1) in three *faṣl,* on mummy (*mūmīā*)

There is a table of contents on fol. 3b. The author wrote this book in the Persian language in order to make these drugs, which he calls اجلّ واشرف ترياقات طبيعيه, known to high and low (*khavāṣṣ va-ʿavāmm*). There had not been, he says, an adequate discussion of the subject in Persian before, and he is going to supply that now (fol. 2a, 4-13). At the same time, he undertook the composition of this work as an act of piety since he could not visit the grave of the eighth imām, Reżā, a second time. He had paid it a visit when, early in his reign, Shāh ʿAbbās II campaigned against Qandahār.[2] A few years before writing this treatise, through the mediation of the *ḥojjāb* at court he had been able to go on pilgrimage to Mecca and Medina and to the tombs of the other eleven imāms (fols. 1b, 8 to 2a, 4). He dedicated his work to Shāh Solaimān Ṣafavī (fol. 2b, 12) and formulated its title as a chronogram: تحفهٔ سليمانى gives the date of 1089/1678 (*hāʾ* to be counted as *tāʾ*; fol. 3a, 12).[3] In the colophon (see above), 8 Moḥarram 1089/2 March 1678 is mentioned as the date of completion.

1. Cf. **No. 124 : MS 49.**
2. Shāh ʿAbbās II (1052-77/1642-66) reconquered Qandahār in 1058/1648. Moḥammad Hāshem's passage reads (fol. 1b, 9-11)

چون ... در اول جلوس ميمنت مانوس بتقريب
مامور گشتن دار القرار قندهار توفيق زيارت ... يافته بود ...

3. In the India Office MS, the title is given as *Toḥfä-ye Solaimān* in this passage, so that the resulting date is 1079/1668 (see Ethé I 1273f., no. 2336 II; PL II 264, no. 451 (3)). If this is the correct date, the colophon in the UCLA manuscript, quoted above, gives the date of its transcription.

PL II 264, no. 451 (3); Monzavī I 403a, no. 3740; Tashkent VIII 101-102, nos. 5683-84 (9269 III and 3383 II, resp.).

No. 124 : MS 49

Moḥammad Hāshem b. Moḥammad Ṭāher Ṭehrānī

ʿAino l-ḥayāt عين الحيوة

MS 49 (ex Coll. Min.), 84 fols., 185 x 115 mm

Bound in flexible sturdy leather of a faded crimson color; simple blind-tooled borders; inner covers bare. Binding worn; original (?). Written on Eastern paper, very thin, transparent, burnished, light beige.

14 lines, 125 x 60 mm, on blind-ruled frame and lines; black with red rubrics; medium-sized copperplate *naskh*. Catchwords in *nastaʿlīq*, partly cut off by trimming. Fols. 1-2, 79-84 blank.

Anonymous, undated copy; ca. 1100/1700.

Marginal notes by scribe, in a small, distinguished *shekastä*, quotations marked منه ; notes on the title, author, and contents on fols. 1a, 2a; scribbles on fols. 1a, 84a.

Incipit, fol. 3b

بسمله. سپاسی چون انفاس عیسوی روح پرور وجان فزا *
سزای بارگاه کبریای خالقیست که بحکمت بالغه * ...
[٤ الف، ٨] ... ودرودی مانند ید بیضای موسوی نوربخش
ودل ارا * شایسته روضه رضوان آسا * ومرقد منور فردوس
سرای طبیبی که موجزی از معالجاتش ...

Explicit, fol. 78a, 13

وصبح وشام باگلاب میل نمایند قدر شربت
بحسب ضعف وقوت مزاج از دو مثقال است
تا چهار پنج مثقال این بود اخر تمامی قول وکلام
واختتام همگی مقصد ومرام که در مقدمه ومقالات
وابواب وفصول این کتاب بیان نمود والحمد لرب
الارباب والصلوة علی خیر من نطق بالصواب
واصحابه خیر ال واصحاب

There follows evidently the author's own colophon (fol. 78b, 4-8):[1]

واین رساله موسومه بعین الحیوة در روز یکشنبه هشتم
ماه یازدهم از ماههای سال ششم از عشر دهم بعد از
الف از هجرت نبویه علی مهاجرها الف الف الثناء والتحیه
سمت اختتام وصورت اتمام پذیرفت یعنی در روز
یکشنبه هشتم ماه ذیقعده الحرام سنه ست وتسعین
بعد الالف * فبک اللهم اعتصم ...

(Pious invocations down to line 12)

Moḥammad Hāshem Ṭabīb-e Ṭehrānī (fol. 6a, 13) wrote his treatise ʿ*Aino l-ḥayāt* (fol. 9b, 3) in a *moqaddemä* and two *maqālä*:[2]

1. *moqaddemä* (begins on fol. 9b, 4) on the discovery of chinaroot (*čub-e čīnī*)
2. *maqālä* 1 (begins on fol. 10b) in nine *bāb,* subdivided into *faṣl,* on chinaroot
3. *maqālä* 2 (begins on fol. 70a, 5) in two *bāb,* subdivided into *faṣl,* on sarsaparilla (ʿ*oshbä-ye maghrebīyä*)

After forty years of medical practice, during which the author tested the therapeutical value of chinaroot, especially for syphilis, he set out to compose this treatise on its merits. He hoped to dispel the controversy about this subject among his contemporaries who did not have an authoritative discussion of it at their disposal. ʿEmādoddīn Maḥmūd[3] had written on the drug, but at the time of its first fame when there had not been much information available as to its *mezāj.* Then Mīrzā Qāżī[4] had devoted a *resālä* to the same topic, but had contradicted ʿEmādoddīn in every respect and had moreover been busy in his office as a judge (*manṣab-e sharʿī*), and so did not exhaustively treat the healing and harmful properties and the *mezāj* of the drug (fols. 5b, 7 to 6b, 2). At the time of Shāh Esmāʿīl, both a new disease, *āteshak,* and a new cure for it, *čūb-e čīnī,* had appeared, on which subjects the ancient authorities were silent (fol. 5b, 2-7). In the introduction to the second *maqālä,* on ʿ*oshbä-ye maghrebīyä,* Moḥammad Hāshem says that the plant is called *saparīna* (سبرینه) in the language of the people of Rūm, and *safarīnā* (سفرینا) in the Franks' tongue;[5] it is called "western herb" because it is imported from the west, or at least it was first discovered there (fol. 70a, 8-10). The author dedicated this work, like his *Toḥfä-ye Solaimānī,*[6] to Shāh Solaimān Ṣafavī, and completed it on Sunday, 8 Ẕū l-qaʿdä 1096/ *Saturday,* 6 October 1685 (see colophon above).

Of the three known works by Moḥammad Hāshem b. Moḥammad Ṭāher Ṭehrānī,[7] ʿ*Aino l-ḥayāt* is the second in order of date: the first, *Toḥfä-ye Solaimānī,* was written in 1089/1678, and the third, *Meftāḥo l-khazāyen va-meṣbāḥo d-dafāyen,* was finished on Thursday, 15 Rajab 1103/*Wednesday,* 2 April 1692.[8] Since the author in 1096/1684 mentions forty years of practice, it appears that he took up writing only toward the end of his career, at an advanced age. His participation in ʿAbbās II's campaign against Qandahār, 1058/1648, thus marks, approximately, the beginning of his practice.[9]

1. The similarity of wording of the colophons in **No. 123 : MS 48** and here suggests a common author; the handwriting appears too different to have been done by the same scribe.
2. There is no third *maqālä* on *jadvār, pādzahr,* etc., in this MS (cf. PL II 264, no. 451 (1)).
3. See **No. 104 : MS 87 II.**

4. See **Nos. 113–114 : MSS 46 VII** and **87 I.**
5. Both forms are probably to represent the Spanish *zarza parilla* (sarsaparilla).
6. See **MS 48.**
7. See PL II 264, no. 451.
8. Nashrīyä III 364a, s.v.
9. Cf. **MS 48.**

PL II 264, no. 451 (1); Monzavī I 438b, no. 4050; Nūrbakhsh I 39, no. 29 III; Charminar, p. 237, nos. 4–5; Osmania Univ., pp. 52–53, nos. 8, 44, resp.

No. 125 : MS 50

Moḥammad Ḥakīm b. Moḥammad Rashīd aṭ-Ṭabīb

Roʾūso l-masāʾel رؤوس المسائل

MS 50 (ex Coll. Min.), 84 fols., 167 x 100 mm

Bound in crimson leather over stiff cardboard, flap; gold-tooled borders, simple pattern; three-medallion design on front, back, and flap: floral scrolls stamped on gold background; inside of covers and flap of grey leather with tooled borders as outside, no medallions; one flyleaf each in front and back, of European paper, medium thin, glazed, beige; no watermark. Binding somewhat worn; later than MS. Written on Eastern paper, medium thick, glazed, cream-colored; fols. 1 and 84 soiled, edges repaired; little other damage.

15 lines, 115 x 65 mm, on blind-ruled frame and lines; borders in black, gold, black, black, red; on fol. 1b a fine *sarlowḥ* in gold, blue, red, and other colors; golden clouds between lines on fols. 1b and 2a; greyish-black with red rubrics; small, thin, fine *shekastä-āmīz*. Catchwords.

Copied, and dated Saturday morning, 11 Rajab 1082/*Friday*, 13 November 1671, by ʿAbdo r-Raḥmān al-Ḥosainī al-Qommī.

Several *tamlīk* on fols. 1a, 84a–b, partly erased; on fol. 84a a note commemorating the birth of a son, ʿAbdo l-Vahhāb, to an owner of the MS, Moḥammad Sharīf b. Moḥammad Ḥosain; on fol. 1a a *tamlīk* of ʿAbdo l-Vahhāb.

On fol. 84b an erased stamp.

Incipit, fol. 1b

ولا حول ولا قوة الا بالله العلی العظیم.
بعد از طی مراتب حمد و ثنای حکیم علی الاطلاق جلّت
آلاؤه وعمت نعماؤه که در خلقت انسان دقایق حکمت
او بی پایان ونعم واحسان او در حق ایشان بیرون از حد وبیانست ...

Explicit, fol. 83b, 4

وبالجمله واجب برطبیب متصف بودن به پنج خصلت عفو از مذنب
وصدق لهجه ورحم برانسان وحیوان ونیکوئی بقدر امکان

قد فرغت من تسويده وانا مؤلفه في يوم السبت السادس
والعشرين من شهر الصفر ختم بالخير والظفر حين مقارنه السعدين
الاكبرين اللذين يسميان بالزهره والمشتري في سنه اثنان [كذا]
وثمانين بعد الالف من الهجرة النبويه عليه من الصلوات افضلها
ومن التحيات اكملها وان اخر لي الله في الاجل وساعدني القدر
نجمع قرابادينا جامعا مشتملا على جميع الامراض بعون الله الملك الفياض
هذا اخر ما اردنا تاليفه واول ما صنفته في عنفوان الشباب مع عدم التميز
بين الخطاء والصواب والحمد لله الحكيم الوهاب تم

Ebn Moḥammad Rashīd Moḥammad Ḥakīm aṭ-Ṭabīb (fol. 2b, 15) finished this, his first work, on Saturday, 26 Ṣafar 1082/4 July 1671, during the conjunction of the two auspicious planets, Venus and Jupiter (see Explicit above). Since it was his first venture as a writer, he called it *Roʾūso l-masāʾel,* "The Prime Questions" (fols. 2b, 15 to 3a, 9). Obviously he intended to dedicate it to the reigning shah (i.e., Shāh Solaimān Safavī), but in this copy, there is no place for his name left after the customary honorific titles of the sovereign and before the eulogies on him (fol. 3a, 15):

... المؤيد من السماء المنصور على الاعداء [ ] خلد الله
ملكه وسلطانه ...

Moḥammad Ḥakīm divided his book into two *fann,* the first, on *kollīyāt,* in a *moqaddemä,* six *maqālä,* and a *khātemä,* and the second, on therapy, in "several" *bāb* (fol. 4a, 4). This MS contains only the first *fann,* all that had been written at the time of its transcription, if the planned second *fann* can be identified with the *qarābāẕīn* mentioned at the end of this MS (see Explicit). It appears that the author's model in composing this treatise was Manṣūr b. Moḥammad b. Aḥmad's *Kefāyä-ye Mojahedīyä,* if the division into two *fann* and the partial identity of the initial eulogies can be taken as evidence (see **No. 32 : MS 12**, etc.).

Not in PL or Monzavī.

No. 126 : MS 47

Jalāloddīn Moḥammad Eṣfahānī

[*Resālä-ye ḥefẓ-e ṣeḥḥat*] [رساله حفظ صحت]

MS 47 (ex Coll. Qāʾenī), 44 fols., 185 x 115 mm

Bound in slightly flexible brown leather; narrow strip of red leather along edges, tooled in gold; spine of brown leather has the same tooling; inner covers rose-colored smooth leather. Binding worm-eaten, worn; too small for MS (original?).

Written on Eastern paper, thin, slightly brittle, transparent, burnished, cream-colored; first two leaves out of binding, later pasted in with tape; first and last fols. stained; some edges torn.

12 lines, 125 x 65 mm, on blind-ruled frame and lines; borders in black, gold, black, black; on fol. 2b *sarlowḥ* with golden floral scrolls; black with red rubrics; medium-small, fine *naskh*. Catchwords. Fols. 1 and 44 blank.

Anonymous, undated copy; ca. 1100/1700.

Entries in different hands on fols. 1–2a (recipes, prayers, poems, title of book); a poem on fol. 44a dated 12 Shaʿbān 1285/28 November 1868; notes in margins, some erased.

On fol. 10a an erased stamp; another stamp, partly legible, on fol. 44b: Muḥammad Jaʿfar.

Incipit, fol. 2b

بسمله. حمد و ثنائی که روایح عطر آن مجالس
خلوت نشینان عالم ملکوترا معطر دارد و شکر
و سپاسی که فوایح نشر آن مجامع ذکر سبحه طرازان
حظایر جبروترا معنبر سازد ذات ذو الجلالی را سزد
که از ترکیب کاف و نون کافه موجوداترا از
کتم عدم بعالم وجود آورد...

Explicit, fol. 43b, 6

و بالجمله حدوث چیزهای غیر معتاد و دوام و کثرت
آن خبر دهد بحدوث مرض سزاوار آنست که اولاً
تحقیق سبب نموده بعد ازان بنحو مناسب معالجه
نمایند تمام شد رسالهٔ حفظ صحت علی سبیل الاستعجال
بعون الله و توفیقه والحمد لله علی کل حال

Jalāloddīn Moḥammad Ṭabīb-e Eṣfahānī (fol. 4a, 5) did not title this treatise on "preventive medicine"; the heading given above appears only in the colophon (see Explicit).[1] The book is divided into a *moqaddemä* and an unnumbered sequence of *faṣl,* some of which are further divided into *faṣl* (fol. 4b, 8). Its topics are the "six causes" (*settä-ye żarūrīyä*) of health or disease.[2] Jalāloddīn dedicated his work to Shāh Solaimān Ṣafavī (fol. 4b, 5). Another book of Jalāloddīn's is *ad-Dastūr al-Jalālī,* or *ar-Risāla al-Jalālīya,* in Arabic;[3] it follows Najīb ad-Dīn as-Samarqandī's *Kitāb al-asbāb wa-l-ʿalāmāt* in its layout, and was composed in Rabīʿ I 1087/14 May–12 June 1676.[4]

1. In the Paris MS, there is also no title except in the colophon; it reads *Ḥefẓ-e ṣeḥḥat-e badano l-ensānīyä* (!) (Blochet IV 316, no. 2389 [from fol. 50a]).
2. On *settä-ye żarūrīyä* see Yūsofī's tract, **MS 25 VII**, etc.
3. See Nashrīyä III 371b s.v. *ad-Dastūr al-Jalālī*; in the Āṣafīya catalogue, this work is described as Persian (PL II 263, no. 450 (1)).
4. Nashrīyä III 371b.

PL II 264, no. 450 (2); not in Monzavī, but cf. ibid., I 535a, no. 4944.

No. 127 : MS 73 II

Mortażāqolī b. Ḥasan Shāmlū

Kherqä خرقه

MS 73 (ex Coll. Min.), 131 fols., 205 x 145 mm; binder's collection of five works in two sections. *Kherqä* on fols. 65–96.

For the description of the MS see **No. 168 : MS 73 I.**

Incipit, fol. 65b

بسمله. سبحان الله رنگ آمیزی بساط حمد و سپاس حکیمی را
که خرقه معرفت را بر قامت صحیح مزاجان درست اعتقاد
بریده ...

Explicit, fol. 95b, 8

نوع دیگر آرد گندمرا با زردهٔ تخم مرغ برهم زده ضماد
نماید خاتمهٔ کتاب موسوم بخرقه ...[۹۶ الف، ۷] چشم
گشوده خار این چمن را گل وجغد این خرابه را بلبل شناسد
مژده که این رقعه بپایان رسید خرقهٔ پیرانه بجوانان رسید
قد وقع الفراغ ...

This is an incomplete copy of *Kherqä* (fol. 66a, 5) by Mortażāqolī b. Ḥasan Shāmlū (fol. 65b, -2); it was dedicated to Shāh Solaimān Ṣafavī, according to the preface (fol. 65b, -4). The text is divided into thirty *bakhyä*; in this MS, there is a lacuna between fols. 67 and 68, so that the text from within the table of contents to within *bakhyä* 18 is missing.

In another group of MSS of *Kherqä*, Moḥammad b. Moḥammad Moʾmen is named as the author.[1] According to Āqā Bozorg, this is the son of the author of *Toḥfato l-moʾmenīn*; he would have dedicated the treatise first to Mortażāqolī and after his death to Amānollāh Khān, who is named as dedicatee in these MSS.[2] The Incipit in this group of copies is different, too:

سبحانك اللهم يا ذا الملك القديم ويا طبيب
كل اليم وسقيم ويا كافي ذي روح وجسيم [3]

The author of *Dharīʿa* thinks it very unlikely that a soldier and statesman such as Mortażāqolī composed a work like *Kherqä*; in his opinion, he merely appropriated the text to himself after it was presented to him by its actual author, Moḥammad b. Moḥammad Moʾmen.[4]

1. PL II 263, no. 449; *Dharīʿa* VII 149, no. 813.
2. See note 1.
3. *Dharīʿa* VII 149, 14; cf. with this wording the Incipit of *Toḥfato l-moʾmenīn*, **No. 115 : MS 115**. Moḥsen *al-madʿūv be*-Āqā Bābā Hamadānī completed his treatise *Toḥfato l-khavānīn* on poisons in 1248/1832; its Incipit corresponds exactly with that quoted from *Dharīʿa* above (PL II 292, no. 524; Monzavī I 488a, no. 4506). The relationship between the texts mentioned here remains subject to further study.
4. See note 1 above.

PL II 263, no. 449; Monzavī I 525a, nos. 4840–59; cf. Monzavī I 473a, no. 4371 (identical with *Kherqä*?); ibid., 481b, no. 4458; Madras IV 1242, no. 1074 I.

No. 128 : MS 51

Moḥammad Kāẓem Qazvīnī

Ḥadīqato l-ḥayāt حديقة الحيوة

MS 51 (ex Coll. Min.), 40 fols., 170 x 110 mm

Bound in flexible plain greenish-brown leather; inner covers pinkish-grey leather. Binding worn; original (?). Written on Eastern paper, slightly transparent, burnished, light beige; some stains and inkblots, some edges torn. For lacunae see below.

16 lines, 120 x 55 mm, on blind-ruled frame and lines; black with red rubrics; medium-sized energetic, even *shekastä-āmīz*. Catchwords.

Collations by scribe.

Anonymous, undated copy (end missing); twelfth/eighteenth century.

Readers' notes on fol. 1a.

Incipit, fol. 1b

بسمله. وبه ثقتي. حمد وستايش * وسپاس بيقياس خالى
از آلايش * كه سواطع روايح ازهار عبوديت شمار آن
محافل عالى منازل قدوسيان عالم ملكوت را معطر ومعنبر
سازد...

Moḥammad Kāẓem Ṭabīb-e Qazvīnī (fol. 2b, 14) divided his treatise *Ḥadīqato l-ḥayāt* (fol. 3a, 4) on "preventive medicine" into a *moqaddemä*, eight *ḥadīqä* subdivided into *shajar*, and a *khātemä* in twelve *raiḥānä* (fols. 3a, 5 and 36b, 11). In this MS, the text breaks off on fol. 40b within *raiḥānä* 10; ca. three leaves are missing. Starting with the initial doxologies, the whole treatise bears close resemblance to Jalāloddīn Moḥammad Eṣfahānī's [*Resālä-ye ḥefẓ-e ṣeḥḥat*].[1] Indeed, Moḥammad Kāẓem may have counted himself among Jalāloddīn's students, if the titles he quotes him by can be understood to mean that:

عالیحضرت استادی جلال الدین محمد اصفهانی طبیب رحمه علیه

He cites a prescription of Jalāloddīn's and adds وبخط خود نوشته که مجرب است (fol. 38b, 5–6). A *noskhä-ye Hendī* for a *rowghan* is quoted from Ḥakīm Moʾmen-e Gīlānī, probably Moḥammad Moʾmen Tonakābonī, the author of *Toḥfato l-moʾmenīn*.[2]

1. See **No. 126 : MS 47.**
2. See **No. 115 : MS 115**, etc.

Not in PL or Monzavī.

No. 129 : MS 55

Moḥammad Kāẓem

Ṣāleḥo l-ʿelāj صالح العلاج

MS 55 (ex Coll. Min.), 63 fols., 220 x 120 mm

Bound recently in slightly flexible cardboard, covered with patterned paper: yellowish-green with pinkish stars; spine pasted with thin cloth of white, pink, blue, black; inner covers pasted with white paper. Binding not original. Written on medium-thick, unburnished, beige Eastern paper; first and last leaves repaired; stains, inkblots; tears, wormholes.
15 lines, 160 x 75 mm; black with red rubrics; medium-sized, extremely hurried, ugly *shekastä-āmīz*. Catchwords.
Anonymous copy, dated 1115/1703.
On back inner cover a *tamlīk* by ʿAbdo r-Rashīd, dated 30 July 1926.
The same stamp on fols. 1a and 63b: huwa s-sulṭān al-ʿalī, 1243/1827.

Incipit, fol. 1b

بسمله. بر ضمیر منیر ارباب دانش وخاطر الباب
بینش پوشیده نماند که نعت جلال احدیت
ووصف کمال صمدیت وشکر مواهب بی نهایت
وذکر لطایف کرم بیغایت مبدعی را که ...

Explicit, fol. 63b, -3

و به ۱۰ م قند سفید شیرین کرده ۲ م روغن زیت
اضافه نمایند و نیم گرم بیاشامند نافع باشد انشاء الله
تعالی با تمام پیوست . . .

Ṣāleḥo l-ʿelāj (fol. 2a, 5) by Moḥammad Kāẓem (fol. 1b, -4) is divided into four *maqalä*: 1) in 18 *bāb*, on theoretical medicine; 2) in 59 *bāb*, on practical medicine, i.e., treatment of diseases; 3) in 28 *bāb* of alphabetical order, on simple drugs; 4) in 22 *bāb*, on compound drugs. The numbers and names of the subdivisions are the same in this text as in Najmoddīn Maḥmūd's *Ghīāṣīyä*;[1] close examination of both works is needed to determine how closely Moḥammad Kāẓem follows his predecessor.

Ṣāleḥo l-ʿelāj was written for, and named after, Ṣāleḥ Khān b. Fedāʾī Khān *mokhāṭab be-kheṭāb-e* Aʿẓam Khānī (fols. 1b, -3 to 2a, 3). Ṣāleḥ Khān was a son of Fedāʾī Khān, a high official during Owrangzēb's reign, who in the course of his career was created Aʿẓam Khān Kōka and died in 1088/1677.[2]

1. See **No. 17 : MS 20.**
2. *Maʾāṣer-e ʿĀlamgīrī* (*M. ʿA., a history of . . . Aurangzib . . . of* Saqi Mustʿad Khan [*sic*], translated into English . . . by Sir Jadu-Nath Sarkar, *Bibl. Ind.*, Work No. 269, Issue No. 1556 [Calcutta 1947]), pp. 90, 104, and index.

Not in PL or Monzavī.

No. 130 : MS 125

Moḥammad Akbar *ʿorf* Moḥammad Arzānī

Qarābāẕīn-e Qāderī قرابادین قادری

MS 125 (ex Coll. Min.), 415 fols., 302 x 197 mm

Bound in crimson leather over thick stiff cardboard; simple blind-tooled borders; three-medallion design with corresponding corner pieces, inlaid with thin gilt leather, blind-stamped with floral scrolls; inner covers pasted with greyish Russian paper; one flyleaf in front and two in back of the same medium-thin, greyish paper. Binding somewhat worn, not original. Written on Eastern paper, medium thin to thin, transparent, burnished, greyish; edges trimmed when MS was rebound.

17 lines, 220 x 100 mm, on blind-ruled frame and lines; black with red rubrics and overlinings; large, even, fine *nastaʿlīq*. Catchwords. Eight fols. (A–H) in front and 407 numbered fols. of text; on fol. Ha table of contents with nos. of fols., not in scribe's hand. Fols. A, Cb, Db, Gb, Hb blank.

Collations by scribe.

Anonymous copy (name of scribe erased in colophon), dated Dāro s-salṭanä-ye Kābol, *dar jolūs-e Tīmūrshāhī*,[1] Thursday, 15 Jomādā II 1203/*Friday*, 13 March 1789.

Medical notes on first eight fols., among them the recipe for a *teryaq-e Tīmūrshāhī*, dated 5 Shaʿbān 1200/3 June 1786.

Incipit, fol. 1b

بسمله. وبه نستعين. رب يسر وتمم بالخير.
ثنائی که شایان جناب مستطاب حضرت الهی تعالی
است بجزوی نباید پس...

Explicit, fol. 407a, 8

من نیز بعمل آوردم در شبانه روزی قریب یکدام میخوردم
بتفاریق فی الواقع اثر کلی پدید آمد مرض زائل شد
باذن الله تعالی واین درویش نیز در اکثر علل مزمنه
تنقیه کامله اثر کلی دارد وهم بامراض سر ونفع دارد هم
بعلل حار سُبْحَانَكَ رَبِّكَ [كذا] رَبِّ الْعِزَّةِ عَمَّا يَصِفُونَ
وَسَلَامٌ عَلَى الْمُرْسَلِينَ وَالْحَمْدُ لِلَّهِ رَبِّ الْعَالَمِينَ تمت...

In this MS, the author is called Moḥammad Akbar *maᶜrūf be-ᶜorf-e* Arzānī (fol. 2a, 2); since he was a spiritual follower of ᶜAbd al-Qādir al-Jīlānī[2] (fol. 2b, 3–6), he called this dispensatory *Qarābāẕīn-e Qāderī.* According to the preface (fol. 2b, 8), it is divided into 22 *bāb,* listing the drugs alphabetically under the diseases for which they are prescribed, *a capite ad calcem* and general diseases. In the course of writing, though, he added another chapter در طریق چوب چینی ومرهمها وحجر التیس وعرقها وسفوفها وقرص وغیره

Moḥammad Arzānī began this book in 1126/1714 (fol. 2a, -6) and finished it in 1130/1717 (fol. 387a, 7). In the preface he lists his previous writings on medical topics, composed to store up credit for good works in the world to come, in what appears to be a chronological order: 1) *Talkhīṣ-e ṭebb-e nabī,* following Shaikh Jalāl ad-Dīn as-Suyūṭī,[3] 2) *Ṭebbo l-Akbar,*[4] 3) *Mofarreḥo l-qolūb,*[5] 4) *Mīzāno ṭ-ṭebb,*[6] 5) *Tafāroqo l-amrāż,*[7] 6) *Mojarrabāt-e Akbarī.*[8] In his *Mofarreḥo l-qolūb,*[9] he mentions *Ṭebbo l-Akbar* and *Ḥudūd al-amrāḍ,* a work written in Arabic.[10] It thus appears that the list in *Qarābāẕīn* is incomplete, since *Talkhīṣ* and *Ḥudūd* cannot be identical, one being written in Persian, the other in Arabic. In consequence, it cannot at present be decided whether the other three books of his not mentioned in *Qarābāẕīn—Vājebo l-ḥefẓ, ᶜElājo ṣ-ṣebyān,* and *Khairo t-tajāreb*[11]—were composed later or not.

Around 1115/1703 Moḥammad Arzānī had sought to become a student of Moᶜtamado l-Molūk Sayyed ᶜAlavī Khān,[12] but upon being refused by him, had gone to Shīrāz to perfect his medical knowledge.[13] He died in Delhi in Rabīᶜ II 1134/19 January–16 February 1722.

1. Tīmūrshāh, son of Aḥmad Shāh Dorrānī, reigned 1187–1207/1773–93.
2. On Qāderī orders see EI² IV 380b, s.v. Ḳādiriyya [Margoliouth].
3. A MS is preserved in Panjāb University; see Shīrānī, p. 396, no. 2147.
4. See **No. 131 : MS 122.**
5. See **No. 132 : MS 123.**

6. See **No. 133 : MS 124 I.**
7. No MS is yet known of this work.
8. See PL II 269, no. 465 (6).
9. See note 5 above.
10. See PL II 268, no. 465 (1); GAL Supp. II 1030.
11. Charminar, p. 242, nos. 154-56, and PL II 268, no. 465 (2, 3), resp.
12. See **No. 142 : MS 124 II.**
13. On Moḥammad Arzānī's biography, see PL II 268, no. 465, with references.

PL II 270, no. 465 (7); Monzavī I 581b, nos. 5419-22; Panjāb P.L., p. 306, no. 232; Charminar, pp. 239-40, nos. 100-102; Eilers-Heinz, p. 70, no. 79; Luzac, p. 38; Miklukho-Maklaĭ, p. 411, nos. 3180-82; Osmania Med. Coll., pp. 111-12, nos. 21 and 30, resp.; Tashkent VI 162-63, nos. 4367-68 (9772 and 9758, resp.); ibid., IX 366-70, nos. 6542-46 (3497, 3513, 3654, 6916 IV, 10810 I, resp.); Yunusov, p. 182, no. 125 (1046).

Ṭebbo n-nabī: Shīrānī II 396, no. 2147; Miklukho-Maklaĭ, p. 374, no. 2864.

Mojarrabāt-e Akbarī: Panjāb P.L., p. 307, no. 233; Eilers-Heinz, p. 92, no. 106; Gujarat I 168-69, 171, no. 104a; Rampur, p. 134, no. 331; Tashkent IX 371, no. 6547 (7362).

Noskhă-ye ṭebb: Rampur, p. 134, no. 332.

An Arabic *risāla*: Tashkent V 279, no. 3936 (2829 II).

No. 131 : MS 122

Moḥammad Akbar ʿ*orf* Moḥammad Arzānī

Ṭebbo l-Akbar طب الاکبر

MS 122 (ex Coll. Min.), 314 fols., 260 x 140 mm

Bound in crimson leather over thick stiff cardboard; three-medallion design with corresponding corners, inlaid in faded grey, thin leather; blind-stamped floral scrolls; tooled lines, painted yellow, connecting medallions and corners; inner covers pasted with greyish paper; one flyleaf in front of much stained, formerly white European paper; watermark: WHATMAN, BALSTON & CO. 1826, and heart emblem. Front cover lost, spine torn; stained and worn; binding not original. Written on Eastern paper, medium thick, burnished, tan; worm-eaten, little wear. For lacunae see below.

22 lines, 190 x 85 mm, on blind-ruled frame and lines; black with red rubrics and overlinings; medium-small, fair *nastaʿlīq*. Catchwords. Fol. 314a blank.

Collations by scribe, dated 23 Shavvāl 1196/1 October 1782 on fol. 1a.

Anonymous, undated copy (end missing); scribe's collation dated 1196/1782 (see above).

Recipes on fol. 314b and in margins.

On fol. 314b a note dated 1198/1783; on fol. 313b an incorrect subscription, naming the book *K-e dastūro l-ʿelāj.*[1]

Incipit, fol. 1a

ترشی بنوشند فواق ساکن کند زراوند مدحرج
کوفته با آب خوردن مفید است ...

Explicit, fol. 313b, 13

وفواید ضروریه که درین مختصر ثبت یافته وآنرا
بخواهند ازین خاتمه نشان موضع او دریابند
واین درویش دل ریش را بفاتحه خیر یاد آرند
تمت [کذا] تمام شد کتاب طب الاکبر ه

In his subscription on fol. 313b (see Explicit), the scribe of this MS calls the text *Ṭebbo l-Akbar.*[2] This identification is supported by a comparison of its organization in *bāb,* subdivided into *faṣl,* and a *khātemä* in two *bāb,* and of their headings with Rieu II 478b, *ad* Egerton 1006-07. In the UCLA manuscript, the *bāb* are not numbered. The first part of the book is missing, and fol. 1a begins within the section on diseases of the stomach; in the *khātemä,* the second *bāb* is not transcribed.

Moḥammad Akbar ʿ*orf* Moḥammad Arzānī gives an expanded translation of *Sharḥ al-Asbāb wa-l-ʿalāmāt* by Nafīs b. ʿIwaḍ al-Kirmānī[3] in his *Ṭebbo l-Akbar*; he composed it in 1112/1700.[4]

1. The best known work of this title was written by Solṭānʿalī Ṭabīb-e Khorāsānī Jonābadī; see PL II 233, no. 404 (but cf. ibid., 315, nos. 37-39).
2. This is obviously the correct title: cf. the author's own citation of his works in **MSS 123** and **125.**
3. See Ullmann, p. 170; Dietrich, p. 122, no. 52.
4. PL II 270, no. 465 (8).

PL II 270, no. 465 (8); Monzavī I 558b, nos. 5206–13; Panjāb P.L., p. 303, nos. 229–31; Charminar, p. 239, nos. 135–39; Miklukho-Maklaĭ, pp. 373–74, nos. 2860–61; Osmania Med. Coll., pp. 110–11, *Persian,* nos. 1 and 25, resp.; Tashkent IX 321-25, nos. 6488–91 (9478, 2629 I, 4759, 3504 X, resp.); Yale, Persian + 101.

No. 132 : MS 123

Moḥammad Akbar ʿ*orf* Moḥammad Arzānī

Mofarreḥo l-qolūb مفرح القلوب

MS 123 (ex Coll. Min.), 266 fols., 343 x 213 mm

Bound in patterned paper of white, grey, blue, and pink over stiff thick cardboard; spine of dark brown leather; inner covers pasted with white paper; one flyleaf in back of medium-thin, off-white paper. Spine much torn, covers nearly off; one quire of the MS out of binding. Written on Eastern paper, thick, burnished, white.

23 lines, 220 x 127 mm, on blind-ruled frame and lines; black with crimson rubrics; different styles of medium-sized good *nastaʿlīq* and *shekastä,* probably by the same scribe. Table of contents on fol. 1b, and headings in top margins (on verso *maqālä,* on recto *faṣl*), in *naskh*; Arabic quotations also in *naskh* or with black overlinings; all by the same scribe. Catchwords. Pagination by scribe (the cataloguer's foliation is quoted here). Fols. 1a, 2a, 264b, 265–266 blank. For lacunae see below.

Collations by scribe.

Anonymous, undated copy (end missing); ca. 1200/1800.

Some marginal notes in small, fine *nastaʿlīq* by ʿAbdollāh b. al-Ḥakīm.

Incipit, fol. 2b, 1

بسمله. و به نستعین. الحمد لله رب العالمین والصلوة
والسّلام علی سید المرسلین وعلی اله واصحابه اجمعین
امّا بعد فقیر حقیر جانی محمّد اکبر عرف محمد ارزانی
مشهور رای صداقت انتمای تالیان این اوراق
وطالبان این مذاق میگرداند که ...

Explicit, fol. 262b, -2

ومعلوم است که اعتدال دم در هر حال مطلوب است
وافراط وتفریط موجب فساد واگر نظر بانکه خون
از درجه اعتدال تنزل نکند تکثیر در غذای خواهند
کرد مزید کرب خواهند شد]

This MS contains the first five *maqālä* of *Mofarreḥo l-qolūb* (fol. 2b, -3) by Moḥammad Akbar, commonly known as (*ʿorf*) Moḥammad Arzānī (fol. 2b, 3):

1. (begins on fol. 3a) in five *faṣl* — فی الامور الطّبیعیة
2. (begins on fol. 38b) in seven *faṣl* — فی التشریح
3. (begins on fol. 71a) in five *faṣl* — فی احوال البدن واسبابها والعلامات الداله علیها
4. (begins on fol. 126a) in six *faṣl* — فی النّبض والتّفسرة
5. (begins on fol. 197b) in ten *faṣl* — فی تدبیر الاصحّاء وعلاج المرضی علی وجه کلّی

In the preface the author explains that after having written *Ṭebbo l-Akbar*[1] and *Ḥudūd al-amrāḍ*,[2] he had planned to compose a book on the *kollīyāt* of medicine, but had not found the time. Then some of his friends studied *Qānūnja* by Maḥmūd b. ʿUmar al-Jaghmīnī,[3] and those of them who were conversant only in Persian asked him to give a commentary on it in this language; he undertook the task hoping to supersede all existing commentaries on *Qānūnja* (fol. 2b, 4–12).

In this MS, there is a long lacuna between fols. 215 and 216 (pp. 428 and 481 resp.), covering *faṣl* 2 to within *faṣl* 6 of *maqālä* 5; pp. 449–451 follow at the end of the MS, after fol. 262. They contain part of *faṣl* 4 of *maqālä* 5.

1. See **No. 131 : MS 122.**
2. See PL II 268, no. 465 (1).
3. In the UCLA manuscript, he is called Moḥammad b. al-Maḥmūdo l-Čaqmīnī; on him see Ullmann, p. 154; Dietrich, p. 85, no. 31. See also **No. 19 : MS 56 II**, note 1.

PL II 219 bottom, no. 377; cf. ibid., 269, no. 465 (5); Monzavī I 601b, nos. 5618–21; Panjāb P.L., p. 308, no. 234; Charminar, p. 239, nos. 85–87; Miklukho-Maklaĭ, p. 559, nos. 4181–82; Osmania Univ., p. 52, no. 22; Rampur, p. 134, no. 333; Tashkent IX 325–28, nos. 6492–96 (1650, 4455, 3501, 9669, 3509 I, resp.); Yunusov, p. 181, no. 124 (608).

No. 133 : MS 124 I

Moḥammad Akbar ʿ*orf* Moḥammad Arzānī

Mīzāno ṭ-ṭebb میزان الطبّ

MS 124 (ex Coll. Min.), 335 fols., 205 x 135 mm; scribe's collection of four Persian works on medicine. (See also **Nos. 142, 155,** and **159**.)
Mīzāno ṭ-ṭebb on fols. 5–172.

Bound in burgundy-colored leather over stiff cardboard; simple blind-tooled borders; inner covers pasted with cream-colored paper; spine partly broken, edges worn, some wormholes. Written on Eastern paper, medium thin, of coarse surface, cream-colored.

12–17 lines, 160 x 90–100 mm, on blind-ruled frame and lines; black with red rubrics and overlinings; medium-large, uneven, undistinguished, but clear *shekastä-āmīz*. Catchwords. Fols. 5a, 173a, 276b, 309a blank.

Collations by scribe.

Copied by Ḥājjī Āqā-ye valad-e Ḥājjī Ghāzī Moḥammad from the quarter of Anzāb of Dāro s-salṭanä-ye Tabrīz at Calcutta in the house, and at the order, of Mīrzā Ḥakīm Moḥammadbakhsh Khān-Ṣāheb Mūsavī b. Moḥammad Reżā Khān Mūsavī, known as Sīādatnasab-Khān Bahādūrshāhī; the scribe dated no. I on 16 Jomādā II 1216/24 October 1801; no. II on Friday, 1 Jomādā I 1216/*Wednesday*, 9 September 1801; no. III on 14 Rabīʿ II 1216/24 August 1801, and left no. IV undated.

Medical notes on fols. 1–4, 173b, 308b, 328b–335b, and in margins.

On fol. 1a a *tamlīk* by Mīrzā ʿAbbāsʿalī Jarrāḥbāshī;[1] on fol. 308a a note dated 26 Shaʿbān 1216/1 January 1802, written by Moḥammad ʿAlī al-Ḥosainī Khorāsānī Qāyenī al-Bīrjandī at the order of a high-ranking person (Moḥammadbakhsh Khān, the first owner of the MS?) درحین داخل شدن دریاء بزرگ; on fol. 308b a note commemorating the successful treatment of Mīrzā ʿEzzoddīn, vizier of Meshgīn,[2] by Ḥaidarqolī Khān Ḥakīm-e Meshgīn, at Lahā,[3] dated 6 Moḥarram 1222/16 March 1807; on front inner cover a note dated 15 Jomādā II 1281/15 November 1864.

Two stamps of Sayyed Moḥammadbakhsh Mūsavī, the first owner of the MS, on fol. 228a, one dated 1199/1784, the other dated 1212/1797.

Incipit, fol. 5b

میزان الطبّ . بسمله . به نستعین .
الحمد لله رب العالمین والصلواة [کذا] والسلام علی سیّد
المرسلین وعلی آله الطّاهرین امّا بعد عبد الجانی محمد ارزانی
المسمی بمحمد اکبر میگوید که چون اطفال فقیر . .

Explicit, fol. 172b, 3

وگفته اند که جگر انسگرا بریان کرده بخورانند نفع تمام
دارد ودرچند نسخه دیده شد تمّت الکتاب [کذا]...

Moḥammad Arzānī, here called Moḥammad Arzānī *al-mosammā be*-Moḥammad Akbar (fol. 5b, 4), wrote his treatise *Mīzāno ṭ-ṭebb* (fol. 2b, -2) in three *maqālä* as a primer in medicine for his adolescent sons.

1. He owned **MS 66**; see also a stamp in **MS 77**.
2. *Farhang-e Joghrāfyā'ī-ye Īrān* IV 498a.
3. Not in *Farhang*.

PL II 268, no. 465 (4); Monzavī I 605b, no. 5652; Panjāb P.L., pp. 309 and 784, nos. 235 and 579, resp.; Shīrānī II 401–402, nos. 2173 and 2175, resp.; Charminar, p. 239, nos. 77–78; Eilers-Heinz, p. 263, no. 337; Gujarat I 128, no. 78; Miklukho-Maklaī, p. 580, no. 4362; Rampur, p. 134, no. 330; Tashkent IX 328–30, nos. 6497–99 (9603 I, 10810 II, 8896 III, resp.).

No. 134 : MS 56 I

Moḥammad Mahdī b. ʿAlī Naqī

Zādo l-mosāferīn زاد المسافرین

MS 56 (ex Coll. Qā'enī), 129 fols., 210 x 122 mm; scribe's collection of one Persian and one Arabic medical text. (See also **No. 19 : MS 56 II**.)
Zādo l-mosāferīn on fols. 2–89.

Bound in sturdy, slightly flexible brown leather; simple blind-tooled borders; inner covers pasted with leaf-patterned cloth of light blue, white, and pink on blue; somewhat worn and torn. Written on Italian papers of different provenance, medium thin, burnished, white; watermarks: 1) reclining nymph with water-jar and name LAVARENNA; 2) six-pointed star, and names BALMIO GHIGLIOTTJ and GHIGLIOTTJ; 3) medallion, showing an eagle displayed, and GIOR MAGNANI; 4) big medallion (? not visible), hanging from it an ensign similar to a Maltese cross; first and last fols. foxed; fol. 1 torn, repaired; some marginal stains.

19–20 lines, 135 x 60, 150 x 60 mm, on blind-ruled frame and lines; black with red rubrics; medium-small undistinguished *naskh*; at end of no. I (fols. 88b–89a) *shekastä-āmīz*. Catchwords.

Anonymous copy, dated (both works) 5 Shavvāl 1261/7 October 1845, corresponding to the Turkish *yılan yıl* (here spelled *'īlān 'īl*), the "year of the snake."

Medical notes on fols. 1, 89b, 90a, 118–123, 126–129 and in margins; partly in Hebrew and partly in Arabic characters.

Incipit, fol. 2b

بسمله. سپاس افزون از خواهش بیماران بشفا وستایش
متجاوز از شوق دردمندان بلقا نثار بارگاه طبیبی است
مهربان که...

Explicit, fol. 88b, 12

وباخود داشتن تریاقاتیکه مذکور شد نیز این اثر دارد
ومار از دارنده زمرد وعقرب از دود گوگرد میگریزند
والله اعلم بحقایق الامور بدانکه از معالجات که در این
اوراق پریشان نگارش یافته اکثر انها موافق دستور
معاصرین است واز دستورات قدماء وانچه در کتب طبّیه
مذکور است حذرا عن الاطناب مسکوت ورزیده ...
[س ۱۸] وچون درحین تسوید این اوراق بعضی از مخادیم
خواهش ذکر علاج بعضی امراض ... این خادم آثم ...
مسئول ایشان نکرده اگر بعضی از موارد با موضوع کتاب
منافی داشته باشد سببش این است قد فرغت ...

Moḥammad Mahdī b. ᶜAlī Naqī (fol. 3a, 4) divided his treatise *Zādo l-mosāferīn* (fol. 3b, 2) into two *maṭlab*: 1) (begins fol. 3b, 6) on the regimen of travelers, 2) (begins fol. 9b, -7) on such cures of diseases *a capite ad calcem*, fevers, and bites of poisonous animals, as could be undertaken in the absence of a doctor. In the concluding paragraph, the author states that most prescriptions mentioned in his book follow contemporary practice rather than that of older authorities (see Explicit), and he apologizes for the brevity of his treatise and possible blunders, referring to the state of turmoil and anxiety that prevailed in Eṣfahān in 1141/1728, not long before the future Nāder Shāh drove the Afghans out and ostensibly restored Ṣafavid rule there in Jomādā I 1142/November 1729.[1]

1. The reference to the situation in Eṣfahān is omitted in this, as in most other, MSS (see PL II 272, no. 471), but see **MS 58 I.**

PL II 272, no. 471; Monzavī I 546a, nos. 5099–5126; cf. ibid., 597b, no. 5585 (?); cf. PL II 334, no. 584 (235) (? cf. **No. 138 : MS 59 I**); al-Khāliṣī, p. 260, no. 8; Nūrbakhsh I 79, no. 54 V; Romaskewicz, p. 10, no. 1094; Tashkent V 283, no. 3948 (2744); ibid., IX 342, no. 6515 (5698 II).

No. 135 : MS 58 I

Moḥammad Mahdī b. ᶜAlī Naqī

Zādo l-mosāferīn زاد المسافرین

MS 58 (ex Coll. Min.), 147 fols., 213 x 153 mm; scribe's collection of (I) Moḥammad Mahdī's *Zād*, (II) and (III) two short tracts on the use of donkey-milk and chinaroot, resp., (IV) very short extracts on compound drugs, alchemical procedures, and of *Ekhtīārāt-e Badīʿī*, (V) an Arabic tract on the secret meaning of the letters of the alphabet, (VI) a primitive sketch of the human skeleton, (VII) an anonymous, untitled treatise on simple and compound drugs, and (VIII) another collection of short extracts on medical subjects. (See also **Nos. 179, 198, 199, 212,** and **213.**)
Zādo l-mosāferīn on fols. 1-99.

Bound in black leather over stiff cardboard; simple blind-tooled borders; front inner cover pasted with white paper, back inner cover bare. Binding torn at spine, worn, warped. Written on two randomly alternating varieties of paper: 1) European, medium thin, burnished, white, no watermark; 2) Russian (?), medium thin, burnished, tan.

Fols. 1-25, 11 lines, fols. 26-147, 17 lines, 135 x 85-90 mm, on blind-ruled frame and lines; black with red rubrics; medium-small ordinary *naskh*. Catchwords. Table of contents on fol. 1a; foliation in letters; rubrics repeated in margins.

Anonymous copy; no. I dated in the hour of the moon, Thursday, 16 (written *15*) Ramażān 1261/18 September 1845; no. III dated Tabrīz, 16 (written *15*) Ramażān 1261; no. IV dated Dāro s-salṭanä-ye Tabrīz, at the beginning of the hour of Jupiter, Thursday (Saturday meant?), 18 Ramażān 1261/20 September 1845. The colophon of III reads as follows (fol. 102a, margin):

تمت التسوید الکتاب [کذا] مقام نیر اعظم در کو درجهٔ
سنبله بود و مقام نیر اصغر در اوایل برج حمل بود س
و یوم ه یه شهر ط فی السنة [کذا] غرسا فی تبریز

and the colophon of IV (fol. 117b, 10):

تمت الکتاب [کذا] بعون الملک الوهاب در دار السلطنه
تبریز با هزار محنت و زحمت و مصیبت در شب مشتری
اول ساعت مشتری یح شهر رمضان مقام شمس کط
درجه سنبله غرسا

Many notes throughout MS.
Owner's stamp on fols. 99b, 102, 103b, reading: ʿAlī Akbar, 1267/1850.

Incipit, fol. 1b

بسمله. سپاس افزون از خواهش بیماران و ستایش
بتجاوز دردمندان بلقا نثار بارگاه طبیبی است مهربان
که ... [۲ الف، س ۶] اما بعد چنین گوید گم گشتهٔ دیار
سرگردانی و مبتلای رنج هیچ مدانی الواثق بالله اللطیف...

Explicit, fol. 99a, 9, as in **MS 56 I**, here followed by the author's epilogue, fol. 99a, -2:

اگر ظاهرا بعضی از موارد با موضوع کتاب منافات داشته
باشد سببش اینست فراغ از تسوید این اوراق در هنگام
پریشانی حال و ضعف بدن و اسیری از وطن و در دار
الأحزان اصفهان در ایام شدّت آفات محنت فی عاشر
صفر المظفر غرما اتفاق افتاد حاضرین این زمان و شرکای
احزان یقین که سهو و نسیان را معذور خواهند داشت

In this MS of Moḥammad Mahdī b. ʿAlī Naqī's (fol. 2a, 7) treatise *Zādo l-mosāferīn* (fol. 3a, 5), the author's own postscript is preserved (see Explicit). The day and month given there conform to the date of completion, 10 Ṣafar 1141/15 September 1728, included in another MS of *Zād,*[1] but the year is at variance: it reads غرما, i.e., 1241/1825, which may be a copyist's blunder for ظرما, 1141/1728-29.

1. Cf. **No. 134 : MS 56 I.**

No. 136 : MS 57 I

Moḥammad Mahdī b. ʿAlī Naqī

Zādo l-mosāferīn زاد المسافرین

MS 57 (ex Coll. Min.), 91 fols., 215 x 172 mm; scribe's collection of three medical texts in Persian. (See also **Nos. 86** and **147 : MSS 57 III** and **57 II**.)
Zādo l-mosāferīn on fols. 1–49.

Bound in slightly flexible black leather; simple blind-tooled borders; inner covers bare; one flyleaf each in front and back of medium-thin, slightly coarse, tan Russian (?) paper; worn and torn, warped. Binding too small for the size of fols.; original? Written on medium-thick, burnished, white Russian paper; blind stamp: oval, a capital *M* in the field, and around the edge *Vyatskoĭ Fabrikiĭ*; fols. 74–79, 81–83, 86–91 of the same paper as flyleaves.

19 lines, 160 x 110 mm, on blind-ruled frame and lines; fols. 61–83 have a written surface of 160 x 140 mm, and the margins written in diagonal lines; black with red rubrics; small to medium-sized fair *shekastä*. Catchwords.

Anonymous copy; nos. I–II dated Jomādā II 1275/6 January–3 February 1859, corresponding to the Turkish *yünt yıl*, the "year of the horse"; no. III is undated.

Many notes on fols. 1a, 83b–91, and in margins.

On fol. 61a a purchase note, saying that the MS was bought from Mīrzā ʿAlī Akbar (is he identical with Mīrzā ʿAlī Akbar Khān, mentioned in PL II 308, no. 569, as teacher at the Dāro l-fonūn and the author of a *Ḥefẓo ṣ-ṣeḥḥä*?).

Incipit, fol. 1b

هو الله تعالى. کتاب زاد المسافرین من تالیفات اقا محمد مهدی
یزدی غفر الله له. بسمله. سپاس افزون از خواهش بیماران بشفا
وستایش متجاوز از شوق بیماران بلقا نثار بارگاه طبیبی است...

Explicit, fol. 49a, 9

مار از زمرد و عقرب از دود کوکرد میگریزد والسلام علیکم
ورحمة الله وبرکاته تمام شد...

Zādo l-mosāferīn by Moḥammad Mahdī b. ᶜAlī an-Naqī ash-Sharīf (fol. 1b, -2).

No. 137 : MS 7 I

Moḥammad Mahdī b. ᶜAlī Naqī

Zādo l-mosāferīn زاد المسافرین

MS 7 (ex Coll. Min.), 214 fols., 176 x 105 mm; binder's collection of two medical texts in Persian. (See also **No. 10 : MS 7 II**.)
Zādo l-mosāferīn on fols. 1–108.

Bound in stiff lacquered cardboard; multicolored borders, panel of pale yellow with a bouquet of flowers in white, pink, yellow, blue, and green; spine of dark brown leather; inner covers pasted with greyish-blue paper, painted (upside down) with a daffodil in watercolors; one flyleaf each in front and back, the former of medium-thick, glazed, white European paper without watermark, and the latter of thin, coarse, greyish-green Eastern (?) paper. Binding worn, battered; spine coming off the covers. I. Fols. 1–108: European paper, medium thick, burnished, tan; II. fols. 109–214: Russian paper, medium thin, burnished, off-white; when MS was mounted, fol. 109 was pasted against a blank leaf (paper like the front flyleaf). Some spots; edges of fol. 1 repaired. On lacunae see below.

I. Fols. 1–108: 14 lines, 120 x 60 mm, on blind-ruled frame and lines; black with red rubrics; medium-small even *nastaᶜlīq*. Catchwords. II. Fols. 109–214: 14 lines, 117 x 65 mm, on blind-ruled frame and lines; black with crimson overlinings and rubrics; medium-small neat *nastaᶜlīq*. Catchwords.

Collations by reader (I) and scribe (II).

I. Copied, and dated Teheran, in the *madrasa* of Āghā Moḥammad Khwājā, Thursday morning, 6 Jomādā I 1258/ *Wednesday*, 15 June 1842, by ᶜAbdo r-Raḥīm b. ᶜAbdo l-Karīm. II. Copied, and dated 1259/1843, by Moḥammad Ebrāhīm Āgūčāk ("Hooklet").

In I, numerous marginal entries; in II, marginal and interlinear glosses, and notes by scribe.

Owner's stamps on fols. 108b and 109b, of ᶜAbd ar-Raḥīm (the scribe of I?) and ᶜabduhū Ismāᶜīl b. Bēgler (?), dated 1256/1840 (?).

Incipit, fol. 1a

اما امام اتقیا معجون ماده الحیواة [کذا] اولیا
و تریاق فاروق سُعدا...

Explicit, fol. 108a, -1

وعقرب از دود کوکرد مگریزد والله اعلم بحقایق الامور
تمت الرساله...

In this copy of Moḥammad Mahdī b. ʿAlī Naqī's *Zādo l-mosāferīn,* one fol. is missing before fol. 1; cf. **No. 134 : MS 56 I.**

No. 138 : MS 59 I

Moḥammad Kāẓem b. Moḥammad Ṣāʾeb al-Khwānsārī

Meftāḥo sh-shefāʾ مفتاح الشفاء

MS 59 (ex Coll. Min.), 142 fols., 208 x 150 mm; scribe's collection of two works. (See also **Nos. 71** and **139 : MSS 59 II** and **59a**.)
Meftāḥo sh-shefāʾ on fols. 3-141.

Bound in flexible plain rust-colored leather; inner covers bare; spine separate, of the same leather; somewhat warped, worn and torn. Binding not original (?), too small for the size of MS. Written on European paper, medium thin, slightly transparent, glazed, white; watermarks: 1) G R; 2) shield, showing an eagle displayed, crested with hooped crown. Fols. 1 and 142 slightly foxed, elsewhere a few inkblots, dog-eared corners, etc.

I. 19-21 lines, 140-50 x 80-90 mm, on blind-ruled frame and lines; black with crimson rubrics and overlinings; medium-small *naskh* of various styles, by one scribe, ranging from careless (last pages) to calligraphic elegance, but always mannered; rubrics occasionally left out, mostly in fine but academic *thuluth,* sometimes in equally distinguished *nastaʿlīq*; rubrics sometimes repeated in margins. Catchwords. II. Margins of fols. 13a, 15b-45a, 46b-124a, diagonal lines; black with crimson rubrics; small *nastaʿlīq* of varying care, by the same scribe as I.

Collations by scribe.

Copied, and dated (I) 1 Zū l-qaʿdä 1265/18 September 1849 and (II) 1265/1848, by Aḥmad b. Moḥammad Bāqer Ṭabīb al-Khwānsārī.

On fol. 1a notes in Armenian, Arabic, and French, the latter two medical terms, all in the same hand; on fols. 1b-3a recipes written in one hand, different from that of fol. 1a; on fols. 141b-142b recipes in hand of fols. 1b-3a, partly rubricated, numbered 1-12, in hand of fol. 1a.

Incipit, fol. 3b

بسمله. الحمد لله رب العالمین الصلوة والسلام علی خیر
خلقه محمد واله اجمعین اما بعد چنین گوید گمگشته

دیار سرگردانی و مبتلاء برنج هیچ مدانی الواثق بالله
ابن محمد صائب محمد کاظم الخوانساری که غرض از
تحریر اینذخیره انست ...

Explicit, fol. 141a, 12

گویند نگاهداشتن زعفران درخانه باعث گریختن
سام ابرص که اورا چلپاسه میگویند اینست
مختصری از سمومات و دفع هوام و حشرات
والله الموفق و هوالمعین و هو شافی الاسقام قد تمت ...

Ebn Moḥammad Ṣāʾeb Moḥammad Kāẓem al-Khwānsārī (fol. 3b, 4) wrote his treatise *Meftāḥo sh-shefāʾ* (fol. 3b, 14) at the instigation of his friends who had asked him to compose a *mokhtaṣar* on the treatment of frequently occurring diseases that could be cured without the help of a physician (fol. 3b, 5-8). The author divided it into two *maṭlab*, the first on the regimen of travelers, and the second on the cure of common diseases not requiring a physician's attendance (fol. 3b, 14-17). Moḥammad Mahdī b. ʿAlī Naqī's *Zādo l-mosāferīn* was obviously the closely followed model for this book.[1] Even the introductory eulogies were imitated here.

1. Cf. **No. 137 : MS 7 I.**

Not in PL or Monzavī, but see PL II 334, no. 584 (235) (? cf. **No. 135 : MS 58 I**).

No. 139 : MS 59a

Moḥammad Kāẓem b. Moḥammad Ṣāʾeb al-Khwānsārī

Meftāḥo sh-shefāʾ מפתאח ל שפא

MS 59a, one loose fol., 135 x 90 mm

This loose leaf, today measuring 135 x 90 mm but originally somewhat larger (the writing is damaged along one side), warrants a separate description, since it represents the first leaf of a MS in Hebrew characters of *Meftāḥo sh-shefāʾ* by Moḥammad Kāẓem b. Moḥammad Ṣāʾeb al-Khwānsārī.

Medium-thin, burnished, light grey Eastern paper; margins frayed.

16 lines, 105 x 70 mm; black; small, good Persian-Hebrew hand, rubrics larger and calligraphic.

Second half thirteenth century/ca. 1835–80.

Interlinear and marginal notes in Hebrew characters; marginal entries also in Arabic script.

Incipit, recto

האזא כתאב מפתאח ל שפא
בשם אלה אלרחמאן ל רחים אל חמד לא[?]
רב א[?] עאלמין אלצלואת אלשלאם עלא
כייר כלקה גנין גויד גם גשתגאן [!] דיאר
סר גדראני ומבתלאיי [בק]נג היץ מדאני
אלואסק בלאה אבן מחמד צאייב מחמד
כאזם כאנסרי כה קרז אז תחריך אין
וגיזה איוסת כה בעזי אז...

This loose leaf contains the beginning of Moḥammad Kāẓem b. Moḥammad Ṣāʾeb al-Khwānsārī's (recto, line 5) treatise *Meftāḥo sh-shefāʾ* (verso, line 6) in Hebrew characters. Unfortunately, no more is preserved of this MS in UCLA's collection.

No. 140 : MS 89

Moḥammad Ḥosain b. Moḥammad Hādī ʿAqīlī ʿAlavī

Makhzano l-advīä va-tazkerä-ye ūlī n-nohā مخزن الادويه وتذكرة اولى النهى

MS 89 (ex Coll. Min.), 429 fols., 306 x 192 mm

Bound in crimson leather over stiff cardboard; covers decorated with two borders and three-medallion design, all inset with blind-stamped floral scrolls, gold in outer border, dark blue in inner border and medallions; inner covers pasted with plain black leather. One flyleaf each in front and back of thin off-white Russian paper; in front, one more flyleaf of medium-thin, glazed, white Italian paper; watermark: crowned shield showing an eagle displayed on top of a tower, and name BIAGGIO. Binding somewhat worn. Written on Italian papers of different provenance, medium thick, glazed, white; watermark visible in fol. 429: leopard rampant sinister in shield and name GIO BATTA; there is a hole in fol. 429, because colophon and, probably, owner's stamp have been effaced.

25 lines, 213 x 125 mm, on blind-ruled frame and lines; borders of black, gold, two black, blue lines; margins framed in black, gold, black; fols. 1b and 2a framed in elaborately illuminated borders in gold, red, and blue; *sarlowḥ* of the same colors on fol. 1b; lines of writing separated by golden clouds on fols. 1b and 2a; black with crimson rubrics; medium-sized good, if a little pedestrian, *naskh*. Catchwords.

Anonymous, undated copy; colophon on fol. 429a thoroughly effaced; of the date, only *alf* is legible (ibid., 16), and of the patron's name only the title *mostowfī l-mamālek* can be read (ibid., 13); first half of thirteenth century/ca. 1785–1835.

Reader's notes on fol. 1a and flyleaves.

On fol. 1a and front flyleaves, several *tamlīk* and stamps erased.

Incipit, fol. 1b

بسمله. وبه نستعين. الحمد لله الذى عرفنا بنفسه وهدينا [كذا] بحمده وجعلنا من امة حبيبة... [س ٣] اما بعد اين مقاله دويم است از كتاب موسوم بمخزن الادويه وتذكرة اولى النبى [كذا. يعنى النهى] در بيان ادويه مركبه مسمى بقرابادين ونسخ انها بطريق اختصار...

Explicit, fol. 429a, 1

تخم خيار گل سرخ از هريك چهار درم گلاب صد مثقال شراب حماض شراب سيب شراب انار شيرين از هريك سى مثقال عسل صاف بقدر حاجت بطريق معهود معجون سازند شربتى يك مثقال بعد چهل روز والله يعلم بالصواب بحكم واراده...

This MS contains the second *maqālä*, the *Qarābāẕīn*, of *Makhzano l-advīä va-tazkerä-ye ūlī n-nohā* (fol. 1b, 3) by Sayyed Moḥammad Ḥosain Khān b. Moḥammad Hādī Khān ʿAqīlī ʿAlavī Khorāsānī Shīrāzī (name not mentioned here).[1] The author divided this *Qarābāẕīn* into a *moqaddemä* in five *faṣl*, on the principles to be followed in compounding medicines; into 28 *bāb*, subdivided into *faṣl*, in alphabetical order (considering also the second and third letters); and a *khātemä* (fol. 1b, 6–8). This part of *Makhzano l-advīä* is an excerpt from Moḥammad Ḥosain's own *qarābāẕīn-e kabīr*, called *Majmaʿo l-javāmeʿ va-ẕakhīrato t-tarākīb*, which he composed in 1185/1771–72.[2]

Moḥammad Ḥosain was a grand-nephew of Moʿtamado l-molūk Ḥakīm Moḥammad Hāshem b. Moḥammad Hādī Sayyed ʿAlavī Khān.[3]

1. PL II 280, no. 492.
2. PL II 281, no. 492 (3).
3. See **No. 159 : MS 124 IV.**

PL II 281, no. 492 (4); Monzavī I 596a, nos. 5574–75; Miklukho-Maklaĭ, p. 538, no. 3984.

No. 141 : MS 104

Moḥammad Mahdī b. Moḥammad Qāsem

Badāyeʿo l-fonūn [*fī tarjamato l-Qānūn*] بدايع الفنون [فى ترجمة القانون]

MS 104, 485 fols., 310 x 210 mm

Bound in black leather over thick cardboard; simple blind-tooled borders; three-medallion design with blind-stamped floral scrolls; inner covers pasted with European paper, dyed light greyish-blue; binding much worn, decoration barely visible. Written on European paper, medium thick, burnished, dyed light blue; watermark: coat of arms, not clear; edges of first and last fols. torn, repaired, and torn again; fols. 4, 5, 398 substituted, paper similar to body of MS, but of more intense blue color. On lacunae see below.

24-25 lines, 240 x 130 mm; black with crimson rubrics and overlinings; medium-sized careful *naskh* leaning to *nastaʿlīq*. Catchwords.

According to the colophon on fol. 484b, -7, this is the author's autograph copy, dated at Borūjerd on Thursday, 15 Rabīʿ I 1215/*Wednesday*, 6 August 1800.

Many marginal notes by author and later owner, Samīʿ (see below on *tamlīk*); recipes on front inner cover and fol. 485b, formulas for amulets on fols. 1b-2a; tract about the numerical value of letters on fol. 485b.

On fol. 2b, *tamlīk* by the writer of many of the marginal entries: al-mālik bi-l-istiḥqāq Samīʿ aṭ-Ṭabīb, dated 1257/1841; on fols. 1a and 485b two *tamlīk* in the same hand and dated on the same day: Friday, 15 (?) Moḥarram, corresponds to 14 Āzarmāh (i.e., A. Yazd. 1304), 1354 *hejrī-ye qamarī*, equals 1314 *hejrī-ye shamsī*/19 April 1935; signature of writer illegible.

Incipit, fol. 2b

بسمله. حمدی که از کیفیت نشأه مفرح راح ریحان
مجمع البیان عباراتش که مبنی بر جرعه جام حقایق
فرجام جامع الفواید منهاج فیوضات نشأتین است ...

Explicit, fol. 484b, -9

وحکه اظفار معالجه کنند انرا بماء البحر که بشویند رایم
انرا باو پس زایل میگردد باو یا بطبیخ عدس وکرسنه
یا بطبیخ خنثی وازاضمده بلبوس وزفت وتین است
مجموع یا فرد تمت الکتاب [کذا] الثالث من کتاب
البدایع الفنون [کذا] فی یوم الخمیس خامس عشر شهر ربیع
الاول علی یده [کذا] المؤلف هذه النمیقه واقل الخلیقه ابن
محمد قاسم محمد مهدی الآثم غفر الله له ولوالدیه فی سنه خمس
عشر مأتین [کذا] والف ١٢١٥ فی بلد البروجرد [کذا] صان
الله عن الافات

After this colophon of *ketāb* 3, there follows the beginning of *ketāb* 4, which breaks off on fol. 484b, -1:

بسمله. الحمد لله ربّ العالمین مقاله اولی ازکتاب الرابع
از بدایع هفت فنون است فن اول مشتمل بر پنج مقاله
مقاله اولی از فن اول ازکتاب الرابع ازکتب بدایع واو مشتمل بر پنج
مقاله مقاله اولی کلام کلی در حمیات]

*Badāye*ʿ*o l-fonūn*[1] (title given in colophon, see above) by Moḥammad Mahdī b. Moḥammad Qāsem (ibid.) is a Persian version of Avicenna's *Qānūn* that was hitherto unknown. It follows the Arabic original rather closely.

1. In the introduction to *ketāb* 4 it is titled *Badāye*ʿ*-e haft fonūn* (see above). The title might be expected to continue *fī tarjamato l-Qānūn*.

Not in PL or Monzavī.

No. 142 : MS 124 II

Ḥājjī Āqā-ye valad-e Ḥājjī Ghāzī Moḥammad

*Kholāṣat-e qavānīno l-*ʿ*elāj* خلاصة قوانین العلاج

MS 124 (ex Coll. Min.), 335 fols., 205 x 135 mm; scribe's collection of four Persian works on medicine. *Kholāṣat-e qavānīno l-*ʿ*elāj* on fols. 174–276.

For the description of the MS see **No. 133 : MS 124 I.**

Incipit, fol. 174a

بسمله. در زکر [کذا] حلاصة القوانین علاج [کذا] امراض
بدن صداع بمعنی درد سر است اگر حدوث آن ازخون
باشد علامتش سرخی رو وچشم ...

Explicit, fol. 276a, 2

واگر معلوم گردد که کدام زهر بوده است انچه مخصوص
انست بآن معالجه کنند در مطولات مذکور است
پس ازکتابها فرا گیرند امّا قد فرغت من تالیف هذا

الکتاب المستطاب المسمی بخلاصة قوانین العلاج ومن
تحریر [کذا] فی یو الجمعه [کذا] غریه جمادی الاوّل [کذا] سنه ۱۲۱۶
درمقام کلکته ...

The title *Kholāṣat-e qavānīno l-ʿelāj* appears at the beginning of the text and in the author's colophon (see above). The treatise discusses the treatment of diseases in the traditional order *a capite ad calcem*, giving a short description of the symptoms and listing various compound medicaments for them.

In the colophon the author says that this tract was written (fol. 276a, -6)

از نسخهٔ علوی خان مرحوم بنام سیّدی سندی سیّد محمد هادی
المخاطب بحکیم معتمد الملوک سیّد علویخان محمّد شاهی

If the word *tālīf* (fol. 276a, 4) can be taken literally, the author must have followed closely a similar treatise of Ḥakīm Moʿtamado l-molūk *Moḥammad Hāshem b.* Moḥammad Hādī, known as Sayyed ʿAlavī Khān.[1] A treatise *Kholāṣato l-qavānīn* by a Moḥammad ʿAlavī Khān is preserved in a MS of Panjāb University;[2] an examination of both texts will be needed to determine their relationship.

1. He was physician to the Mughal prince Moḥammad Aʿẓam, a son of Owrangzēb, and to the emperors Bahādor Shāh and Moḥammad Shāh, and died in Delhi in 1160/1747 or 1162/1748; on his biography see PL II 273–74, no. 475, with references.
2. PL II 274, no. 475 (2).

Not in PL or Monzavī.

No. 143 : MS 63

Moḥammad Moʾmen an-Nakhaʿī al-Āshtīānī "Mīrzā Bābā"

Tazkerato l-ʿelāj تذکرة العلاج

MS 63 (ex Coll. Min.), 171 fols., 195 x 125 mm

Bound in black leather over stiff cardboard; blind-tooled patterned borders; three-medallion design with blind-stamped floral scrolls; inner covers pasted with off-white paper; one flyleaf in front of medium-thin, yellowish Russian (?) paper; binding somewhat worn. Written on medium-thin, burnished, tan Russian (?) paper; fol. 1 and a few other leaves of medium-thick, burnished, white European paper; watermark obscure; water stains and inkblots.

16 lines, 145 x 70 mm, on blind-ruled frame and lines; on fols. 2b–4a and the following tables, borders of grey, crimson, and rust; greyish-black with crimson rubrics; small to medium-small thin, fair, sometimes very dense *shekastä-āmīz*; rubrics often in separate line. Catchwords.

Collations and marginal notes by scribe.

Anonymous, undated copy; second half of thirteenth century/ca. 1835–80.

Recipes on fols. 1b, 2a, 164b, 165.

On fol. 1a a former owner's illegible stamp.

Incipit, fol. 2b

بسمله. ستایش بیقیاس تحفه بارگاه حکیمی که کلیات
عالم اسباب از مفردات مشیتش مختصر نمونه ایست ...
[۳ الف، س ۱٤] اما بعد چنین گوید اقل واحقر ناس واضعف
عباد محمد مؤمن شهیر بمیرزا بابا ابن محمد حسین النخعی
الاشتیانی غفر الله لهما ولوالدیهما که چون غرض اصلی ...

Explicit, fol. 171a, 12

نهایت جالینوس دوای کندر را بهتر از این لا ذوق
[کذا. یعنی لزوق] میدانند صفت ان کندر صاف را
سحق و صلایه بلیغ نموده و با سفید و تخم مرغ سرشته
بطریق مسطور استعمال نمایند

Moḥammad Mo᾽men *shahīr be*-Mīrzā Bābā ebn Moḥammad Ḥosain an-Nakha῾ī al-Āshtīānī (fol. 3a, -3) dedicated this book, *Tazkerato l-῾elāj* (fol. 3b, 13), to ῾Abbās Mīrzā, Fatḥ῾alī Shāh Qājār's son and heir apparent (fol. 4a, -3). It is divided into unnumbered *tazkerä*; in the first, in tabular form, the pulse, urine, and other symptoms (*῾alāmāt*) of the state of health are discussed; the following deal with therapy in the usual order *a capite ad calcem*, general diseases, skin disorders, syphilis (*āteshak*), fevers, poisons, and simple and compound drugs.

Not in PL; Monzavī I 494b, nos. 4594–95.

No. 144 : MS Ar. 96 I

Moḥammad b. ῾Abdo ṣ-Ṣabūr Khū᾽ī Tabrīzī "Ṭabīb"

Morakkabāt-e jowharīyä مرکّبات جوهریّه

MS Ar. 96 (ex Coll. Min.), 159 fols., 212 x 150 mm; binder's collection of two Arabic (nos. III and V [fragments of al-Jaghmīnī's *Qānūnja*]) and six Persian texts. No. IV non-medical, not catalogued here (*Mer᾽āto s-samā᾽* by Moḥammad Mahdī b. Moḥammad Sa῾īd al-Jīlānī, copied by Mīrzā ῾Abdo l-Karīm valad-e Mīrzā Kāẓem Ṭabīb-e Khwānsārī and dated by him 6 Ẕū l-ḥejjä 1257/19 January 1842). (See also **Nos. 101, 145, 185,** and **217.**)
Morakkabāt-e jowharīyä on fols. 1–34.

Bound in black leather over stiff thick cardboard; simple blind-tooled borders. Written on different varieties of European and Eastern (?) papers: 1) fols. 1-34: European paper, thin, burnished, white; watermark—coat of arms—obscure; 2) fols. 35-44, different European papers, thin, burnished, white; watermarks obscure; 3) fols. 101-155 and five loose fols. at the back of the MS: Eastern (?) paper, medium thin, lightly burnished, white; 4) fols. 156-159: Russian (?) paper, medium thin, coarse surface, beige.

A. Fols. 1-34 (no. I): 18-24 lines, 135-60 x 80 mm, on blind-ruled frame and lines; black with red rubrics; medium-sized, even, but undistinguished *shekastä-āmīz*. Catchwords. B. Fols. 35-44 (no. II): 15-18 lines, 140 x 95 mm, on blind-ruled frame and lines; black; medium-sized undistinguished *shekastä-āmīz*. Catchwords. Fols. 45, 46a blank. C. Fols. 123-139a (almost through no. VI): 14-15 lines, 170 x 120 mm, on blind-ruled frame and lines; black with some rubrics in crimson; small to medium-small, uneven, unattractive *shekastä*; partly in larger aggressive *shekastä*, partly in smallish *naskh*, but one hand. Catchwords. D. Fols. 139b-158b (end of no. VI, no. VII): 13-14 lines, 150-65 x 115 mm, on blind-ruled frame and lines; black, until fol. 144a with crimson or black rubrics and crimson overlinings; small to medium-large, partly spidery, neat *naskh*, sometimes leaning to *nastaʿlīq*. Catchwords. E. Five loose leaves: 14 lines, 150 x 90 mm, on blind-ruled frame and lines; black; medium-sized unattractive *shekastä-āmīz*. Same hand as in C? Catchwords.

Anonymous, undated copies (end of nos. II and VIII missing), except no. IV (see above); second half of thirteenth century/ca. 1835-80. Scribe C may be Mīrzā ʿAbdo l-Karīm, who copied no. IV and dated it 1257/1842 (see above).

Notes on fols. 46b and 101a.

Owner's stamp on fol. 1a, legible only: Maḥmūd; on fol. 46a two illegible owner's stamps.

Incipit, fol. 1b

بسمله . سبحانك اللهم یا من یداوی الارواح بطب
الحقیقه ویعالج القلوب بحکمة الطریقه ...

Explicit, fol. 34b, top margin, line 6 from left

تا اینکه از برکت توجه والتاف [کذا. یعنی التفات]
شاهزاده در صفحه عالم یادگار بماند

After the customary reference to the reigning sovereign, Fatḥʿalī Shāh Qājār (fol. 1b, -1), Moḥammad b. ʿAbdo ṣ-Ṣabūr Khūʾī *al-aṣl* Tabrīzī *al-vaṭan mashhūr be-*Ṭabīb (fol. 3a, 8) praises the interest taken by the heir apparent, ʿAbbās Mīrzā (fol. 2b, 1), in the development of arts and sciences. He paid special attention to the training of physicians in both Galenic and Paracelsian medicine (fol. 2b, -6, etc.), and since the mineral drugs used by European doctors in the "seven kingdoms" (*haft qīrāl*) were not readily available in Iran, he ordered the author to translate the Latin (*zabān-e lāṭīn*) of European pharmacopoeias into Persian (fol. 3a, 1-10). Moḥammad b. ʿAbdo ṣ-Ṣabūr called his work accordingly *Morakkabāt-e jowharīyä* (fol. 3a, -2). It is divided into a *moqaddemä*, 320 prescriptions, and a *khātemä* (ibid.). The *khatemä* appears to be missing in this MS. In another treatise begun by order of ʿAbbās Mīrzā, the author attempts to combine traditional and modern European medicine: *Jāmeʿo l-ḥekmatain va-majmaʿo ṭ-ṭebbain*, in a *moqaddemä*, 44 *qānūn*, and a *khātemä* (see PL II 291, no. 520).

This title not in PL or Monzavī; cf. PL II 291, no. 520; Monzavī I 579b, nos. 5388-89; ibid., 594b, nos. 5565-66.

No. 145 : MS Ar. 96 II

[Moḥammad b. ʿAbdo ṣ-Ṣabūr Khūʾī Tabrīzī "Ṭabīb"]

[*Morakkabāt-e jowharīyä*], Index [مركّبات جوهريّة]

MS Ar. 96 (ex Coll. Min.), 159 fols., 212 x 150 mm; binder's collection of eight Arabic and Persian texts. Index to *Morakkabāt-e jowharīyä* on fols. 35–44.

For the description of the MS see **No. 144 : MS Ar. 96 I.**

Incipit, fol. 35a

بسمله . دواهاى كه نافعند درامراض صفراوى حب ٦٧
سكنجبين ٧ معجون ٥٨ درامراض حارّه حقنه او٢ و٣
سكنجبين ١ شراب ٤٢ ...

Explicit, fol. 44b, -1

وجوارش ١١ دوآء ١ روغن معجون ٢ ٤٢ سياه كننده موى
خضاب [...

This is an index to *Morakkabāt-e jowharīyä,* listing the recipes by number according to their indication. No author of the index is named in this MS, which is incomplete at the end.

See **No. 144 : MS Ar. 96 I** for references.

No. 146 : MS 65

Moḥammad ʿAlī al-Fānī b. Mollā Eskandar Shervānī

Kīmīāʾo sh-shefā كيمياء الشفا

MS 65 (ex Coll. Min.), 68 fols., 210 x 150 mm

Bound in crimson leather over stiff cardboard; simple blind-tooled borders; inner covers pasted with green paper. Outside of binding worn, MS loose in binding. Written on Italian paper, medium thin, glazed, off-white; watermark: coat of arms and motto IL GRAN MASSO. A few stains and smears in MS, one fol. torn.

16 lines, blind-ruled within borders of red, gold, black, and blue, measuring 156 x 91 mm; black, with crimson rubrics and overlinings; small, neat *shekastä-āmīz*. Catchwords. On fol. 1b *sarlowḥ*: a simple panel of parallel red lines; an outer *jadval* of two hair-thin black lines frames all pages, measuring 198 x 133 mm.

Copied, and dated Eṣfahān, 25 Rabīʿ I 1252/10 July 1836, by Moḥammad Karīm al-Eṣfahānī for Moḥammad Esmāʿīl Khān Qājār.

Recipes on fol. 68b.

Incipit, fol. 1b

بسمله. بر مبتدیان ترکیب معاجین جواهر انشا
اهم وواجب وبر متصدیان تخمیر خمیرهٔ
زواهر معنی لازم ولاذب حمد حکیم
ابدی وشکر چاره ساز سرمدیست ...

fol. 2a, 1

اما بعد چنین گوید اقل فقرا واضعف ضعفا
المدعو محمد علی الفانی ابن ملا اسکندر شروانی
غفر الله له ولوالدیه ...

Explicit, fol. 68a, -6

چنانچه توتیا وافیتمون وسرمه ومرقشیثا واقلیمیا
واسهال اینها ادویه مجربه را باین قانون بسایند
که غبار محض وهبا باشد والسلام

Moḥammad ʿAlī al-Fānī b. Mollā Eskandar Shervānī (fol. 2a, 1) wrote his dispensatory in alphabetical order, *Kīmīāʾo sh-shefā* (fol. 2a, -1), following the new, *chemical* system of Paracelsus. Judging by the titles of the books he left,[1] his main interest was in alchemy/chemistry and its application to medicine. An abridged version of his preface to *Kīmīāʾo sh-shefā* (fols. 2a-3a) follows here because of its contribution to the history of Middle Eastern medicine in the nineteenth century:

... ولوالدیه که مدتی مدید وعهدی بعید بود که
خوشه چین خرمن حکمت ومعرفت علم طبابت

بودم تا که بتاریخ سنه ١٢٣٣ بعنوان سیاحت
بدار السلطنه قسطنطیه [کذا] رسید [کذا] ودرانجا
چندی قصد اقامت کرده بمذهب ومشرب ایشان
متشبه شده درطلب مطلب خود وسیاحت مشرب
ایشان بوده وبا عرفا وحکما واطبا ملاقات ومراوده
میکرده تا اینکه برئیس الاطباء العثمانی [کذا] السید
محمد خراسانی که اباء... ان... درخدمت سلاطین
ال عثمان سالهای سال بوده با ان بزرگوار بنده‌را الفت
ومحبت کلی بهم رسید وفقیررا بمنزل خود دعوت
نمود بنابر اخلاق حمیده... ایشان دعوتش را
اجابت کرده... روزی بطریق محبت... فرمودند
که والد مرحوم درایام شبابش جهت تحصیل
وتکمیل علم طب بفرنگستان رفته ومدت شصت
سال تمام فرنگستانرا سیاحت وعلوم طب وتشریحرا
کما هو حقه تحصیل بالتخصیص طب کیمیویرا در
خدمت حکیم خرمانس که افلاطون وقت
وسرامد اطباء فرنگستان وحکمای انزمان بود تکمیل
کرد ولب لباب... ان معانیرا انتخاب نموده
از زبان فرنگی بلسان ترکی تحویل کرده بکیمیاء
2b الشفا نام نهاد بعد المراجعت | من السفر بنظر
فیض اثر سلطان مصطفی رسانید سلطان مرحوم
نیز ارباب این صنعت واصحاب این حکمت را جمع
کرده برغبت تمام ومحبت تام بتجربه نسخ ان کتاب
کوشید فی الواقع اغلب نسخ اورا برؤ الساعة یافت ان
کتابرا نسخ متعدد نویسانیده درخزانه نهاد فقیر
چون این... شنیدم... بشوق... طالب... شده اذن

استنساخ گرفته ... نسخهٔ از روی نسخه اصل نوشتم
وگاگاهی عند الحاجة. بعض نسخه اورا تجربه میکردم
وبر اکثر طبایع وامزجه مطابق ... میدیدم ... الحاصل ان
کتاب بهمراه فقیر بود تا بتاریخ سنه ۱۲۵۲ باقلیم
ایران وشهر اصفهان وارد گردید ... اسماعیل خان ابن
ابراهیم خان فرمان فرمای ملك کرمان .. بفقیر داعی
فرمود جانا از مرز بوم روم دوستانرا چه تحفه ...
3a اوردی ... | فقیر ذکر کتاب را من الباب الی المحراب
بیان نمود درجواب فرمودند ... اگر این کتاب فارسی
العباره میبود ... فوائدش تمامتر بود چه شود اگر ...
شاهدان ... عبارات رومیرا بالبسه ... فارسی حلوه دهی ...
بحسب الامر ... این فقیر حقیر در همان روز بترجمه
این کتاب ... شروع نموده ... بنای این کتابرا
بطریق حروف مقطعه ترتیب کرده ...
آبزن جزئی از ترکیبات موسیطانوس طبیب است ...

The information given in this preface concerning the place and date of translation from the Turkish version is at variance with the Teheran Med. Fac. MS which has Baghdad, 1246/1830.[2] It seems possible that the copyist of this MS altered the text to flatter the patron for whom he transcribed it. His patron was apparently the son of the governor who was supposed to have commissioned the translation.

1. *Qānūno sh-shefā* (Monzavī I 579a, no. 5385; MS dated 1250/1834); *Kīmiā* (ibid., 633b, no. 5885; MS dated 1265/1848); *Meftāḥo l-ḥayāt fī asrāro n-nabāt* (ibid., 642b, no. 5994; MS dated 1248/1832). On further works of his see PL II 292, no. 523.
2. Rahāvard, pp. 411–12, no. 261 III; PL II 292, no. 523.

PL II 292, no. 523; Monzavī I 564a, nos. 5271–74.

No. 147 : MS 57 II

Moḥammad b. Zakarīyāʾ ar-Rāzī/Aḥmad b. Moḥammad Ḥosain Tonakābonī

[*Tarjamä-ye Borʾo s-sāʿä*] [ترجمهٔ برء الساعه]

MS 57 (ex Coll. Min.), 91 fols., 215 x 172 mm; scribe's collection of three medical texts in Persian. [*Tarjamä-ye Borʾo s-sāʿä*] on fols. 49–61.

For the description of the MS see **No. 136 : MS 57 I.**

Incipit, fol. 49b

ترجمه کتاب برء الساعه محمد زکریا رازی .
بسمله. حمد بیحد وستایش لا تحصی ولا تعد نثار بارگاه
وایثار پیشگاه کبریای حکیمی است جلّ قدرته که طبیعت
نوع انسان ازچار طبع مختلف الطبیعه باقتصار حکمت شامله
وقدرت کامله الفت ترکیب داده ...

Explicit, fol. 61a, 2

وسیر وپیاز وتخم تره تیزک مساوی هم پخته مرهم سازند
وبکار دارند والسلام علی من اتبع الهدی تمام ...

In the introduction, ebn Moḥammad Ḥosain Aḥmad ash-Sharīf aṭ-Ṭabīb at-Tonakābonī (fol. 49b, -5) says that he translated *Burʾ as-sāʿa* by Muḥammad b. Zakarīyāʾ ar-Rāzī into Persian at the order of Fatḥʿalī Shāh Qājār (fols. 49b, -1 to 50a, 8), without giving his version a title;[1] he supplemented its 23 *bāb* by seven. In fact, *bāb* 24, on sore muscles, is also by ar-Rāzī, and only the last six were written by Aḥmad at-Tonakābonī; in them, he discusses the dyeing of hair, depilation without the use of lime, deodorization of sweat, diet for emaciation, and antidotes for poisons in general and arsenic in particular.

Aḥmad b. Moḥammad Ḥosain Tonakābonī was one of the *ḥakīmbāshī* officeholders in the reign of Fatḥʿalī Shāh.[2]

1. Monzavī quotes this version under the title *Toḥfä-ye shāhī* (I 488b), but cf. PL II 197, no. 351 (1c), where this is given as the title of a Persian translation prepared for Owrangzēb's son Moḥammad Aʿẓam.
2. PL II 293, no. 525.

PL II 198, no. 351 (1 e); ibid., 293, no. 525 (1); Monzavī I 488b, nos. 4508–15.

No. 148 : MS 61 III

Moḥammad Bāqer b. Moḥammad Ḥosain al-Ḥosainī al-Monajjem

Majmaʿo t-tajāreb مجمع التجارب

MS 61 (ex Coll. Min.), 247 fols., 215 x 150 mm; scribe's collection of three works.
Majmaʿo t-tajāreb on fols. 200–243.

For the description of the MS see **No. 41 : MS 61 I.**

Incipit, fol. 200b

بسمله. وبه نستعين. الحمد لله الحكيم العليم الذى يشفى بلطفه
السقيم والصلوة والسلام على من اوتى بالدين القويم وعلى آله
واولاده الذين...

Explicit, fol. 243a

واگر وجعى در عضوى از اعضا باقى باشد روغن ناردين
بر بدن طلا نمايد انگاه داخل آب گرم حمّام شود
اينست شرايط كليه كه در استعمال

The MS is an unfinished copy—fol. 243b is blank—of Moḥammad Bāqer b. Moḥammad Ḥosain al-Ḥosainī al-Monajjem's treatise on syphilis (*āteshak*), *Majmaʿo t-tajāreb* (fols. 200b, 6; 201a, 1), in the author's own hand. He wrote it to give the subject of *āteshak* the full and detailed discussion it deserved as a widespread disease of recent occurrence: the ancients did not deal with it, since it was unknown at the time, and even later authors who gave it their attention, such as Amīr Bahāʾo d-dowlä Nūrbakhshī,[1] ʿEmādoddīn Maḥmūd,[2] and Jalāloddīn Moḥammad Ṭabīb,[3] had done so only briefly; among contemporary physicians, there was nobody prepared to write on *āteshak* (fols. 200b–201a). *Majmaʿo t-tajāreb* is divided into a *moqaddemä,* seven *bāb,* and a *khātemä*:

moqaddemä (begins on fol. 201a, 8)

در ذكر وقت ظهور وسبب حدوث واسامى ناخوشى
مزبور على اختلاف الروايات

bāb 1 (begins on fol. 202a, -6)

در ذكر تعريف واسباب حصول اين مرض اعم
از اسباب داخلى وخارجى على اختلاف الاقوال والآرا

bāb 2 (begins on fol. 205b, 6)

در ذكر علامات اين ناخوشى مطلقا اعم از انكه از سوداء
محرق بهمرسد يا از ساير اخلاط محرقه

bāb 3 (begins on fol. 207b, 6)

در ذکر معالجات این مرض بطریق کلّیه که شامل جمیع
اقسام باشد وبطریق جزؤیت که معالجه هریك از
اقسام بوده باشد

bāb 4 (begins on fol. 215a, -3)

اما معالجه این مرض برسبیل جزئیت هرکاماد اورا سودای
محترق از دم بوده باشد [لیس هذا بعنوان الباب الرابع: لاعنوان هنا]

bāb 5 (begins on fol. 220a, 3)

در ذکر تاثیر زیبق ونفع وفایده که ازاو محسوس وبتجربه
رسیده است

bāb 6 (begins on fol. 221b, 7; written in the margins of fols. 221b and 222a)

در ذکر حلّ سیماب وتکلیس زیبق

bāb 7 (begins on fol. 221b, 7)

در ذکر معالجه ناخوشی اتشك از زیبق بطریق مختلفه
وانحاء متفاوته

khātemä (begins on fol. 238b, -2)

در ذکر طریق خوردن بیخ چینی بطریق قهوه

1. See **No. 46 : MS 23.**
2. See **No. 99 : MS 46 II** and references to other MSS there.
3. See **No. 126 : MS 47.**

Not in PL or Monzavī.

No. 149 : MS Ar. 53 III

Joseph Désiré Tholozan and Moṣṭafā b. ᶜAqīl ᶜAlavī Eṣfahānī

Badāyeᶜo l-ḥekmato n-Nāṣerī بدايع الحكمة الناصرى

MS Ar. 53 (ex Coll. Min.), 138 fols., 165 x 100 mm; binder's collection of several Arabic and two Persian medical texts. *Badāyeᶜo l-ḥekmato n-Nāṣerī* on pp. 151–263.

For the description of the MS see **No. 221 : MS Ar. 53 II.**

Incipit, p. 151, 1

بدایع [کذا] الحکمة الناصری. بسملة. چون بزورگار
دولت ابد مدت اعلیحضرت سلطان ... [س ۹] ابو المظفر
سلطان ناصر الدین شاه نمازکه دولتش ماننده و حشمتش
فزاینده باد حکیمان افلاطون دها از ممالک اروپا ...

Explicit, p. 263, 5

و باید دانست که کامل بدون وجود علتی قلب
و اراتی [؟ آیا یعنی آورتی؟] کامل بدون

This medical text, titled *Badāyeᶜo l-ḥekmato n-Nāṣerī* by the scribe (p. 151), appears to be identical with *Badāyeᶜo l-ḥekam-e Nāṣerī* by Joseph Désiré Tholozan and Moṣṭafā b. ᶜAqīl ᶜAlavī Eṣfahānī, on auscultation and palpation.[1] In this MS, the text breaks off on p. 263, 6, in the middle of a page.

1. See PL II 298, no. 545, and 299, no. 545 (2).

PL II 299, no. 545 (2); Monzavī I 482a, no. 4459.

No. 150 : MS 62

Muḥammad b. Zakarīyāʾ ar-Rāzī

Borʾo s-sāᶜä برء الساعه

MS 62 (ex Coll. Min.), 5 fols., 215 x 135 mm; **MSS 62, 80–83** are obviously parts of a scribe's collection of medical treatises that was only recently taken apart and bound separately.

Modern brochure of thin, flexible, plain green (**MSS 62, 80–82**) or blue (**MS 83**) fading cardboard; one flyleaf each in front and back of modern thin, smooth, white paper. Written on Eastern paper, thin to medium thin, transparent, burnished, beige; worm-eaten throughout, partly mouse-eaten; trimmed and repaired when rebound.

15 lines, 170 x 95 mm, on blind-ruled frame and lines; black with red rubrics; large, neat, but unattractive *nastaᶜlīq*. Catchwords. Fol. 5b blank.

Anonymous copy, dated Thursday [no month given] 1240; the other parts of this unnamed scribe's collection are dated Jomādā I 1240/22 December 1824–20 January 1825 (**MS 80**) and simply 1240/1824 (**MSS 81–83**), resp.

Incipit, fol. 1a

بسمله. آغاز کتاب برء الساعت از مقوله حکیم فیلسوف.
چنین گوید حکیم کامل فیلسوف فاضل محمد بن ذکریاء
[کذا] الزاری تغمده الله تعالی روزی در خدمت ابو
القاسم که از وزرای عصر بود نشسته بودم سخن از
علم طب میگذشت...

Explicit, fol. 5a, -3

و در زمستن در آب گرم شدید درآمده ایستادن نیز
عجیب النفع است در حال ماندگی و تعب برطرف شود
باذن الله تعالی تمام شد...

This Persian version of Muḥammad b. Zakarīyāʾ ar-Rāzī's (fol. 1a, 3) *Burʾ as-sāʿa* (fol. 1b, 3) is obviously the same as one represented in a Tabrīz MS that was copied in 1083/1672;[1] a Bankipore MS, transcribed in the nineteenth century, also appears to contain *Borʾ* in this version.[2]

1. Tabrīz I 253–54, no. 193 (*shomārä-ye daftar* 3414 V).
2. Bankipore, Supp. II 177, no. 2275.

Cf. PL II 197, no. 351 (1); Monzavī I 496a, nos. 4608–15; ibid., 533a, no. 4931; Cambridge, *Supp.*, p. 267, no. 1596 (a, p), Trinity, R. 13.45; Tashkent VIII 99, no. 5680 (8312 II).

No. 151 : MS 29 X

abū Bakr Muḥammad b. Zakarīyāʾ ar-Rāzī

Borʾo s-sāʿä برء الساعه

MS 29 (ex Coll. Min.), 119 fols., 200 x 135 mm; scribe's collection of ten works.
Borʾo s-sāʿä on fols. 111b–118b.

For the description of the MS see **No. 79 : MS 29 I.**

Incipit, fol. 111b, -4

چنین گوید محمد بن زکریّای رازی طبیب که در وقتی
از اوقات در مجلس ابو القاسم بن عبدالله حاضر بودم
که در آنحضرت ذکر ... از معالجات طبی میگذاشت

Explicit, fol. 118b, 10

آب بسیار گرم و یك کف نمك بران ریزد
و یکساعت دست و پارا درمیان آب گذارد
انشاء الله نافع می افتد و الله اعلم بالصواب تمت [کذا]
الکتاب ...

In this MS of a Persian version of Muḥammad b. Zakarīyāʾ ar-Rāzī's (see Incipit) *Burʾ as-sāʿa*, no title is mentioned. As far as can be gathered from Elgood's English version of the Incipit in his copy, as quoted by Storey,[1] this MS may contain the same translation as that in his MS. In *Dharīʿa* (III 84, no. 253), a translation of *Burʾ as-sāʿa* is quoted as beginning

چنین گوید ابوبکر محمد بن زکریا

It does not appear rash to conclude that the version quoted in *Dharīʿa* is at least very close to those in the UCLA and Elgood MSS, resp.

1. PL II 198, no. 351 (1 i); the MS was transcribed in 1266/1849. It is identical with the MS in the Royal Coll. of Physicians (JRAS [1951], p. 188, no. 41 VI), listed in PL II 198, no. 351 (1 j) as "inadequately described."

No. 152 : MS 103

Anonymous

Basāyeṭo n-nabż بسایط النبض

MS 103 (ex Coll. Min.), 40 fols., 150 x 100 mm

Bound in flexible crimson leather; simple blind-tooled borders, three-medallion design with corresponding corners, blind-stamped with floral scrolls; inner covers dark grey leather; one flyleaf each in front and back of thin, burnished, cream-colored European paper; no watermarks. Top and bottom of spine lightly worn, binding otherwise in fine condition. Written on Italian paper of two varieties, medium thin, glazed, cream-colored; watermarks: 1) GIO BATTA and coat of arms; 2) DE FERRARI 19, and coat of arms; ink smears on fols. 11a and 39b.

Fols. 1–10: 100 x 58 mm, 4 x 4 fields in tables; fols. 11–39: 15 lines, 95 x 50 mm, on blind-ruled frame and lines; black with crimson rubrics and overlinings; small neat *naskh*. Catchwords. Fols. 11a and 40 blank.

Anonymous, undated copy: colophon erased on fol. 39b; thirteenth/nineteenth century.

Incipit, fol. 1b

بسایط النبض طویل دلّ علی کثرة الحرارة
ضیق دلّ علی قلّة الرطوبة قصیر دلّ علی قلّة الحرارة ...

Explicit, fol. 39b, 6

وامثال اینها باعث هلاکت میشود هم بجهة عدم
دفع ابخره وهم بجهة عدم ایصال هوا بروح از مسام
ضیّقه جلدیّه والله اعلم بحقیقة الحال تمّ

Beginning of text on fol. 11b

بسمله وبه نثقی . الحمد لله ربّ العالمین : والصّلوة والسّلام
علی خیر خلقه محمد واله الطاهرین قال الشیخ رحمه الله الجملة
الاولی من الفنّ الثانی فی النبض : بدانکه طالب هر علمی را
لازم است که ...

This treatise on the pulse is divided into two parts: fols. 1b–10b are taken up by a survey of the different modes of the pulse in tabular form, the text being in Arabic; on fol. 11b, there follows a Persian adaptation of the section of the *Qānūn* dealing with the pulse: *kitāb* 1, *fann* 2, *jumla* 1.[1] The scribe of this MS titled the whole *Basāyeṭo n-nabż* on fol. 1b.

1. Ed. Būlāq I 123–35; the first six *faṣl*, on generalities, on pp. 123–29.

Not in PL or Monzavī.

No. 153 : MS 64

Anonymous

[*Tashrīḥo l-amᶜā*] [تشریح الامعا]

MS 64 (ex Coll. Min.), 43 fols., 153 x 105 mm

Bound in stiff cardboard, covered with marbled paper in blue, grey, pink; corners and spine brown and red, resp., leather; inner covers pasted with grey paper; MS out of binding. Binding original? Written on European paper, medium thin, slightly transparent, burnished, white; watermark: shield with a star (only partly visible), crested with a hooped crown, name AL M[ASSO?].

15 lines, 100 x 63 mm, on blind-ruled frame and lines; black with rubrics overlined in black; small copperplate *naskh*. Catchwords. Rubrics repeated in margins by scribe (?).

Copied, and dated Tuesday, 8 Jomādā II 1254/*Wednesday*, 29 August 1838, by al-Ḥājj ʿAlī Moḥammad b. Moḥammad Ḥasan.

Incipit, fol. 1b

بسمله. يا مسهّل الصعاب سهل لنا سلوك طريق الصواب...
وارزق لنا خير العاقبة وحسن الماب بمحمد واله الاحباب
انك الوهّاب وبعد اما تشريح امعا بر سبيل اجمال چون
در علاج هر عضوى از اعضا چنانچه در موضع خود
بيان كرده اند...

Explicit, fol. 43b, 2

با سه برابر اجزا عسل بعد از شش ماه استعمال [...]
متفاوتنست واز غايت شهرت احتياج
بتقييس نيست تمّت...

The text of this anonymous, untitled treatise does not discuss the anatomy of the intestines, as is mentioned in the preface (see Incipit), but the treatment of diseases affecting them. There are apparently no divisions into sections, although on fol. 4a, 10 a "first" *faṣl* begins. In the whole text, the corresponding passages of Avicenna's ***Qānūn*** are closely followed,[1] but the exact relationship between Avicenna's text and this MS will have to be determined by further study.

1. Cf. *Qānūn* (ed. Būlāq) II 418, etc.

Not in PL or Monzavī.

No. 154 : MS 74 II

ʿAlī b. ʿĪsā al-Kaḥḥāl

Tazkerato l-kaḥḥālīn

تذكرة الكحّالين

MS 74 (ex Coll. Min.), 284 fols., 175 x 133 mm; scribe's collection of two works.
Tazkerato l-kaḥḥālīn on fols. 223–284.

For the description of the MS see **No. 1 : MS 74 I.**

Incipit, fol. 223b

بسمله. الحمد لله رب العالمين وصلوته على محمد واله اجمعين. گفتار نخستين ياد كنيم حد چشم و شرح دهيم انرا كه چگونه است...

Explicit, fol. 284a

وطبع هريك را جدا بگفتم تا اسان باشد بركسى كه طلب اين علم كند والله الموفق للصواب...

The title of this text is given, in the scribe's hand, as *Tazkerato l-kaḥḥālīn* on fol. 223a; in the text itself neither author nor title is mentioned. The work is divided into three *goftār*: 1) (begins on fol. 223b, 2) on the anatomy of the eye in 21 *bāb* (in the MS sometimes mistakenly called *goftār*); 2) (begins on fol. 229a, -10) on diseases of the eye that can be perceived by the senses, in 73 *dar*, as they are called in the introductory remark; and 3) (begins on fol. 271a, -4) on diseases that cannot be perceived by the senses, in 28 *bāb*. This organization of the contents identifies the text as ᶜAlī b. ᶜĪsā's work.[1] Which, if any, of its known Persian translations in three *goftār* is represented here cannot be determined without an actual comparison of the MSS, especially since a preface is lacking in this copy. It seems to be a version similar to those in Teheran Med. Fac., corresponding to the Arabic original in the number of *bāb* and *goftār* (*maqāla*), except that in this MS, *goftār* 3 is divided into 28, not 26, *bāb*.[2]

1. Ullmann, p. 208; Rahāvard, pp. 136–39.
2. See note 1, and cf. PL II 204, no. 357 (f).

Cf. PL II 203, no. 357; Monzavī I 494b, nos. 4596–4603, 4604.

No. 155 : MS 124 III

Maḥmūd b. ᶜOmar Čaghmīnī

Resālä-ye Qānūnčä-ye Fārsī رسالهٔ قانونچهٔ فارسى

MS 124 (ex Coll. Min.), 335 fols., 205 x 135 mm; scribe's collection of four Persian works on medicine. *Resālä-ye Qānūnčä-ye Fārsī* on fols. 277–308.

For the description of the MS see **No. 133 : MS 124 I.**

Incipit, fol. 277a

یا علی مدد . رسالهٔ قانونچهٔ فارسی
وبه نستعین . بسمله . این رساله مرتّب گشته بر ده مقاله
مقاله اوّل در امور طبیعی باید دانست که طبیعت چیست ...

Explicit, fol. 308a, 1

امّا راسب پس دلالت میکند در رسوب طبیعی بر تمامی
پختگی وغیر طبیعی بر بدحالی این چند کلمه در بلده کلکته ...

This MS obviously represents the same Persian version of *Qānūnja* by Maḥmūd b. ʿUmar al-Jaghmīnī[1] as Bankipore MS no. 967.[2] In neither MS, however, is title or author's name mentioned in the text itself. In the UCLA copy, the text ends after the fourth *maqālä* on the pulse and urine.

1. Cf. **No. 19 : MS 56 II** and **No. 132 : MS 123,** note 3.
2. *Cat.* XI 9.

PL II 219, no. 377 (c); cf. Monzavī I 504a, nos. 4667–68.

No. 156 : MS 67 IV

Excerpts from various authors

[*Taẕkerä-ye ṭabīb*] [تذکرهٔ طبیب]

MS 67 (ex Coll. Min.), 145 fols., 215 x 140 mm; scribe's collection of medical texts and charms in Arabic and Persian; nos. I-III in Arabic: I. (fols. 4–10) *ar-Risala adh-dhahabīya* by Pseudo-ʿAlī b. Mūsā ar-Riḍā; II. (fols. 11–14) *Burʾ as-sāʿa* by Muḥammad b. Zakarīyāʾ ar-Rāzī; III. (fols. 15–26b, 10) charms.
Untitled excerpts from various authors in Arabic and Persian on fols. 26b, 11 to 144b.

Bound in flexible dark brown leather, stiffened inside by dark grey cardboard; simple blind-tooled borders, panels decorated with diagonal, blind-tooled lines; one flyleaf in back of thin, green, Eastern (?) paper; many fols. out of binding. Written on papers of different provenance: 1) fols. 1–28: medium thin, burnished, white; Russian, with two different illegible blind stamps; 2) fols. 29–145: Eastern (?), medium thin, burnished, beige; some spots and stains. For lacunae see below.

160–70 x 80–85 mm, on blind-ruled frame and lines; the number of lines differs according to their direction: on some pages there are paragraphs in horizontal and in diagonal lines; greyish-black with crimson overlinings; medium-large, neat *nastaʿlīq*; rubrics in margins. Catchwords. Fols. 1–3, 4a blank.

Anonymous, undated copy (end missing); thirteenth/nineteenth century.
Recipes by readers on fol. 145a.

Incipit, fol. 26b, 11

فاضل زکریا در کتاب حفظ الصّحة خود می فرماید ایزد
تبارك وتعالی سپرزرا بیافرید خاکدان تن گردانید تا هر
فسادی که اندرتن باشد از خون سوخته ...

Explicit, fol. 144b, -2

وهم این کسان را بسیار بُوده است که اندر میانه
شراب که هنوز مزه شراب همی یافته است وبه نقل
دهان خوش می کرده]

This section of **MS 67** appears to be a doctor's *vade mecum,* a collection of excerpts from different authors, such as Hippocrates (Boqrāṭ),[1] Dioscorides (Dīsqūrīdūs),[2] Galen (Jālīnūs),[3] ar-Rāzī, ibn Sīnā, abū l-Faraj,[4] ʿAllāmā-ye Meṣrī,[5] Fāżel-e Hendī,[6] Malaṭī,[7] and Ḥakīm Moʾmen,[8] in Arabic and Persian. There is a lacuna between fols. 28 and 29, and the text breaks off on fol. 144b.

1. See Ullmann, pp. 25–35; GAS III 23–47; PL II 193, no. 345.
2. See Ullmann, pp. 257–63; GAS III 58–60; PL II 194, no. 347.
3. See Ullmann, pp. 35–68 and index; GAS III 68–140.
4. It is not clear which abū l-Faraj is meant here: ibn Hindū (Ullmann, p. 152; GAS III 334–35), ibn al-Quff (Ullmann, pp. 176–77 and index, s.v.), or a third physician of this name; if "Malaṭī" further down really does refer to Barhebraeus, it is unlikely that he is meant here.
5. Not identified.
6. This is probably Bahāʾoddīn Moḥammad b. Tājoddīn Ḥasan Eṣfahānī (1062–1137/1652–1725), the author of *Baḥro l-mavvāj* on the Koran, *Ḥekmat-e khānīyā* on logic, natural science, and metaphysics, and of other works; see PL I 216f., no. 279, and index; Monzavī I 8a, nos. 65–66, s.v. *Baḥro l-mavvāj,* and 662b, no. 6186, s.v. *Ḥekmat-e khānīyā.*
7. Perhaps Barhebraeus is meant here, who was born at Malatya (see EI² III 804b–805b [J. B. Segal]; cf. Ullmann, pp. 232, 277).
8. This might be Moḥammad Moʾmen b. Moḥammad Zamān Tonakābonī, the author of *Toḥfato l-moʾmenīn*; cf. **MSS 115–121.**

No. 157 : MS Ar. 60 II

ʿAbdo r-Razzāq

Kholāṣato t-tashrīḥ خلاصة التشريح

MS Ar. 60 (ex Coll. Min.), 56 fols., 254 x 167 mm; binder's collection of one Arabic and three Persian works: I (fols. 3–48), a fragment of *Kāmil aṣ-ṣināʿa* by ʿAlī b. al-ʿAbbās, in Arabic; II, *Kholāṣato t-tashrīḥ*; III, on music, not catalogued; IV, *Zakhīrā-ye Khwārezmshāhī* (see **No. 7 : MS Ar. 60 IV**).
Kholāṣato t-tashrīḥ on fols. 49–56.

Bound in thick, flexible, plain black leather; some wear, some leaves out of binding. Binding too small for MS, not original. Fols. 49–56 written on Eastern paper, medium thin, burnished, cream colored; fols. 1–2, added when binding was done, of Eastern paper, medium thin, burnished, beige. Fol. 49a rather soiled: before being bound into present volume, was first fol. of a volume. For lacunae see below.

21 lines, 162 x 102 mm, on blind-ruled frame and lines; black with red rubrics and punctuation; medium-sized, even, fine *naskh*. Margins written by different hand: diagonal lines, greyish-black with red rubrics; medium-sized, fair to fine *naskh*, sometimes leaning to *nastaᶜlīq*. Catchwords throughout.

Sketches in black and red on fol. 55b; on fol. 56a room left for anatomical illustration, but not filled.

Collations by scribe.

Anonymous, undated copies (end missing); ca. 1000/1600.

Notes by reader on fol. 1 and in margins.

On fol. 2a a note dated Tuesday, 27 Rabīᶜ II, the year left out.

On fols. 50a, 55a, within the written surface a stamp reading: waqf Luṭf Allāh.

Incipit, fol. 49b

بسمله هست زاسباب شفای سقیم.
لطایف حمد وثنا حکیمی را سزد که بهر تشریح ابدان
انسان وترویح اجسام ایشان انوار حکمتش چون روح
در مجاری شرایین جاریست واثار نعمتش چون
خون در موارد اورده ساری ...

Explicit, fol. 56b, -2

وسبب استحکام مفصل ان شده ودر بعضی شش زایده
ودر بعضی هشت زایده میباشد که آنرا شواخص خوانند
وبغیر ازین شواخص زایدهای دیگر هست که بر پشت]

The MS contains the beginning of a treatise on anatomy, *Kholāṣato t-tashrīḥ* (fol. 51b, 2), by ᶜAbdo r-Razzāq (fol. 49b, -4). It is divided into a *moqaddemä*, دربیان اعضا وتکون آن, and six *faṣl*:

1. در تشریح عظام وغضروف
2. در تشریح اعصاب
3. در تشریح شرایین
4. در تشریح اورده

5. در تشريح عضله

6. در تشريح اعضای مركّب

and a *khātemä* در تكون جنين (fol. 51b, 3-6). The work is dedicated to Moʿezzo d-dowlä va-s-salṭanä va-l-khelāfä Khosrav-e ghāzī Homāyūn[1] (fol. 51a, -6). In the long and elaborate introduction (fols. 49b, -2 to 50a, -7) the author praises his teacher and mentor Qoṭboddīn Moḥammad Ādam, who had appointed him physician and teacher at the hospital founded by the late sultan (*solṭāno l-marḥūm*). As his sources he mentions تشريح قانون وكامل الصناعة وذخيره وتشريح قرشي وغيرآن and adds that he translated from them into Persian to make them accessible to *khavaṣṣ va-ʿavāmm* (fol. 51a, 2-3). Of these authorities, ʿAlī b. ʿAbbās al-Majūsī and ibn Sīnā are well known; *Zakhīrä* is certainly Esmāʿīl Jorjānī's famous work,[2] and *Tashrīḥ-e Qorashī* are the anatomical sections of ibn an-Nafīs's great commentary on the *Qānūn*.[3] This MS breaks off within *faṣl* 1, on bones.

1. It cannot at present be determined whether this is the Mughal *pādshāh* or another ruler of this name, such as ʿAlāʾoddīn Homāyūn Shāh Bahmanī (862-67/1457-62). Homāyūn b. Bābar's *laqab* was Nāṣeroddīn, not formed with Moʿezz either. ʿAbdo r-Razzāq does call him *pādshāh* (fol. 51a, 4), but not as a formal title.
2. Cf. **MSS 1-5**. In Pseudo-Thābit b. Qurra's *K. adh-dhakhīra* anatomy is not discussed, cf. Ullmann, p. 136.
3. See Ullmann, p. 173.

PL II 320, no. 584 (93); Monzavī I 529a, no. 4895; Osmania Med. Coll., p. 111, no. 17.

No. 158 : MS 120 III

Anonymous

[*Dar rūzhā-ye boḥrān*] [در روزهای بحران]

MS 120 (ex Coll. Min.), 187 fols., 222 x 120 mm; binder's collection of four works, nos. I-III copied by the same scribe. [*Dar rūzhā-ye boḥrān*] on fols. 39b-40a.

For the description of the MS see **No. 120 : MS 120 I.**

Incipit, fol. 39b

باسامی. بسمله. روز اول و روز دوم. روز سيّم
بسيار باشد كه بيماريها باشد كه بغايت گرم و سوزان
بود اندرين روز بحران كند...

Explicit, fol. 40a, left bottom field

روز چهلم این روز بحران است و بحرانی که بعد ازین
روز باشد ضعیف خواهد بود

This tract on the crisis-days of diseases is written in the form of tables; author's name and title are missing.

No. 159 : MS 124 IV

Moḥammad Bēg

Dastūro l-faṣd دستور الفصد

MS 124 (ex Coll. Min.), 335 fols., 205 x 135 mm; scribe's collection of four Persian works on medicine. *Dastūro l-faṣd* on fols. 309–328.

For the description of the MS see **No. 133 : MS 124 I.**

Incipit, fol. 309b

رسالهٔ فصّادی المسمّی بدستور
الفصد من تألیف مرزا محمد بیگ غفر الله له تعالی. بسمله.
وبه نستعین. تمم بالخیر.
سپاس بیکران وستایش بی پایان مر حکیم مطلق را سزد
که وجود بشر را از کارخانه عنایت خلعت لقد خلقنا الانسان
فی احسن التقویم کرامت فرموده...

Explicit, fol. 328a, 1

گرداگرد جراحت را بروغن بنفشه یا یاسمین چرب دارند
واز روغن کنجد گرم کرده نیز چرب کنند خالی از منفعت
نخواهد بود والله اعلم بالصواب

Moḥammad Bēg (fol. 310a, 1) excerpted this treatise on bloodletting, *Dastūro l-faṣd* (ibid., 4), from Esmāʿīl Jorjānī's *Zakhīrä-ye Khwārezmshāhī* and other "reliable treatises" and divided it into six *bāb*. The period of the author's lifetime cannot at present be determined.[1]

1. See PL II 315, no. 36.

PL II 315, no. 584 (36); Monzavī I 574b, no. 5346; Osmania Univ., p. 53, no. 34.

No. 160 : MS 26 XI

Saifoddīn b. Qoṭboddīn al-Badakhshī

[*Ḥefẓo ṣ-ṣeḥḥä*] [حفظ الصحه]

MS 26 (ex Coll. Min.), 103 fols., 178 x 120 mm; binder's collection of eleven works. Al-Badakhshī's untitled treatise on fols. 82b to 103b, 4.

For the description of the MS see **No. 62 : MS 26 I.**

Incipit, fol. 82b, 6

بسمله. الحمد لله الذی ارسل بالهدی من قال العلم علمان ...
[۸۲ ب، ۱۰] اما بعد چنین گوید بندهٔ محتاج بخداوند ... سیف
الدین بن قطب الدین البدخشی ...

Explicit, fol. 103b, 2

اگر درد غالب بود یکدوی حجامت ان درد را بکشند
وغذا کشك جو خورند وبجای آب دوغ بیاشامند

This untitled treatise on diet and hygiene by Saifoddīn b. Qoṭboddīn al-Badakhshī (fol. 82b, 11) is divided into irregular *faṣl*. There is a lacuna between fols. 98 and 99, and the text breaks off on fol. 103b, 4; the lower part of the page is blank. Probably this MS was transcribed from a defective copy.

Not in PL or Monzavī.

No. 161 : MS 18

Anonymous

Mūjez-e Kommī موجز کمّی

MS 18 (ex Coll. Min.), 132 fols., 178 x 115 mm

Bound in flexible dark brown leather; three-medallion design with blind-stamped floral scrolls. One flyleaf each in front and back of thin, off-white, Russian (?) paper. Outside of binding badly damaged, except along edges. Binding too small for MS, not original. Written on Eastern paper, medium thin, layered, burnished, beige. First fols. stained and foxed, some mended with the same paper used for flyleaves; one blank fol. of the same paper substituted for two missing leaves between fols. 3 and 5. On other damage to the text see below.

14 lines, 132 x 67 mm, on blind-ruled frame and lines; black with red rubrics and overlining, these sometimes omitted; medium-small, neat, fine *nastaʿlīq*. Catchwords.

Collations by scribe.

Copied, and dated 24 Jomādā II 1084/6 October 1673, by Aḥmad b. Shamsoddīn (there follow four undecipherable words).

Marginal notes by readers; recipes in various hands on fols. 124b–131.

On fol. 1a *tamlīk* saying that the book was sent through the mediation of Mashhadī Moṣṭafā on 28 Rabīʿ I 1224/13 May 1809.

Incipit, fol. 5a

هر دو چشم را با حریر بمالد ومثانه بچه را بمالد
تا میزیدن آسان شود وپیوندها را گل سرخ وبرگ
مورد را نرم بکوبد وبپاشد . . .

Explicit, fol. 124a

واگر کسی را باید تا تمام شبهت درین دو علم
از پیش خاطر وی برخیزد بکتاب نبض وتفسره
قانون بازگردد وبقراط وجالینوس درین دو علم
کتابها جدا کرده اند وشرح وسط تمام داده اند تا
بدین اختصار عیب نکند والله اعلم بالصواب

The MS contains an anonymous, untitled treatise in 38 *bāb*, further divided into *faṣl*, on pediatrics, hygiene, treatment of diseases (*a capite ad calcem*, and general diseases), bleeding, cupping, pulse, and urine. Its identification as *Mūjez-e Kommī* rests on a comparison with Rieu II 476a. In the UCLA manuscript, introduction, beginning of the table of contents (two fols.), end of the table of contents, and the beginnning of the first *bāb* are missing.

According to the introduction quoted by Rieu (loc. cit.), this book was compiled as an abridgment (*mokhtaṣar*) of " 'the most esteemed Arabic and Persian works' "; the author lists as the latter abū Bakr Rabīʿ b. Aḥmad al-Akhavainī al-Bokhārī's *Hedāyato l-motaʿallemīn fī ṭ-ṭebb*,[1] Aḥmad-e Farrokh's *Kefāyä*,[2] and Esmāʿīl Jorjānī's *Zakhīrä*, *K. al-aghrāż*, and *Khoffī-ye ʿAlāʾī*. The explicit quotations found in this MS present a slightly different picture of the author's Persian sources: Akhavainī Bokhārī is quoted seven times,[3] Esmāʿīl is cited once with his name alone, once with his *Zakhīrä*, and three times with his book *at-Tuḥfa as-saʿdīya*.[4] There is no quotation from Aḥmad-e Farrokh; but most of the explicit quotations occur in sections on the treatment of diseases with compound medicines, not in passages discussing symptoms and diagnosis. It cannot be ruled out that these passages are taken without acknowledgment from the other sources listed in the introduction.

As to Greek and Arabic sources, the whole syllabus of medical learning is represented in the quotations; in the following list, only authors from ar-Rāzī on are named, on the assumption that earlier (and probably also many later) sources were not directly used by this author: ar-Rāzī,[5] Thābit b. Qurra, i.e., Pseudo-Thābit,[6] Aḥmad b. Muḥammad aṭ-Ṭabarī,[7] ʿAlī b. al-ʿAbbās al-Majūsī,[8] abū ʿAlī b. Sīnā,[9] Badr ad-Dīn al-Qalānisī,[10] Najīb ad-Dīn as-Samarqandī.[11]

Two sources could not be identified: abū l-Ḥakīm ʿAbd al-Masīḥ ad-Dimashqī, with his book *al-Jāmiʿ*,[12] and a work called *K. al-Kāfī*.[13] A book of this title was written by ar-Rāzī,[14] Jibrīl b. ʿUbaidallāh b. Bukhtīshūʿ,[15] and abū Naṣr ʿAdnān b. Naṣr al-ʿAinzarbī,[16] and *al-Kāfī fī l-kuḥl* by Khalīfa b. abī l-maḥāsin al-Ḥalabī.[17]

Since the identity of Saifoddīn Nūrī, whom the author calls *ostād-e man emām-e fāżel*,[18] has not been established, the date of composition remains uncertain; Najīb ad-Dīn as-Samarqandī, the latest source mentioned and thus serving as *terminus a quo*, was killed during the Mongol conquest of Herāt in 619/1222.[19] It is tempting, however, to understand the title *Mūjez-e Kommī*, "Sleeve-Book,"[20] as an allusion not only to Esmāʿīl Jorjānī's *Khoffī-ye ʿAlāʾī*, "ʿAlāʾ[o d-dowlä]'s Boot-Book," but also to ibn an-Nafīs's famous *Mūjiz al-Qānūn*. That would move its date forward to the very end of the seventh/thirteenth century at least.[21]

1. This is the earliest medical compendium written in Neo-Persian; its author was at one remove a student of ar-Rāzī; see *Hedāyä*, ed. J. Matīnī, *Enteshārāt-e Dāneshgāh-e Mashhad, sh.* 9 (Mashhad 1344), esp. p. *panjāh va-noh*.
2. Esmāʿīl Jorjānī quoted this author in his *Zakhīrä-ye Khwārezmshāhī*; see **No. 2 : MS 1.**
3. Fols. 24a, 3; 42a, -3; 42b, 3; 83a, 5, 8, -2; 83b, 4.
4. Fol. 99a, 3; fol. 48a, 3; and fols. 62a, -7; 71a, -4; 97a, -3, resp.
5. Fols. 15b, 2; 48b, 2; 50b, 5; 56a, 1; 64b, 2; 67a, -4; 72a, 1; 82b, -7; 100b, 1; 111b, -3.
6. *K. adh-dhakhīra*, fols. 24b, -3; 52a, 8; 56b, 3; 59a, 3; 62b, 6; 64a, 1; 78a, 6; 117a, -6.
7. *K. al-muʿālajāt al-Buqrāṭīya*, here quoted as *Moʿālajāt-e Boqrāṭ*, fol. 7b, 2.
8. *Kāmil aṣ-ṣināʿa*, fols. 23b, -4; 64a, 3; 84b, -5.
9. Fols. 58b, 6; 119a, -3.
10. *Aqrābādhīn*, fol. 66b, -2.
11. Fol. 65b, 5 and *al-Asbāb wa-l-ʿalāmāt*, fol. 109b, -2.
12. Fols. 59a, 7; 60b, 5; 70b, -7; 85a, 1; ibn a. Uṣaibiʿa mentions an abū ʿAlī Yūḥannā b. ʿAbd al-Masīḥ (I 243, 28), but he appears to have lived in Mesopotamia rather than in Syria, which makes it unlikely that abū l-Ḥakīm was his father (cf. Dietrich, p. 232, no. 117; GAS III 337). Nor can it be at present more than a guess to relate him to ʿAbd al-Masīḥ b. ʿAbdallāh al-Ḥimṣī "ibn Nāʿima," the translator (ibn a. Uṣaibiʿa, I 214, 15).
13. Fol. 71a, -4.
14. See Ullmann, p. 132.
15. Died A.D. 1006; see Ullmann, p. 110.
16. Died A.D. 1153; see Ullmann, p. 161.

17. Composed between A.D. 1266 and 1275; see Ullmann, p. 212.
18. Fol. 18a, -1.
19. See Ullmann, p. 170.
20. Strictly speaking, a compendium small enough to be carried about in the sleeve.
21. Ibn an-Nafīs died in 687/1288; see Ullmann, p. 172.

PL II 327, no. 584 (158); Monzavī I 605a, no. 5650.

No. 162 : MS 19

Anonymous

Mūjez-e Kommī موجز كمّى

MS 19 (ex Coll. Min.), 110 fols., 191 x 122 mm

Bound in cream-colored paper over stiff cardboard, spine of dark brown leather. Two flyleaves in front, one in back added later in European paper; fols. 111 and 112 not part of the original MS. Front cover missing, outside of binding stained. Binding not original. Written on Eastern paper, medium thick, burnished, beige. Heavy water stains in lower part of many fols.; margins of some mended; MS trimmed down from original size. On lacunae see below.

16 lines, 145 x 72 mm, on blind-ruled frame and lines; black with red rubrics; medium-sized fair *nastaʿlīq*. Catchwords. Fol. 110 blank.

Collations, by scribe with *ṣaḥḥa* and *nuskha*, by reader without mark.

Anonymous, undated copy (end missing); twelfth/eighteenth century.

Occasional marginal notes.

An earthquake is mentioned in a note dated 25 Rajab 1249/8 December 1833. On fol. 3a a note, dated 1252/1836, on the purchase of this MS from Mīrzā Kūček during his lifetime; close to it a stamp (belonging to the writer of this note?), reading ʿabduhū Muḥammad b. Muḥammad b. ʿAbd al-Bāqī al-Ḥusainī; only the century, 12(00), of its date is legible. On fols. 35a, etc., older stamp with pious formula. On fol. 68a stamp reading: māl Mūsā.

An old foliation of this MS shows that two fols. are missing in front, one at the end (after fol. 108), and one after fol. 101; fols. 15 and 16 are misbound between fols. 106 and 107.

No. 163 : MS 95

Anonymous

[*Ṭebb*] [طبّ]

MS 95, 24 fols., 175 x 115 mm

Unbound, leaves held together by crude stapling. Written on Eastern paper, medium thin, burnished, greyish-white; heavily soiled, foxed, stained, torn along edges. On lacunae see below.

14–18 lines, 140–45 x 75–80 mm; black; small, careful *nastaʿlīq* of two styles (by same scribe?). Catchwords.

Anonymous, undated copy (end missing); ca. 1100/1700?

The order of fols. is disrupted in this fragmentary copy of an unidentified medical compendium; the correct order is as follows: beginning missing, 19-24, lacuna, 11-18, lacuna, 1-4, lacuna, 5-10, end missing. As far as can be gathered from this MS, the text is divided into *faṣl*:

1. (beginning missing; starts here on fol. 19a) on the faculties, *qovā*, "spirits," *arvāḥ*, and parts, *aʿżāʾ*, of the body in general
2. (begins on fol. 19b, 3)

در بیان خلقت وماهیت هریك از اعضای مفرده ومرکبه

3. (begins on fol. 24b, -3)

در بیان کیفیت ورود غذا به بدن وتولد هریك از اخلاط اربعه

4. (begins on fol. 12b, -8) در بیان حفظ صحت وتدبیر سته ضروریه

(5.?) (begins on fol. 4b, -2), unnumbered

در تدبیر مسافر

(6.?) (begins on fol. 8a, 7), unnumbered

در کیفیت حدوث حمیات واقسام تبها

No. 164 : MS 54 I

Moḥammad Mojīr

ʿAino l-ḥayāt عین الحیات [کذا]

MS 54, 125 fols., 215 x 120 mm; binder's collection of seven works; V-VII, on interpretation of dreams and astrology, not catalogued. (See also **Nos. 190, 200,** and **201.**)
ʿAino l-ḥayāt on fols. 4-77.

Bound in marbled cardboard, spine of cloth; MS partly loose in binding. Binding not original. Written on Eastern paper, thin, burnished, beige. Many wormholes; fols. 37, 43, 45 loose; water stains; edges repaired; hole cut into fol. 35, note torn out of fol. 124.

I. Fols. 4b-77a: 18-21 lines, 175-95 x 80-90 mm, on blind-ruled frame and lines; black with red rubrics; careless *nastaʿlīq*. Catchwords. II. Fols. 78-122: 22-26 lines, 190 x 100 mm, on blind-ruled frame and lines; greyish-black with red rubrics; small, careless *shekastä-āmīz*. Catchwords. Apparently different scribe from I.

Collations by scribe on fols. 4b-103b (top); no collations on fols. 103b (bottom) to 112b.

I. Fols. 4-77: anonymous copy, dated at noon on Sunday, 8 Jomādā II 1136/*Saturday*, 4 March 1724. II. Fols. 78-122: anonymous, undated copy; of approximately the same period as I.

Modern bookdealer notes on fols. 1a, 4b.

Incipit, fol. 4b

بسمله. رب یسر وتمم بالخیر. الحمد لله رب العالمین والصلوة
[کذا] علی رسوله محمد واله اجمعین. بدانکه حق سبحانه

وتعالی علم طب در کلام مجید خویش فرمود کلو[کذا]
واشربوا ...

Explicit, fol. 77a, 9

سلام علی نوح فی العالمین وصلی الله علی خیر خلقه محمد
وآله اجمعین بمب[کذا] تمام شد هذا الکتاب مسمی
[کذا] عین الحیات [کذا] ...

The MS contains a treatise on treatment of diseases *a capite ad calcem* and the bezoar stone in 91 *bāb* by Moḥammad Mojīr (fol. 5a). Its title is given as *ʿAino l-ḥayāt* in the colophon (fol. 77a, -2). A *terminus ad quem* for its composition is furnished by a Mashhad MS of 1058/1648.[1]

1. PL II 311, no. 584 (4).

PL II 311, no. 584 (4); Monzavī I 570a, no. 5307.

No. 165 : MS 66 II

Anonymous

[*Moʿālajāt*] [معالجات]

MS 66 (ex Coll. Min.), 130 fols., 310 x 215 mm; owner's collection of four medical works. Untitled treatise on pathology and therapy on fols. 2–63, margin.

For the description of the MS see **No. 194 : MS 66 I.**

Incipit, fol. 2a

باب در امراض اذن وجع اذن چند نوع است نوع اول حادث
میشود از ریاح حاره حاده بخاریه ممکن در عصو علامت
ان بودن وجع ...

Explicit, fol. 63b

و بعد از انفجار خروج مده نمایند و تصنیف حرحر و بعد
از استعمال مراهم منبته لحم قابضه مجففه و ذرورات
جالیه و هرگاه بسیار رطوبت داشته باشد

This anonymous, untitled work on pathology and treatment of diseases is divided into 363 short *bāb*, arranged in the usual order *a capite ad calcem*, and general diseases. It begins abruptly with the section on disorders of the ear, and ends equally abruptly (see Incipit and Explicit).

No. 166 : MS 66 III

Anonymous

Mokhtaṣarato l-ʿavāmm مختصرة العوام

MS 66 (ex Coll. Min.), 130 fols., 310 x 215 mm; owner's collection of four medical works. *Mokhtaṣarato l-ʿavāmm* on fols. 76–81a, margin.

For the description of the MS see **No. 194 : MS 66 I.**

Incipit, fol. 76a, margin

هذا الکتاب مختصرة العوام فی الطب. بسمله. الحمد لله
الذّی خلق السموات والارض وصلی الله علی خیر خلقه
محمد و اله اجمعین الطیبین الطاهرین اما بعد فی امراض
البدن من الراس الی القدم
زامراض سر میکنم ابتدا   عدد لفظ کد آمده جمله را
سرسام واورام سر   دوار وسدر بسی سبات سپهر

Explicit, fol. 81a, margin

مرضهای مسری که هفت آمده جذام بهق سل رمد آبله
دیگر حصبه وان حمیات وبا نگه‌دار بادت از اینها خدا
خدایا منم حیرت برگناه بنزد تو شرمند مدو سیاه [؟]
چه من عاصیم تو رحمی رحیم بیامرز عصیان من ای کریم
ببخشا گناه خفی وجلی بنور محمد [آیا یعنی محض ؟] براست علی
حسب الفرمایش [کذا] عالیجاه میرزا عباسعلی جراح باشی ...

In this short tract, the diseases of the body, *a capite ad calcem,* and general diseases are listed in *maṣnavī* verses. The title, *Mokhtaṣarato l-ʿavāmm,* is mentioned only in the heading (see Incipit).

Not in PL or Monzavī.

No. 167 : MS 68 IV

Anonymous

[*Moʿālajāt*] [معالجات]

MS 68 (ex Coll. Min.), 132 fols., 205 x 145 mm; binder's collection of seven works in two sections. [*Moʿālajāt*] on fols. 74a, -5, 76b.

For the description of the MS see **No. 184 : MS 68 I.**

Incipit, fol. 74a, -5

بسمله. در نشانهای هر مرضی که صاحب علت را بتوان
شناخت لقوه لقوه مرضی را گویند ...

Explicit, fol. 76b, -1

قدری کلح [؟] را گرفته و پخته داخل اجزا کند قرص
سازند و ریش را بشویند

It is not clear whether this short anonymous, untitled tract on therapy is incomplete at the end or not: there is no catchword written on fol. 76b, as against all the other leaves, but the text appears to be incomplete.

No. 168 : MS 73 I

Anonymous

[*Moᶜālajāt*] [معالجات]

MS 73 (ex Coll. Min.), 131 fols., 205 x 145 mm; binder's collection of five works in two sections: A) nos. I–IV (fols. 1–99), and B) no. V (fols. 100–131), each section written by one scribe; no. V, the alchemical treatise *Majmūᶜato ṣ-ṣanāyeᶜ*, not catalogued. (See also **Nos. 127, 197,** and **203**.)
[*Moᶜālajāt*] on fols. 1–64.

Bound in thick, slightly flexible, plain burgundy-colored leather; inner covers pasted with tan paper; binding somewhat worn. Written on European paper, medium thin, burnished, white; watermark obscure; edges torn, heavily stained. On lacunae see below.

A) Fols. 1–99: 15 lines, 140 x 85 mm, on blind-ruled frame and lines; black with black overlinings; different styles of *naskh*, leaning to *nastaᶜlīq*, and *nastaᶜlīq* by one scribe. Catchwords. On fol. 65a text scratched out.

Collations by scribe.

Anonymous copy, no. II dated 9 Rabīᶜ II 1123/27 May 1711, and no. IV, Shavvāl 1094/23 September–21 October 1683.

On fols. 96b, 97b, 99b, and in margins many recipes copied by scribe and quoted among other sources from *Toḥfato l-moʾmenīn*; one patient for whom compound medicines from *Toḥfä* was prepared is called Ākhond Mollā Moḥammad Ṣāleḥ.

On fol. 66a owner's stamp reading Ṣāliḥ walad al-muʾmin, 1125/1713.

Incipit, fol. 1a

درمری و حنجره وبسا باشد که مادهٔ فالج بیك عصب ریخته
عضوی که بآن متصل است مفلوج گردد وسایر اعضا
صحیح باشد ...

Explicit, fol. 64b, -1

اما انچه صاحب کامل درامراض اناث فرموده ازانجمله
یکی از تلا مذه استعلامات[؟] افراط]

This acephalous, anonymous, untitled treatise on treatment of diseases in the usual order *a capite ad calcem* begins in this MS within the first *maqṣad*, on diseases of the head, and breaks off on fol. 64b within *maqṣad* 14, on diseases of the female genital tract.

No. 169 : MS 85 I

Mohannā b. Doqāq (?)

[*Mo*ʿ*ālajāt*] [معالجات]

MS 85 (ex Coll. Min.), 51 fols., 190 x 110 mm; scribe's collection of two works on medicine. (See also **No. 98 : MS 85 II**.) [*Mo*ʿ*ālajāt-e Mohannā b. Doqāq*] on fols. 1-3 et al. (see below).

Bound in flexible black leather; simple blind-tooled borders, three-medallion design, inlaid with thin brown leather, blind-stamped in floral scrolls; inner covers pasted with European paper, now heavily foxed; one flyleaf each in front and back, of thin yellow cardboard in front, and in back of thin yellow paper. Binding warped, worn, worm-eaten; not original. Written on European papers of different provenance, of varying thickness, coarse and smooth surface, white; watermarks obscure; heavily stained, margins sometimes cut off, often repaired; all leaves trimmed for present binding. On lacunae see below.

12 lines, 130 x 70 mm, on blind-ruled frame and lines; black with crimson rubrics and overlinings; large, fine *naskh*, except on fols. 36 and 47 (later substitutions): large, undistinguished *naskh*. Catchwords, often partly trimmed off.

Collations by scribe.

Anonymous, undated copy (end missing); twelfth/eighteenth century.

Marginal notes by one reader.

The verso of all fols. is inscribed *vaqf*; on fol. 3b an owner's stamp reading Muḥammad ʿAlī al-Ḥusainī, dated 1168/1754.

Incipit, fol. 47a

قلاع از بلغم مالح حادث شود علامت آن سفیدی
زبان بود و قلت عطش و وجع علاج گلقند
و رازیانه و بیخ مهک جلابی سازند...

A note on the front flyleaf, not written by the scribe, gives *Mo*ʿ*ālajāt-e Mohannā b. Doqāq* as title and author of this fragmentary treatise on the treatment of diseases *a capite ad calcem* and of general ailments. In this MS, the order of fols. is disrupted; it is to be corrected as follows: beginning missing, fol. 47 (on *qelā*ʿ), lacuna, 1-3 (*gordä* to *maṣānä*), lacuna, 42, 37-38, 43 (*mafāṣel, dā*ʾ*o l-fīl,* etc.), lacuna, 12-26, 48, lacuna (?), 32 (all on *ḥommayāt*), lacuna, 27-31, 33 (*owrām, boṣūr*), end missing.

Not in PL or Monzavī.

No. 170 : MS 94

Anonymous

[*Moʿālajāt*] [معالجات]

MS 94 (ex Coll. Min.), 93 [77] fols., 207 x 135 mm

Bound in plain black leather over stiff, thick cardboard; inner covers pasted with greyish-pink dyed European paper; one flyleaf in back of medium-thick, glazed, white Eastern paper; binding worn and torn, spine broken; nearly the entire MS is out of binding. Written on medium-thin, slightly transparent, burnished, off-white European paper; watermark: PORRATA and indiscernible emblem; few traces of use. On lacunae see below.

19 lines, 152 x 78 mm, on blind-ruled frame and lines; black with red rubrics; I. fols. 1-77: medium-small, fine *nastaʿlīq*; II. fols. 78-93: small, not as fine *nastaʿlīq*, rubrics left out; scribe different from I? Catchwords.

Anonymous, undated copy; thirteenth/nineteenth century.

Recipes and poetical quotations (Saʿdī) on fol. 1a; medical notes also on fol. 78a and inner covers.

On back inner cover one erased and two legible *tamlīk*, one by Aḥmad Khān, dated 13 Jomādā I 1254 /5 August 1838, and the other by Āqā Mīrzā Asadollāh Shīrāzī, dated Tuesday, 22 (?) Rabīʿ I 1273/*Thursday*, 21 November 1856.

Incipit, fol. 1b

معجون دواء السنته ودواء الملوك نیز گویند و معجون
بزرگیست واین معجونرا برای پادشاهان فارس وعرب ترکیب
نموده اند

The MS contains an untitled, anonymous *vade mecum* of medicine, excerpted from different sources, without numbered subdivisions. On fol. 1a a reader's hand has written ذخيره طب, but that appears to be an indication of contents rather than a title. The first part of the text consists of a number of compound medications, without any apparent order as to their preparation or indication; some are quoted from *Moʿālajāt-e Boqrāṭ*.[1] On fol. 7a, a discussion of the pulse begins, following the *Qānūn*;[2] first the Arabic passage is quoted, then a Persian translation and commentary are given. In the same format, a discussion of urine opens on fol. 14b, -5: color (ibid.), consistency (fol. 16b, -7), odor (fol. 17a, 8), clearness (fol. 17a, -1), sediments (fol. 18a, 5).[3] On fols. 19a, 3 to 21b, 5, *bāb* 7-11 of *maqālā* 5 of *ketāb* 2 of *Zakhīrā-ye Khwārezmshāhī*[4] are quoted. Fols. 21b, 5 to 31a, 6 contain a list of simple and compound drugs in no particular order. Fols. 31a, 6 to 73b, -6 discuss the treatment of diseases, roughly *a capite ad calcem*, then skin disorders and cosmetics; there is a long lacuna between fols. 43 and 44 (from *khafaqān* to diseases of the male genitals). There is no mention of *āteshak* (due to the choice of sources?). On fol. 73b, -6 a discussion of excessive thirst in infants and of other pediatric problems begins. On fol. 75a, 7 a section on love-sickness, *ʿeshq*.

A "*mokhtaṣar*" from *Ekhtīārāt-e Badīʿī*, on simple drugs, opens on fol. 75b, 6; it breaks off within the section on *esqīl* on fol. 77b; fols. 78b-93 repeat the text of fols. 1b to 21a, 6.

1. Is this Aḥmad b. Muḥammad aṭ-Ṭabarī at-Turunjī's famous *K. al-muʿālajāt al-buqrāṭīya* (see Ullmann, p. 140) or perhaps ʿEmādoddīn Maḥmūd Shīrāzī's book (PL II 242, no. 411 (3))?
2. Cf. *Qānūn* I 123-28, *faṣl* 1-3 of the section on *nabḍ*.
3. Cf. *Qānūn* I 135-45, *faṣl* 1-6 of the section on *baul*.
4. Cf. **Nos. 2-4 : MSS 1-3.**

No. 171 : MS 99

Anonymous

[*Ṭebb*] [طبّ]

MS 99 (ex Coll. Min.), 63 fols., 240 x 115 mm

Bound in flexible leather; covers patched together out of small pieces, mostly burgundy-colored, with simple blind-tooled borders; inner covers bare leather, partly pasted with pink paper; one flyleaf each in front and back, added after MS was copied: medium-thick, glazed, light blue dyed European paper; watermark: coat of arms. Written on burnished Eastern paper of varying thickness and color: yellow, pink, brown, off-white. Lower inner corner of most fols., containing catch-words, lost because of acid stains (?). On lacunae see below.

19 lines, 175 x 70 mm, on blind-ruled frame and lines; black with red rubrics; different styles of medium-sized good to fair *nasta'līq*. Catchwords lost (see above).

Anonymous, undated copy (end missing); ca. 1200/1800.

Beginning of text (as far as preserved), fol. 10a, 1

[ودر برج جوزا وفروردین واردی بهشت وخردادماه پادشاهی اندرتن مردم گرمی ونرمی سرخ وروشن است پس همچنانکه خون اندرین سرماه برتن آدمی قوة اندردشت وباغ همرآن رنگ پیدا کند گل وشقایق شکوفه کند ...

The MS contains an unidentified compendium of medicine that is divided into 65 *bāb*. Of these, there are extant parts from *bāb* 1 to *bāb* 50. The order of fols. is disrupted and is to be restored as follows: lacuna, 10, 1–2, lacuna, 9 (correct place?), 3–4, lacuna, 6, lacuna, 39–43, 13, 45–46, lacuna, 61, lacuna, 62, lacuna, 49, 50, 26, lacuna, 27, 20 (or lacuna between 27 and 20?), 19, 5, 22–23, lacuna, 48, 32–38, 44, 51, 47, 54–57, 18, lacuna, 8 (correct place?), lacuna, 11, 7, 52–53, 16–17, 24–25, 21, lacuna, 58, lacuna, 14–15, lacuna; the correct position of fols. 59 and 60 could not be determined. It appears that the MS was transcribed from a disordered copy since what logically belongs at the beginning of the text, the table of contents, starts on fol. 10b, -6, while the rest of fol. 10 is taken up by part of *bāb* 4.

Fols. 10b, -6 to end and 1a to 2a, -6 contain the table of contents. As far as preserved (the lower third of fol. 1 is torn out), it reads:

bāb 1. در آفرینش مردم

2. در صفت اندامها وابتداء چشم

3. اندر آفرینش دل

bāb 4. اندر طبایع عالم و ماهها و اختیار شرابها

5. اندر کودکی تا پیری

6. اندر چهار طبایع داروها

7. اندر مجها[؟ آیا یعنی مزاجها؟] شناختن

8. در سناختن آبها

9. در مقالت سکته از هر نوع

10. اندر بحرانهای نیك و بد

11. در علامت مرگ بیماران

12. در رسیدن طعام دهان بیماران

13. از پرهیز کردن بیماران زقی

14. در داروها که خطرست از خوردن

15. در آرزوی بیمار و منع او

16. در حبات[؟] ابجد و معرفه عقاقیرها

17. در بیان مطبوخات

18. ایارجات فقرا [کذا]

19. در مقالت حبها

20. در قرصها که سود دارد

21. در مقالت گوارشها

22. در اطریفلهای بزرگ

23. در بیان معجون شهریاران

24. طلاهای گرم و ضمادها

25. در بیان تب گوناگون

26. در شراب

27. در بیان زهرها

(28.-35. lost)

bāb 36. در بیان دا لثعلب [کذا]

37. در لقوه و فالج و رعشه واختلاج

38. اندر بهق و ابرص [کذا] وجذام

39. درد پشت وعرق النسا

40. اندر صرع وعلاج آن

41. در دیوانگی و وسواس عشق

42. اندر یرقان ودق

43. اندر اسپتسقا

44. اندر دردهای معده

45. اندر دردهای دل

46. اندر درد جگر وذات الریه

47. اندر ذات الجنب

48. اندر دردهای سپرز

49. در گرده وسنگهای مثانه وقضیب وخایه

(50.-54. lost)

55. در بادها که پدید آید

56. اندر مقالت فربهی مردم

57. اندر شقاق وبواسیر واشتقاء مواض [؟]

58. در داء الفیل ودا للحیه [کذا]

59. در طاعون

60. از آتش وآب گرم وروغن ورحم
وآبکینه رسیدن از نیرو

61. [در] ناخن کژ وشکافتن زیرپا ودرد ناخن وحارس

62. در رگها که خون گیرد وخاصیت نبض [؟] وحجامه

bāb 63. در خاصیت گرمابه

64. در چربی [؟] وشیرینی وترشی وتلخی وشوری

65. اندر طبایع حلواها

The first *bāb* begins on fol. 2a, -7:

چنین گوید محمد بن [   ] المنصوری رحمة الله علیه
که چون مردم از مادر بزایند [   ] اندر تن مردم پانزده
سال وچندین ماه را [   ] مردم گرم بود وهرچه بیاموزند
بتوانند آموخت

Since part of fol. 2 is torn out, the name of the father of the quoted authority is missing. It cannot now be determined whether this Moḥammad b. . . . al-Manṣūrī[1] is the author of a following short quotation or, possibly, of the whole treatise in **MS 99.**

1. It would be tempting to read Moḥammad b. Zakarīyāʾ and [*Ketāb*] *al-Manṣūrī* out of this, but the evidence does not bear it out.

No. 172 : MS 93 IV

Anonymous

[*Maṣnavī dar ṭebb*] [مثنوی در طبّ]

MS 93 (ex Coll. Min.), 81 fols., 110 x 210 mm (*jong*); binder's collection in six sections. [*Maṣnavī dar ṭebb*] on fols. 49a–52b.

For the description of the MS see **No. 74 : MS 93 II.**

Incipit, fol. 49a

بحکمت همه حالها بگذران   نگهدار تواند دان
که اشراف درجملهٔ کارها براست   نشایسته مردم بخرد است
زبقراط دیگر چنین پاسخ است   نکو شنو این نکته بس نازک است
هرانکه باشراف ماهی خورد   صداع اورا قوّت شد برد

Explicit, fol. 52b, 8

بکوبند نرگس بگیرند آب   بوقتی که خفتند [؟] در جامه خاب[1]
کند بینند [؟] زان آب تر   بشوهر رسد گیر اگیر [؟] بسر

This anonymous, untitled *masnavī* contains 121 verses. A MS in Teheran[2] which contains the same text[3] is also anonymous and does not provide any information on the date of composition.[4]

1. In the second hemistich, the meter is obviously incorrect.
2. Rahāvard, p. 6, no. 259 V.
3. It lacks the first two *bait* of the UCLA manuscript, but appears to be longer. Its last verse reads:

این نصیحت ز بوعلی بشنو   تا شوی از حیات برخوردار

4. It was copied by Moḥammad ʿAlī Enābat (Rahāvard writes "Etābat" with a question mark) in 1329/1911.

PL II 311, no. 584 (2); not in Monzavī.

No. 173 : MS 29 VIII

Anonymous

[*Qeṭʿä dar ṭaʿm-e bad*]   [قطعه در طعم بد]

MS 29 (ex Coll. Min.), 119 fols., 200 x 135 mm; scribe's collection of ten works.
[*Qeṭʿä dar ṭaʿm-e bad*] on fols. 108b–109a.

For the description of the MS see **No. 79 : MS 29 I.**

Incipit, fol. 108b (center)

هر آن کوی بدرد [؟] زخواب برخست
بود طعم دهانش نیك پیدا

Explicit, fol. 109a (top)

دوای جملهٔ خلقان همین است
غرض میگوید از قول اطبّا

These anonymous *qeṭʿä* verses discuss the treatment of foul taste in the mouth in twelve couplets.

No. 174 : MS 53

Ebrāhīmo l-Ḥosainī

Menhājo l-mobtadeʾīn منهاج المبتدئين

MS 53 (ex Coll. Min.), 171 fols., 200 x 145 mm

Bound in plain crimson leather over stiff cardboard; inner covers pasted with dark green paper. Binding worn and stained. Written on European paper, medium thin, glazed, white; watermark: sun motif; some stains, fol. 1 loose.

20 lines, 137 x 91 mm, on blind-ruled frame and lines; black with red rubrics and overlinings; small even *shekastä-āmīz*; chapter headings repeated in large crimson *naskh* in top margins. Catchwords.

Copied, and dated Monday, 23 Jomādā II 1230/*Friday*, 2 June 1815, by Moḥammad Jaʿfar "Jarrāḥ-e Shīrāzī."

Marginal notes by readers; recipes, dated Rajab 1270/30 March–28 April 1854, on fols. 170b and 171a.

Incipit, fol. 1b

هذا كتاب منهاج المبتدئين.
بسمله. وبه نستعين. منهاج ادويه شفا حمد مسبب
الاسباب است ... [س ٢١] وبر ال اطهار او خصوصا ...
[٢ الف، س ١] امام العالمين ويعسوب الدين ابو الحسين على ابن
[كذا] ابى طالب ... وعلى اولاده المعصومين الطيبين
اما بعد برارباب فطنت پوشيده نماند كه فقير حقير
ابراهيم الحسينى را درحين معالجه مرضى مركبات مناسب
هر مرض ... به منهاج المبتدئين مسمى ساخت ...
واين كتاب را برچهل ودو باب وخاتمه مشتمل ساخت

Explicit, fol. 170a, 3

سطرون [كذا. يعنى مسطرون] صغير شش درخمى
است كرمه دركناش اوطوس ميگويند يك دانگ
ونيم يا دو دانگ تمت الكتاب [كذا] ...

The MS contains Ebrāhīmo l-Ḥosainī's (fol. 2a, 3) *Menhājo l-mobtadeʾīn* (fol. 2a, 7), a dispensatory in 42 *bāb* and a *khātemä* (ibid.); in the first *bāb* a list of commonly used compound medicines is given according to the *abjad* alphabet; the following chapters list them according to their indication: fevers, diseases *a capite ad calcem*, skin disorders, poisons (table of contents on fol. 2a, 8 to 2b, 9); the *khātemä* gives a survey of weights and measures used in pharmacy (begins on fol. 169a, -6). The author's most widely used sources appear to be ar-Rāzī and Pseudo-Thābit b. Qurra among Islamic writers, and Galen among Greek authors; among the other physicians quoted are Aḥmad b. Muḥammad aṭ-Ṭabarī, abū l-Faraj b. Hindū, ibn Sīnā, abū l-Barakāt al-Baghdādī, and "aṭebbā-ye Hend."[1] In the *khātemä* on weights and measures, he quotes abū l-Faraj b. Hindū with his *Miftāḥ aṭ-Ṭibb*[2] and the *Kunnāsh* by Sāhir.[3]

The latest among these authorities is abū l-Barakāt, who died after 560/1164.[4] Persian medical authors are noticeably absent from the list of sources quoted. The evidence thus gathered would point to a rather early date of composition, if it were not for the very markedly Shīʿite eulogies in the preface. Ebrāhīm's silence on the subject of syphilis seems to rule out a date later than 900/1494. Possibly the book was written during the second half of the ninth/fifteenth century after the Ṣafavids had adopted Shīʿism, but before the year 900/1494. If this hypothesis is correct, then a certain Moḥammad Ebrāhīm al-Ḥosainī, mentioned in Naniana II 242, no. CIX, as the author of a *Mojmalo l-moʿālajāt* in 44 chapters, cannot be identified as Ebrāhīmo l-Ḥosainī since Moḥammad Ebrāhīm copied and signed a MS of his work in 1105/1693.

1. Some earlier writers, almost certainly quoted from ar-Rāzī's *K. al-ḥāwī* and other standard works, have been omitted from this list.
2. Ullmann, p. 152.
3. Ullmann, pp. 124, 319. The metrological passages from his *Kunnāsh* were quoted by Avicenna at the end of his *Qānūn*.
4. Ullmann, p. 138.

PL II 325, no. 584 (131); Monzavī I 604b, nos. 5641–49; Osmania Univ., p. 52, no. 23.

No. 175 : MS 52

Sharafoddīn b. Shāh Ḥosain Bairamī Lārī

Merṣādo l-aṭebbāʾ مرصاد الاطبّاء

MS 52 (ex Coll. Min.), 431 fols., 290 x 195 mm

Bound in crimson leather over stiff cardboard; simple blind-tooled borders; inner covers pasted with blue-marbled paper; two flyleaves each in front and back, of European paper: (in front) thin, unburnished, cream-colored; (in back) medium thin, burnished, cream-colored. Binding not original. Written on Eastern paper, medium thin, slightly transparent, burnished, beige; fols. 1 and 431 restored by pasting together with other paper, soiled; otherwise little wear; margins intact, trimmed when MS was bound in present binding.

21 lines, 195 x 110 mm, on blind-ruled frame and lines; black with red rubrics; medium-sized fair *nastaʿlīq*, quotations from Qorʾān and Ḥadīth in *naskh*. Catchwords.

Collations by scribe.

Copied, and dated Monday, 28 Rajab 1122/22 September 1710, by ʿAṭāʾollāh b. Mollā Moḥammad Kāteb-e Lārī b. Ostādmandī b. Nākhodā ʿAlī Hormūzī.

Readers' notes in margins.

On fol. 1b an illegible stamp; on fol. 431a a *tamlīk* and stamp of Fażlollāh b. Gholāmreżā Eṣfahānī; his stamp is dated 1164/1750 (?).

Incipit, fol. 1b

بسمله و به نستعین. لالی تسبیح لباسی * که موجب تحلیه
و تحلّی سامعه تکرار اذکار ساکنان عالم بالا * و یواقیت
تمجید تقدیس اساسی که باعث تصفیه و تجلّی باصره وافکار
ابکار متوطّنان کرهٔ غبرا باشد * ...

Explicit, fol. 431a, 10

و وصف طریق ترکیب هریك از این مرکبات در فصل
سئم از مطلب اول مذکور گشت خواهنده بدان
رجوع و تحقیق نماید تمّت [کذا] الکتاب ...

Ebn Shāh Ḥosain Sharafoddīn Bairamī Lārī (fol. 2a, -3) named this combined pharmacopoeia and dispensatory *Merṣādo l-aṭebbā*ʾ (fol. 3a, 13). He divided it into a *moqaddemä*, three *maṭlab*, and a *khātemä*, each with subdivisions:

1. *moqaddemä* (begins on fol. 10b, 11) in four *faṣl*, subdivided alternately into *qesm* and *now*ʿ:

در تعریف بعضی الفاظ ولغات که در کتب طبّی
دربیان اعضا وامزجه وارواح واخلاط وامراض
وغیر آن مذکور میشود ... وبیان برخی علامات دالة
بر صحت وفساد بدن وغیر آن.

2. *maṭlab* 1 (begins on fol. 35b, 7) in three *faṣl*; *faṣl* 1 is divided into six *baḥs*, *faṣl* 2 and 3 are organized in chapters according to the alphabet (بترتیب حروف هجا):

دربیان طریق تحصیل ادویه وکیفیت ترکیب آن وبیان اسامی
وصفات وطبایع هریك از ادویه مفرده وغیره

3. *maṭlab* 2 (begins on fol. 184a, 4) in 29 *bāb*, following the order of particular diseases *a capite ad calcem*; the *bāb* are subdivided into *faṣl* and *baḥs*, or into *maqṣad* and *baḥs*:

دربیان ادویه امراضی که بعضوهای خاص مضاف
میشود بالفاظ عربی مثل وجع الکبد والامعا ومانند

اینها یا بلغت فارسی مثل صداع وشقیقه که
بفارسی درد سر ونیمسر گویند ...

4. *maṭlab* 3 (begins on fol. 304a, 11) in 25 *bāb*, on general diseases, in alphabetical order:

دربیان ادویه امراضی که هریك را اسم خاصی هست
واضافه بعضوی مخصوص نمیباشد

5. *khātemä* (begins on fol. 396a, -4) in 20 *maqṣad*, discussing prescriptions for hygienic and cosmetic medications, for antidotes, aphrodisiacs, magic drugs, etc.; some *maqṣad* are further divided into *faṣl* and *baḥṣ*:

در ذکر فواید ومنافع چند متفرقه :

۱) در ادویه که جهت بزرگی درنظر خلق وشجاعت
وبرخصم غالب آمدن نافع است
۲) درادویه که نافعست جهت اشتهاء طعام وهضم آن
۳) درادویه که نافعست جهت تقویت بدن وفربه
شدن ودفع چشم زخم
٤) درادویهٔ که جهت زیادتی حافظه وتیزی ذهن
نفع دارد
٥) درادویه که نافعست جهت حصول نشاط ورفع غم
٦) درادویه که تعلق بموی دارد
٧) درادویه که منع احتلام وشهوت بکند
٨) درادویه که تعلق ومناسبت بزنان دارد
٩) درادویه که رفتن خون را منع کند
١٠) درادویه که جهت حصول دوستی نافع است
١١) درادویه که نافع است جهت اطفال

۱۲) در ادویه که نافع است جهت سموم

۱۳) در ادویه که تعلق بهوام و طیور و حیوان
وجن دارد

۱۴) در اشیائی که جهت رفع خستگی و تعبی
که از راه رفتن حاصل شده باشد نفع دارد

۱۵) در اشیائی که جهت تدارك شکستگی
اعضا نافع بود

۱۶) در چیزی چند که جهت بیرون آوردن خار
و پیکان مفید بود

۱۷) در اشیائی که دفع درد سوختگی آتش کند

۱۸) در اشیائی که دفع مستی و خمار و سحر کند

۱۹) در اشیائی که خواب اورد

۲۰) در اشیائی چند متفرق ودران شش فصل بود
فصل اول در ادویه که جهت محافظت ثمره
و زراعت مفید بود فصل دوم در اشیائی که
منع تگرگ کند فصل سئم در اشیائی که عشق
واختلاج طرف کند فصل چهارم در اشیائی که
درمیان دو شخص یا بیشتر عداوت افکند
فصل پنجم در اشیائی که جهت رفع لکه واثرها
از بدن و اعضا نفع دارد و رنگ بدن وصدر
صاف گرداند... فصل ششم در ذکر
بعضی معالجات وادویه متفرقه

The author of this work remains unknown; his name suggests that he, or at least his family, came from Bairam in the province of Lār.[1] The period of his life can so far only be approximated by the date of the MS, 1122/1710 (see above), and by quotations from earlier authors. In the introduction (fol. 3a, 8–16), he lists the following books as his sources, and to make quoting easier, adds a sign to each of them: 1) *Ekhtīārāt-e Badīʿī* (no sign in this MS),[2] 2) *Morakkabāt-e* Shefāʾī (مر),[3] 3) *Morakkabāt-e* Qalānesī (قل),[4] *Ḥayāt al-ḥayawān* (ح),[5] 5) *Nozhatnāmä-ye ʿAlāʾī* (ن),[6] 6) *Resālä-ye ṣaidīyä* (ص),[7] 7) *Nūro l-ʿoyūn* (نو),[8] 8) *Tadhkirat al-kaḥḥālīn* (تذ),[9] 9) *Zakhīrä-ye Khwārezmshāhī* (ذ),[10] 10) *Ḥaqāʾiq asrār aṭ-ṭibb* (حق),[11] 11) *Kefāyä-ye Manṣūrī* (كف).[12] The latest of these is Shefāʾī's dispensatory; he died in 963/1555.[13] Sharafoddīn says that he updated the style of his sources written in فرس قديم (*sic*!), simplified it if it was very involved and mannered, and translated what was Arabic into Persian (fol. 3a, 10–12). He expresses the hope that his book will prove useful to everybody, but especially to Shīʿites (fol. 3a, 2).

1. Bairam is the center of the village district of the same name in the province of Lār (*Farhang-e Joghrāfyāʾī-ye Īrān* VII 44a, s.v. Bairam).
2. See **MS 36**, etc.
3. See **MS 105 III**, etc.
4. Compiled in 590/1193 (see Ullmann, p. 307).
5. This title appears to imply that the author of *Merṣād* used the Arabic original of ad-Damīrī's book (Damīrī died in 808/1405; see EI² II, s.v.), since the Persian translations of it have different titles; the earliest of these, it seems, was done by Ghiāsoddīn Manṣūr b. ʿEmādoddīn Ḥosain b. Ebrāhīm Ījī Shabānkārāʾī in 903/1497 or 930/1523 and titled *Khavāṣṣo l-ḥayavān* (or *Ṣefāto l-ḥayavān*; see Nashrīyä III 311b, s.v. *Khavāṣṣo l-ḥayavān*). Another version, titled *Ḥayāto l-ensān*, was dedicated to the Ottoman sultan Soliman the Magnificent (Sulaimān b. Salīm; see Blochet II 80, no. 816). The title *Khavāṣṣo l-ḥayavān* was also given to a Persian translation dating from the time of Shāh ʿAbbās II (1052–77/1642–66); its author is Mīrzā Taqī b. Khwājä Moḥammad Tabrīzī (Nashrīyä III 18a, s.v.). The latest Persian version, done in 1249/1833, cannot have served as a source for Sharafoddīn (Nashrīyä III 311b, s.v. *Khavāṣṣo l-ḥayavān*).
6. By Shahmardān b. abī l-Khair for ʿAlāʾo d-dowlä Garshāsp, the Kākūyid ruler of Yazd (488–513 / 1095–1119), written shortly before 513/1119 (see Gilbert Lazard, "Un amateur de sciences . . . ," in *Mélanges Massé* [Teheran 1963], pp. 219–28).
7. Not identified, unless this title is a misspelling for al-Bīrūnī's *Kitāb/Risālat aṣ-ṣaidana* (or *ṣaidala*), cf. **No. 114 : MS 87 I.**
8. See **No. 1 : MS 74 I.**
9. See **No. 154 : MS 74 II.**
10. See **No. 2 : MS 1**, etc.
11. By Masʿūd b. Muḥammad as-Sijzī on medical terminology, written before 734/1333, the date of a MS of this work (see Ullmann, p. 237).
12. See **No. 32 : MS 12**, etc.
13. See note 2 above.

Not in PL or Monzavī.

No. 176 : MS 92

Anonymous

[*Moʿālajāt*] [معالجات]

MS 92 (ex Coll. Min.), 239 fols., 273 x 162 mm

Bound in thin flexible brown leather; simple blind-tooled borders; inner covers pasted with dark blue dyed European paper; one flyleaf each of thin, coarse, grey paper; three more blank leaves in front of European paper, medium thin, burnished, white (now foxed); watermarks: on the first and third FABIANI, on the second a shield (hill with tower, crested with a six-pointed star) and in three lines C B, F, E. M. VEDOVA, resp.; one blank fol. in back, paper as in front, but heavily stained; watermarks: ornamented shield crested with a count's coronet, and GIUSEPPE. Binding not original. Written on Eastern paper of varying thickness, burnished, cream-colored; fol. 239 substituted in European paper as above; stained and foxed, especially first and last fols.; edges torn and repaired with European paper; edges of whole MS stained. On lacunae see below.

15 lines, 170 x 85 mm, on blind-ruled frame and lines; black with red rubrics; medium-small to medium-large neat *naskh* of different styles (by the same scribe?); fol. 239, substituted later, written by reader who also left marginal notes. Catchwords. All fols. are numbered in Indian numerals.

Collations by scribe.

Anonymous, undated copy (end missing); *terminus ad quem* given by a *tamlīk* on fol. 2a, dated 1165/1751.

Marginal notes by reader.

On fol. 2a a *tamlīk* by Moḥammad Salīm, dated 1165/1751; on fol. 64b, a note dated 1185/1771.

On fol. 1a, two erased stamps; on fol. 2a two stamps by Moḥammad Salīm; on fols. 5a and 6a illegible owner's stamp, dated 1131/1718.

Incipit, fol. 1a

فندق و بادام شیرین و نارکل خائیدن نافع بود شمع و قیر بخایند
نیکو بود

Explicit, fol. 239a, 4

و در زمستان دو روز بعد از آن بپالایند و با غذا تناول نمایند
باب هشتم در ادویهٔ مسهله و ملیّنه آنچه

The MS contains part of a very detailed *qarābāẕīn*; according to the foliation (see above), only one fol. is missing in front, which does not appear likely, given the length of the two extant *bāb* in this copy. The subjects are arranged according to the diseases for which the drugs are prescribed:

bāb 5 (beginning missing) on dental medicines (see Incipit)
bāb 6 (begins on fol. 10a, 8; according to foliation, fol. 11)

در ادویه امراض حلق و سینه و آلت دم زدن

bāb 7 (begins on fol. 110a, -2; numbered as fol. 111)

در بیان داروها که در بیماری معده و جگر و سپرز بکار آید

bāb 8 (begins on fol. 239a, 5; numbered fol. 240), see Explicit.

No. 177 : MS 60 II

Anonymous

Montakhabo l-aṭebbā' منتخب الاطباء

MS 60 (ex Coll. Min.), 74 fols., 240 x 150 mm; binder's collection of five Persian texts, nos. II–V medical, and *Majmū'ä-ye maṣnū'āt*, here ascribed to Moḥammad Morād (in the text, fol. 1a, 5; not catalogued). (See also **Nos. 60, 178,** and **193.**) *Montakhabo l-aṭebbā'* on fols. 29–52.

Bound in pinkish-grey, blue, green marbled paper over thin, flexible cardboard; inner covers pasted with cream-colored paper; spine of beige cloth; spine torn, MS out of binding, falling apart. Written on different varieties of Eastern paper: 1) fols. 1–52, 65–75: thin to thick, rough, beige; 2) fols. 53–60: medium thin, rough, tan; 3) fols. 61–64: medium thin, rough, blueish-grey; worm-eaten; stained; margins torn, loose leaves. On lacunae see below.

I. Fols. 29–52: 19 lines, 190 x 105 mm; black with red rubrics; ordinary Indian *shekastä-āmīz*. Catchwords. Foliation. II. Fols. 53–64: a) fols. 53–60: 17 lines, 190 x 105 mm; black with red rubrics; medium-small good *nasta'līq*. Catchwords. b) fols. 61–64: 21 lines, 210 x 120 mm; black with red rubrics; medium-sized ordinary *shekastä-āmīz*; scribe different from II a) ? Catchwords. III. Fols. 65–73b, 2: ca. 175 x 105 mm; black with black overlinings; medium-large, hasty, ugly *shekastä*. Catchwords.

The different sections of the MS have old foliations that help determine lacunae.

Collations by scribe I, in no. II (fols. 29–52).

Anonymous copies; nos. I, III–V undated (incomplete); no. II dated Monday, 21 Rabī' II 1103/*Friday*, 11 January 1692.

On fols. 31b–32b, 73b, and 74 recipes, charms, *fāl*, etc.

On fol. 1a, etc. *tamlīk* by Nāṣer 'Alī Dabīrmāher; on fol. 73b in English: This book belongs to Nasir 'Ali Bahrainy (Dabirmahir).

Explicit, fol. 30b, 10

اگر رنك اسب سرخه باشد یا سبزه باشد رنق کرده در
ازمایش امده است تمام شد نسخه منتخب الاطبا ...

The title, *Montakhabo l-aṭebbā'*, of this dispensatory in 29 *bāb* appears only in the colophon (see Explicit); no author's name is mentioned, but that may be the result of damage to this MS. The order of fols. is disrupted and there are several lacunae, the extent of which is shown by an old foliation; the MS has to be reordered as follows: 6 fols. missing, 33–48, 9 fols. missing, 49–52, 1 fol. missing, 29–32. The text begins on fol. 33a within *bāb* 7, on compound medicines for toothaches, earaches, etc. There follow:

bāb 8. (begins on fol. 33b, 7) در معالجات بواسیر خونی

9. (begins on fol. 34b, 7) در معالجات آتشك

10. (begins on fol. 35b, 8) در معالجات جزام [كذا] و برص

bāb 11. (begins on fol. 36a, -6) در معالجات جهی [؟] ذوق

12. (begins on fol. 37a, 4)

در معالجات سنگرانتی [؟ آیا یعنی سنگدانگی ؟] اینست که هرچه بخورد هضم نشود

13. (begins on fol. 38a, -8) در معالجات داد [؟] و بهق

14. (begins on fol. 38b, -3) در معالجات حلق زده

15. (begins on fol. 40b, 5) در معالجات لذتی [؟]

16. (begins on fol. 41b, 9) در معالجات قوت باه و امساک

17. (begins on fol. 46a, -7)

در معالجات افلاطونی و دفعه هفت امراض باد فالج و عرق نسا

18. (begins on fol. 48b, -2) در معالجات استسقا

(lacuna between fols. 48 and 49)

26. (beginning missing), on various ailments

27. (begins on fol. 50b, -4) در معالجات ضیق النفس و سنگ مثانه

28. (begins on fol. 52a, -2) در بیان کشتن فلزات و ساختن مروارید

29. (begins on fol. 30a, 9) در بیان صید جانوران چارپایه و پرندگان

A medical work titled *Montakhabo l-aṭebbā*ʾ is listed in PL II 328 (166); two MSS of it are preserved in Indian libraries; in one the author is called ʿAbbādollāh Khairābādī, and in the other, Khairollāh Allāhābādī. It remains to be determined whether the text in the UCLA manuscript is identical with either of these works.

See above for reference in PL; not in Monzavī.

No. 178 : MS 60 III

Anonymous

[*Moʿālajāt*] [معالجات]

MS 60 (ex Coll. Min.), 74 fols., 240 x 150 mm; binder's collection in five sections.
[*Moʿālajāt*] on fols. 53–60.

For the description of the MS see **No. 177 : MS 60 II.**

This fragment of an unidentified dispensatory is divided into unnumbered *bāb* according to the prescriptions of the various drugs; the text begins on fol. 53a within a section on different diseases. There follow:

(fol. 53a, -7) باب، در بیماریهای پشت

(fol. 54a, -2) باب در امراض مادی چون لقوه و تشنج و عرق النساء

(fol. 56a, 2) باب اندر ادویه سینی

(fol. 58a, -3) باب در هکهک ان را فواق گویند

(fol. 58b, 10) باب ادویه بادکوله سکر و اروغ

(fol. 58b, -1) باب در ادویه اسهال

The text breaks off within this last *bāb* on fol. 60b.

No. 179 : MS 58 VII

Anonymous

[*Moʿālajāt*] [معالجات]

MS 58 (ex Coll. Min.), 147 fols., 213 x 153 mm; scribe's collection.
[*Moʿālajāt*] on fols. 123–133.

For the description of the MS see **No. 135 : MS 58 I.**

Incipit, fol. 123b

بسمله. بنام نگارندهٔ تحت فوق [كذا] كه شد منبت
عقل جان مست شوق حكمی [؟] كه آدم ز خاك آفرید
ز نور خودش روح در تن دمید

In this MS, the treatise breaks off on fol. 133b, 2, within *bāb* 8. The headings of the first eight *bāb* are:

1. (fol. 123b, -2) دربیان اندامهای مردم وصفات ان
2. (fol. 125a, -6) ازکودکی یا پیری شدن
3. (fol. 125b, 1) اندر مقالات طبع
4. (fol. 126b, 3) درعقاقیرها بحروف ابجد الف اسارون
5. (fol. 128a, -7) اندر مقالت حبّها
6. (fol. 128b, -6) درمقالت قرصها
7. (fol. 129a, 4) درمقالت گوارشها
8. (fol. 129b, 6) اندر مقالات [کذا] معاجین

This last *bāb* is, contrary to its heading, a miscellany of formulas for various compound medicines, not all of them *maᶜājīn*. Fol. 131b is blank. In the introduction on fol. 123b, the names of Boqrāṭ, Loqmān, and Jāmās are mentioned.

No. 180 : MS 86 IV

ᶜAbdollāh b. ᶜAbdo ṣ-Ṣamad

Zobdato t-tejārāt زبدت التجارات

MS 86, 140 fols., 260 x 150 mm; scribe's collection in five sections.
Zobdato t-tejārāt on fols. 105–109.

For the description of the MS see **No. 187 : MS 86 II.**

Incipit, fol. 105a, -2

ربّ یسر وتمم بالخیر. بسمله. الحمد اللّه [کذا] ربّ العالمین
والعاقبت للمتقین. والصلواة [کذا] والسّلام علی رسوله

محمّد و اله و اصحابه اجمعین امّا احقر عباد الله عبد الله بن عبد
الصّمد آنجا که جمیع کتب طبیب [کذا] هندی یونانی
از روی تجربه امتحان مکرّر بعمل آوردند و فایدهٔ مفخر
ازان حاصل شده ...

Explicit, fol. 109a, -2

چون پسد شود برابر سرمه درچشم کشند چشم بسیار
روشن شود

The text of this short tract on compound drugs, titled *Zobdato t-tejārāt* (or *Badīyato t-tejārāt*? fol. 105b, 8) by ʿAbdollāh b. ʿAbdo ṣ-Ṣamad (fol. 105b, 2), appears to be incomplete in this copy. After the preface, there immediately follows the rubric *nowʿ-e dīgar* (fol. 105b, -4).

On fol. 140a, 4-11, immediately after the end of *Mofradāt-e ṣaḥīḥ* (see **No. 108 : MS 86 V**), the introduction to another (?) work by ʿAbdollāh b. ʿAbdo ṣ-Ṣamad is copied, breaking off with the last line on fol. 140a:

امّا بعد فقیر عباد الله عبد الله ابن [کذا] عبد الصّمد آنچه
کتب هندی یونانی چون جالینوس جاماسپ
بقراط ابوعلی سینا از روی تجربه که فایداش [کذا]
عام نفعش عامست تا بنده‌گان حق سبحانه وتعالی
برسید تا بهره‌مند گردند ...

From the close resemblance to the introduction to *Zobdato t-tejārāt*, it might be concluded that this is a gloss on it, copied in the wrong place.

Not in PL or Monzavī.

No. 181 : MS 75

Anonymous

[*Kaḥḥālī*] [کحّالی]

MS 75 (ex Coll. Min.), 89 fols., 226 x 125 mm

Bound in strong brown suede leather of one piece; binding smaller than MS, carelessly stitched to MS; stained. Binding not original. Written on Eastern paper of two varieties, one being the original MS, the other later substitutions, medium-thick to thick, slightly coarse, beige; stains, cuts, holes especially in fols. close to covers; some fols. badly fragmented, many loose in binding; MS trimmed down from original size. On lacunae see below.

Written in two different hands: I. body of MS: 18 lines, 165 x 85 mm, on blind-ruled frame and lines; black with red rubrics and punctuation; medium-sized, open, fair *nastaʿlīq* leaning to *naskh*. Catchwords. II. Later substitutions (fols. 12-13, 21-22, 38, 51-54, 61-63, 69-77, 80-84): 15-18 lines, 160-70 x 80-85 mm, on blind-ruled frame and lines; black with red rubrics and punctuation; medium-sized, dense, neat, but undistinguished *naskh*.

On some fols. drawings of the eyes, eyebrows, and nose *en face*, transferred to this copy by puncturing; while most are in black outlines only, those on fols. 14b and 15a are finished in colors, showing where to operate on the eye; on the substituted fol. 82b a pen-drawing of the same subject.

Anonymous, undated copy (end missing); ca. 1000/1500.

Marginal notes by scribe and readers, some giving birth dates in 1254/1838, 1258/1842, and 1260/1844.

The MS contains an anonymous, untitled treatise on ophthalmology; the beginning and end are missing, and there is a lacuna between fols. 78 and 79. The text consists of (at least) seven *maqālä*, further divided into *bāb*; at the end of each *bāb* a few mnemonic verses, a *maṣnavī* or *qeṭʿä*, sum up the subject discussed. A table of contents is prefixed to each *maqālä*:

I. In nineteen *bāb* on the anatomy and physiology of the eye; this MS begins within *bāb* 13 on the uvea.
II. (begins on fol. 5b, 10) in two *jozv*, in six and thirty *bāb* resp. The first *jozv* deals with general principles to be followed in the treatment of the eye, the second (begins on fol. 12a, 7) with the diseases of the lid, one in each *bāb*.
III. (begins on fol. 33b, 6) in three *bāb*, on the diseases of the lachrymal duct
IV. (begins on fol. 37b, 7) in thirteen *bāb*, on as many diseases of the conjunctiva
V. (begins on fol. 59b, 1) in thirteen *bāb*, on the same number of diseases of the cornea
VI. (begins on fol. 71a, 7) in five *bāb*, on five diseases of the uvea, including cataract
VII. (begins on fol. 84a, -6) in thirteen *bāb*, on various other diseases of the eye:

1. phantoms in vision not related to cataract
2. diseases of the albuminoid humor
3. diseases of the ice-like (crystalline) humor
4. diseases of the visual spirit
5. night-blindness
6. day-blindness
7. the blinding effect of coldness on the eye
8. diseases of the vitreous humor
9. diseases of the retina
10. diseases of the hollow nerve
11. diseases of the muscles of the hollow nerve
12. exophthalmus because of paralysis
13. amblyopia

The MS breaks off on fol. 89b within *bāb* 5 of this *maqālä*.

The division of this text into seven discourses (*maqālä*) conforms with the section on ophthalmology of Esmāʿīl Jorjānī's *Ẕakhīrä*; from *jozv* 2 of *maqālä* II on, this MS is even identical with Esmāʿīl's text, except for the mnemonic verses inserted at the end of each *bāb*. Therefore it is reasonable to assume that this work did not have more than the seven discourses extant in this MS, unless it included one or two more on simple and compound drugs. The sequence of, and division into, chapters differs from *Ẕakhīrä* in a few cases, and *bāb* 1 of *maqālä* VII is not represented there. A major source for the first discourse, and for the first *jozv* of the second, appears to be ʿAlī b. ʿĪsā's *Tadhkirat al-kaḥḥālīn*; the text represents a Persian version different from that of **No. 154 : MS 74 II**; cf. *bāb* 14-16 of *maqālä* I with *bāb* 16-18 of *goftār* I there (**MS 74**, fols. 227a, -6 to 227b, -2), *bāb* 1-3 and 6 of *jozv* 1 of *maqālä* II with parts of *bāb* 1, and *bāb* 2 of *goftār* II (**MS 74**, fols. 230a, -5 to 235a, -8).

Authors quoted in the sections not taken from *Zakhīrä* are Hippocrates, Galen, and ʿAlī b. ʿĪsā; elsewhere the same quotations as in *Zakhīrä* are to be found. Hippocrates' aphorisms are quoted in Arabic, followed by a Persian translation (fols. 6a, 2; 10b, -8).

The author's name and title of this treatise remain unknown; certain features of the orthography, such as انك for انكه and aspirate *d* in postvocalic position, point to a date no later than 700/1300.

The following are samples of the mnemonic verses mentioned above:

1. (fol. 33b, 5–12), MS title "*masnavī*" (on whiteness of the eyelashes):

چون سپیدی درمژه پیدا شود
از تری باشد که درانجا شود

تری باشد لزج ای هوشمند
اصل مو اورده ان تری ببند

تنقیه باید در اول بعد ازان
لال دشتی طلا کردن بران

پیه بز با روغن زیتون بیار
و زیبائی پیه خوش ای هوشیار

حل کن وانجا طلا کردن بشب
پس طلا دیگر ازحلزون طلب

روشنائی سرد دارد گاه گاه
زانك این دارو مژه دارد سیاه

بیست ونه علة که جالینوس گفت
درجفون وازسیا سیوس [کذا] گفت

هر یکی برجای خود اورده ام
کاندرین صنعت بسی خون خورده ام

2. (fol. 50a, -7 to -3), untitled *qeṭʿä* (on induration of the conjunctiva)

سختی بچشم نام جسا گفت اوستاد [کذا]
این نوع رنج ملتحمه چونك اوفتاد
ممکن نگردد انك بگردد بخانه چشم
بیدار گر شود نتوان دیده برگشاد
سرخست رنگ او وزخشکیست رنج او
با درد گفت باشد انکس که طب نهاد
خلط بد غلیظ بچشم اندرش بود
ورطبع نرم کردی بیمار گشت شاد
گرمابهٔ دوامی وسر بر بخار اب
باید که دارد انکس برنه گذار باد

Not in PL or Monzavī.

No. 182 : MS 76

Anonymous

Kanzo l-kaḥḥālīn

کنز الکحّالین

MS 76 (ex Coll. Min.), 395 fols., 240 x 182 mm

Bound in black leather over stiff thick cardboard; simple blind-tooled borders; inner covers pasted with dark blue paper with faded golden floral scrolls *à la chinoise*. Binding worn, corners torn. Binding not original. Written on Eastern and different varieties of European paper: 1) body of MS: Eastern paper, medium thin to very thin, transparent, burnished, greyish; 2) fols. 1, 4–7, substituted later for missing fols.: European paper, medium thin, burnished, cream-colored; 3) final restoration of MS (together with binding), blank fols. 2, 3, 11, and lower third of fol. 10, substituted for missing fols.: Italian paper, medium thin, burnished, white; watermarks: coat of arms and names AL MASSO and GIORG. MAGNANI. First and last fols. torn, mended; cuts in other fols. mended; some stains and smears; fol. 395 partly torn out. On lacunae see below.

I. Fols. 8–20: 23 lines, 185 x 105 mm, on blind-ruled frame and lines; black; medium-large, energetic *naskh*; later overlinings in crimson. Catchwords. II. Fols. 21–395a: 13–16 lines, 130–60 x 90–100 mm, on blind-ruled frame and lines; light grey to black with red rubrics; medium-sized clear but undistinguished *naskh*; rubrics and overlining added later as in I, on fols. 75b–92a also in black and green. III. Fols. 1b and 4–7: varying number of lines, 175 x 105 mm; black with red rubrics and punctuation; medium-sized, neat, fair *naskh*. Catchwords.

Collations by scribe (fols. 8-20) and readers (fols. 8–395).

Copied by Moḥammad Ḥosain b. Aḥmad . . . (destroyed); the date is also destroyed; ca. 1100/1700.

Notes in margins and on fol. 395b.

A previous owner's stamp was erased on fols. 22a and 222a.

Incipit, fol. 1b

بسمله وبه نستعين . هذا كتاب كنز الكحالين
سپاس بیقیاس بصیری را که دیده بصیرت اولی
الابصار در ادراک الوان مصنوعات واشکال انواع
مخلوقات ... اما بعد بعد از حمد افریدگار وثنای
پروردگار صد هزارات ...

Explicit, fol. 395a

وغلظ امراض طبقه صلبه مشترکه اقسام سوء المزاج
وقدم والتوا واسترخا ونفوق الابصار است والله
اعلم بالصواب

The MS is a slightly incomplete copy of *Kanzo l-kaḥḥālin* (title mentioned, e.g., fol. 273b, -2). If its author named himself in the introduction, it was in the missing part for which the blank fols. 2 and 3 have been substituted. The book is little more than a collection of quotations from works on ophthalmology, arranged in 250 *faṣl*; all of these are listed in the table of contents.[1] Here is a short account of the contents:

- *faṣl* 1–6 (begin on fol. 8a, -5), introduction: subject of ophthalmology, definition of the eye, the oculist's duties, etc.
- *faṣl* 7–25 (begin on fol. 12b, 10), anatomy and physiology of the eye, its tunics, the optic nerve, the colors of the eye
- *faṣl* 26–45 (begin on fol. 37b, 3), diseases of the eye and their treatment in general
- *faṣl* 46–52 (begin on fol. 56a, -1), simple drugs
- *faṣl* 53–66 (begin on fol. 102b, 5), diseases of the conjunctiva
- *faṣl* 67–78 (begin on fol. 135a, 7), diseases of the cornea
- *faṣl* 79–83 (begin on fol. 152a, -4), diseases of the uvea
- *faṣl* 84–85 (begin on fol. 163a, 7), cataract
- *faṣl* 86–88 (begin on fol. 175b, -7), diseases of the visual spirit, night-blindness, etc.
- *faṣl* 89–96 (begin on fol. 180a, 3), diseases of the optic nerve
- *faṣl* 97 (begins on fol. 186a, 2), diseases of the arachnoid tunic
- *faṣl* 98 (begins on fol. 187a, -7), diseases of the albuminoid humor
- *faṣl* 99 (begins on fol. 189a, -4) diseases of the ice-like (crystalline) humor
- *faṣl* 100 (begins on fol. 192a, 8), diseases of the vitreous humor
- *faṣl* 101 (begins on fol. 195b, 5), diseases of the retina

faṣl 102 (begins on fol. 198a, 2), diseases of the choroid tunic
faṣl 103 (begins on fol. 199a, -1), diseases of the sclera
faṣl 104–157 (begin on fol. 200b, -5), other diseases of the eye, trachoma (*jarab*), exophthalmus (*joḥūẓ*), diseases of the lid
faṣl 158–182 (begin on fol. 273b, -3), compound drugs according to their preparation
faṣl 183–249 (begin on fol. 328b, -5), drugs according to their indication
faṣl 250 (begins on fol. 394a, 6), diseases that affect the lid, tunica, and humors of the eye simultaneously

This list shows clearly that more than a third of the book is given over to a discussion of drugs. Naturally enough, in these sections virtually the whole text consists of quotations, but in the other chapters it is quite the same. It is interesting that the list of great oculists of the past, given in the introduction (fol. 8b, 13), does not nearly reflect the extent to which the author excerpted older texts, nor does it even give the most important sources of his work. It serves rather to illustrate the author's notion of the age and rank of his field, since he places its roots in antiquity and links it to the most prominent names in pre-Islamic science and philosophy:

ارطاطاليس [كذا] وهرمس وروفس و افلاطون
وبقراط وارخيجانس وزرده گليم وانطليس

It is surprising to see Zardä-Gelīm[2] included in this list of exalted names. From the number of quotations in the text itself it appears that apart from the standard works on general medicine and *materia medica*, his most thoroughly used sources[3] were ʿAlī b. ʿĪsā's *Tadhkirat al-kaḥḥālīn*,[4] abū Rowḥ Moḥammad b. Manṣūr Zarrīndast's *Nūro l-ʿoyūn*,[5] ibn al-Baiṭār's *Tajribat al-kaḥḥālīn*,[6] and ibn an-Nafīs's *Miftāḥ ash-shifāʾ*.[7] The last two of these were hitherto unknown.[8] The author's own date remains uncertain. A *terminus a quo* is given by a quotation from ʿEzzoddīn Masʿūd Shīrāzī, who died in 813/1410.[9] If Shāreḥ-e Asbāb[10] is indeed Nafīs b. ʿIwaḍ al-Kirmānī, who died in 853/1449, the *terminus a quo* would move forward even further.[11]

1. Fols. 4–7. The substituted text of fol. 7 overlaps partly with fol. 8: 7b, -1 corresponds to 8b, -11.
2. Known only from a MS of his *Mokhtaṣar andar ʿelm-e ṭabīb* in Leiden; there his name is written Zard Gelīm. The date of the Leiden MS, 563/1167, is a *terminus ad quem* for his book (Leiden *Cat.* III 273–74, Cod 604 C (I) Warn.).
3. To list all authors quoted would not give an adequate picture, given the wealth of quotations in ibn al-Baiṭār's works and others of this author's immediate sources.
4. Fols. 9b, -3; 299b, 9 et passim.
5. Fols. 25b, 1; 127a, -1; 128b, 6; 292a, 2 et passim.
6. Fols. 16a, 8; 291b, 7; 292b, 4, etc.: *Tajribat al-kaḥḥālīn*; fols. 344b, 8, -4; 345a, 6, 8: Mālaqī.
7. Fols. 9b, -1; 128b, 7; 152b, 2; 288b, 4 et passim.
8. They are not listed in GAL, EI² (s.v. al-Baiṭār and ibn an-Nafīs, resp.), or Ullmann, who mentions a book on ophthalmology by the latter author, titled *K. al-muhadhdhab fī l-kuḥl* (p. 213; see Sellheim, pp. 213–16, no. 56).
9. This physician is mentioned by Aḥmad b. Zainoddīn ʿAlī Anṣārī "Ḥājjī Zaino l-ʿAṭṭār," in his untitled book on the lives and sayings of philosophers and sages (Rieu II 873a, -9), as having died in 813/1410; his name is also quoted in the anonymous *Qarābāẓīn* for Timur's grandson Jalāloddīn Eskandar (see **No. 40 : MS 24 VIII**).
10. Fols. 200b, -4; 212a, 3; 219a, -1.
11. Ullmann, p. 170. A number of authors quoted could not be identified: abū l-Ḥasan b. Nuʿmān, who supposedly lived in the fourth/tenth century (fol. 305b, -2); ibn Sarīḥ (fol. 324a, 8); Madāʾinī (fol. 345a, -5. A *K. fī ʿilm al-khawāṣṣ* was written by abū l-Ḥasan ʿAlī b. Muḥammad b. Shuʿaib al-Madāʾinī in the fourth/tenth century; see GAS III 378); ibn Jahm (fol. 274b, 6. Al-Jāḥiẓ in *K. al-ḥayawān* quotes from Muḥammad b. al-Jahm al-Barmakī; see GAS III 362); Amīn ad-Dīn (fol. 345a, -3. See **No. 15 : MS 84**, on Amīno d-dowlä al-Ūtājī); Jamāl ad-Dīn ʿArab Kaḥḥāl (fol. 336a, 6); Muʿīn ad-Dīn (fol. 336a, -3). Some books are quoted whose authors remain unknown: *K. ejmāl-e jamālī* (fol. 325b, 4; a *K. aṭ-Ṭibb al-Jamālī* was written by ibn Hubal for the vizier Jamāl ad-Dīn Muḥammad, see ibn a. Uṣaibiʿa I 306, 6), *K. farādīs al-kuḥl* (fol. 302b, 7), and *K. mokhleṣ* (fol. 292b, 7). The transcription of these names as according to Arabic or Persian pronunciation remains necessarily uncertain.

Not in PL or Monzavī.

No. 183 : MS 78 III

Anonymous

[*Kaḥḥālī*] [کحّالی]

MS 78 (ex Coll. Min.), 117 fols., 115 x 230 mm (*jong*); scribe's collection of three medical texts and prayers, etc. [*Kaḥḥālī*] on fols. 59–95.

For the description of the MS see **No. 186 : MS 78 I.**

Incipit, fol. 59b

فصل یازدهم در امراض کنج چشم که باقر اکبر گویند
بدانکه یك امراض کنج چشم غرب است و غرب
ناصور کنج چشم را گویند وسبب او ماده حاده
باشد که ...

Explicit, fol. 95a, 1

چون در دهان گیرند خوشحالی بخشد این است داروهای
که استعمال کنند اندر علاج چشم و قوت طبیعی هر یك را
جدا جدا گفتم تا باتمام رسید والله اعلم بالصواب

Neither the title nor the author's name is mentioned in this acephalous MS of a treatise on ophthalmology in four *bāb* (of thirteen, five, four, and eight *faṣl* resp.) and a *khātemä* (begins on fol. 78b, 8), in two *nowᶜ*, on ophthalmic drugs, listed in alphabetical order. In this MS, the text begins with *faṣl* 11 of *bāb* 1.

Further study will have to determine the relationship between this text and *Żīā-ye ᶜoyūn*, an anonymous treatise on ophthalmology in four *bāb* and a *khātemä*, preserved in Tashkent (*Cat.* X 120, no. 6867 [10299], dated 978/1570).

Not in PL or Monzavī.

No. 184 : MS 68 I

Anonymous

[*Kaḥḥālī*] [کحّالی]

MS 68 (ex Coll. Min.), 132 fols., 205 x 145 mm; binder's collection of seven works in two sections: A) nos. I-II (fols. 1-52), and B) nos. III-VII (fols. 53-132), each written by one scribe; nos. V-VII (fols. 77-132) non-medical, not catalogued. (See also **Nos. 167, 210,** and **216**.)
[*Kaḥḥālī*] on fols. 1-46.

Bound in flexible black leather; simple blind-tooled borders; inner covers bare; one flyleaf each in front and back of thin, burnished, white Russian paper; binding torn, warped; part of MS out of binding. Written on two different papers: A) fols. 1-52: thin, burnished, light blue and white, Russian; blind stamps illegible; B) fols. 53-132: thin, burnished, cream-colored, European; watermarks obscure; margins of fol. 53 (fol. 1 in an earlier MS) soiled; some wear in B).

A) Fols. 1-52: 17-18 lines, 140 x 80-105 mm; greyish-black, rubrics overlined; ordinary *shekastä*. Catchwords. Fol. 16a blank. B) Fols. 53-132: 16 lines, 145 x 75 mm, on blind-ruled frame and lines; black with red rubrics; medium-small, fair *shekastä-āmīz*. Catchwords.

A) and B) anonymous copies; no. I dated 17 Ramażān 1287/11 December 1870, no. II dated 6 Jomādā I 1297/16 April 1880; B) undated, also thirteenth/nineteenth century, but somewhat older than A).

Notes by scribe and readers on fol. 53a and in margins of B).

Tamlīk on back flyleaf written by one Moḥammad ʿAlī; owner's name illegible.

Incipit, fol. 1a

بسمله . الحمد لله [کذا] رب العالمس والصلاه والسلام
علی خیر خلقه محمد واله الطاهرین اما بعد این رساله
ایست در کحالی ومشتمل است بر مقدمه ودوازده
باب اما مقدمه چون قوه باصره از برای انسانی [کذا]
از جمیع حواس ...

Explicit, fol. 46b, 10

وچون در این کتاب محتاج به نسخهٔ شوند که بتفصیل
ذکر نگشته است باید بکتاب قرابادین فرنگی
رجوع نمایند که دراینجا هر نسخهٔ به تفصیل نوشته
شده واین کتاب را چون خواستیم مختصر نوشته
شود لهذا بذکر انها نپرداخته وبهمان رسم [؟]
مختصری که مسطور گشت اکتفا نمودیم تمت الکتاب [کذا]

This MS contains an anonymous, untitled tract on ophthalmology in a *moqaddemä* and twelve *bāb* (see Incipit):

bāb 1. (begins on fol. 1b, -7) in three *faṣl* در شرح عین و عمل ابصار

2. (begins on fol. 5a, -9) در طریقه امتحان نمودن چشم

3. (begins on fol. 6b, -7) in several *faṣl* در جراحات وارده بر چشم

4. (begins on fol. 9a, 3)
در بیان اشیاء خارجه متوقعه در چشم واثر انها

5. (begins on fol. 9b, -2) in several *faṣl* در اورام چشم

6. (begins on fol. 22a, -5) در اورام مرکبه بصر بامراض مزاجی

7. (begins on fol. 24b, -5) در قرحات قرنیه

8. (begins on fol. 25b, -3)
در تغیر هیات وشکل چشم از حالت طبیعی

9. (begins on fol. 32a, -3) in three *faṣl* در التصاقات چشم

10. (begins on fol. 37a, 1) in two *bayān*
در تغییر یافتن الات چشم ازسوی محور خود

11. (begins on fol. 38a, -7)
در انفقاد الات باره [؟ آیا یعنی باره؟] در چشم

12. (begins on fol. 39a, -7) در امراض سازجه وعصبانی بصر

If *qarābāzīn-e Farangī* (see Explicit) can be understood to mean a modern European dispensatory, the period of composition of this text must be mid- to late thirteenth/middle third of nineteenth century. This internal evidence would be supported by a manuscript in al-Khāliṣī library (*Cat.* p. 264, no. 15 III), if a comparison of the two texts showed their common identity. In the Khāliṣī copy, Dr. Polak is named as author.[1] In the UCLA manuscript, fol. 33 is misbound: it belongs between fols. 27 and 28.

1. See PL II 294, no. 530 (1).

See note 1; not in Monzavī.

No. 185 : MS Ar. 96 VI

Anonymous

[*Kaḥḥālī*] [کحّالی]

MS Ar. 96 (ex Coll. Min.), 159 fols., 212 x 150 mm; binder's collection of eight Arabic and Persian texts. [*Kaḥḥālī*] on fols. 123–144.

For the description of the MS see **No. 144 : MS Ar. 96 I.**

Incipit, fol. 123b

رساله است در کهلی [کذا. یعنی کحّالی]. بسمله. هد [کذا]
رسالهٔ نافعه. در علاج چشم نوع الاول که از خون باشد
اول تلطیف خون کنند بعد ازان خون از رگ قیفال
بگیرند

Explicit, fol. 144a, 7

وصبر و کندر سوده بر جراحت میگذارند تا خشك میسازد
ریم انر[؟ آیا یعنی آنرا؟] می بندد باذن الله تعالی والله اعلم
بحقایق [البیاض صحیح] العلا ت

This anonymous, untitled treatise on ophthalmology discusses the treatment of eye diseases in 25 *faṣl*, subdivided into *nowᶜ*. This MS apparently begins within *faṣl* 3 and ends after (?) *faṣl* 25, misnumbered 26, the section on medicines for inflammation of the lachrymal duct.

Not in PL or Monzavī.

No. 186 : MS 78 I

Anonymous

[***Ketāb-e nozhato l-molūk***] [کتاب نزهة الملوك]

MS 78 (ex Coll. Min.), 117 fols., 115 x 230 mm (*jong*); scribe's collection of three medical texts (nos. I, III, IV) and prayers, etc. (no. II, not catalogued). (See also **Nos. 73** and **183 : MSS 78 IV** and **78 III**.)
[*Ketāb-e nozhato l-molūk*] on fols. 1–18.

Bound in flexible plain dark brown leather; inner covers bare. Binding badly warped, too short for the size of the MS, so the first and last fols. are heavily damaged. Written on Eastern paper, medium thin, of coarse surface (worn?), dark brown (soiled?). For lacunae see below.

18 lines, written over the whole surface of fols.; black with black overlinings; medium-small even, fine *nastaʿlīq* alternating with medium-sized awkward *naskh*. Written by the same scribe?

Anonymous, undated copy (end missing); ca. 1200/1800.

Fols. 1-18a, 11 of this MS contain a text on sexual medicine. It begins on fol. 1 within *bāb* 5; there is a lacuna between fols. 5 and 6, from within *bāb* 9 to within *bāb* 11; and on fol. 7b, 9 *bāb* 16 begins, in two *faṣl*, on simple and compound medicines. The text breaks off within this *bāb* on fol. 18a, 11. The identification of this MS as *Ketāb-e nozhato l-molūk* rests on a comparison of its chapter headings with the information given in Bodleian I 974 on no. 1622 (c).

Cf. PL II 217, no. 372 (c); Monzavī I 478a, nos. 4426–30; ibid., 479b, nos. 4439–40.

No. 187 : MS 86 II

Anonymous

[*Nozhato l-molūk*] [نزهة الملوك]

MS 86, 140 fols., 260 x 150 mm; scribe's collection of prayers in Arabic and Persian (no. I, not catalogued) and four Persian medical texts. (See also **Nos. 108, 180,** and **205**.)
[*Nozhato l-molūk*] on fols. 32–69.

Bound in dark brown leather over slightly flexible cardboard; covers partly pasted with cigarette wrappers, Turkish brands with text in Ottoman Turkish; inner covers pasted with scrap paper (used envelopes); three flyleaves in front of off-white Eastern paper, one in back, pasted together out of an old letter and a used envelope. Binding original? Written on Eastern paper, thin to medium thin, burnished, tan; some margins repaired; little wear.

12 lines, 190 x 100 mm; black with red rubrics; medium-sized ordinary *naskh* leaning to *nastaʿlīq*. Catchwords. Fols. 70a, 140b and verso of front flyleaves blank.

Anonymous, undated copy; ca. 1200/1800.

Some marginal entries in Turkish.

Incipit, fol. 32a

بسمله. الحمد لله ربّ العالمين والعاقبة للمتقين الصّلواه
[كذا] والسّلام على رسوله محمّد وآله اجمعين بدانكه
حکماء درین اجازت نکاح دادند از فعل...

The identification of this treatise on sexual intercourse as *Nozhato l-molūk* rests on a comparison with **No. 186 : MS 78 I**. In this MS, there follow some short *faṣl* on various subjects after *bāb* 16 (from fol. 56b, 3).

No. 188 : MS 26 X

Anonymous

Resālä-ye bāhīyä رسالهٔ باهیّه

MS 26 (ex Coll. Min.), 103 fols., 178 x 120 mm; binder's collection of eleven works.
Resālä-ye bāhīyä on fols. 80–81.

For the description of the MS see **No. 62 : MS 26 I.**

Incipit, fol. 80a

و طبیعت از پی دفع منی شود مثل بول و براز
و اگر بادی باو جمع شود قوت مجامعت پیدا آید...

Explicit, fol. 81a

این مقصود از چیزهای ترش پرهیز کند و چیزهای
مخدر ضرر دارد ملتمس از ناظران این اوراق...

Virtually the whole text of this treatise on sexual medicine is missing in this MS. In the colophon (fol. 81a, 6) it is called *ar-Risāla al-bāhīya*. It appears very possible that this is the treatise *Bāhīyä* by Shamsoddīn Moḥammad Ṭabīb that Sālekoddīn Moḥammad Ḥamavī copied in his collection *Ḥajalato l-ʿarāyes.*[1]

1. See Nashrīyä III 15b, no. 20. For chronological reasons, the fragment in **MS 26 X** cannot be part of *Bāhīyä* by Neẓāmoddīn Aḥmad Gīlānī, who died in 1059/1649: this copy was transcribed in 981/1573 (see **MS 26 I**; Monzavī I 480b).

No. 189 : MS 72 I

Anonymous

Toḥfato s-solṭān تحفة السلطان

MS 72 (ex Coll. Min.), 182 fols., 173 x 105 mm; scribe's collection in four sections; nos. II–IV (fols. 25–182) non-medical, not catalogued: II. *Nūshāfrīn va-Gowhartāj*; III. *Majmūʿä-ye tarassol*; IV. *Robāʿīyāt-e* abū Saʿīd-e abū l-Khair. *Tohfato s-soltān* on fols. 1–24.

Bound in flexible black leather; simple blind-tooled borders; inner covers bare; binding somewhat worn. Written on Russian papers of different provenance (different blind stamps), medium thin to medium thick, burnished, off-white to white; fols. 122–123 of English paper, dyed light blue; watermark: C. Millington, London 1863; first and last fols. soiled; worn and torn, stained.

I. Fols. 1–24: 13 lines, 120 x 65 mm, on blind-ruled frame and lines; black with black overlinings, rubrics often left out; medium-sized fair *shekastä-āmīz*. Catchwords.

Copied, and dated 3 Jomādā I 1276/28 November 1859, by Bahrām b. Eqbāl.

Marginal notes by scribe.

On fol. 182b *tamlīk* by Moḥammad Esmāʿīl-e Moḥammad Ebrāhīm.

Incipit, fol. 1b

بسمله. این مختصریست درباه ملتقط از کتب طبی
مشتمل بر چند فصل در بیان وصیت حکماء
واطباء [و] یونان چون افلاطون وارسطو وبقراط
وجالینوس واطباء اسلام چون محمد ذکریا [کذا]
وحنین ابن اسحق [کذا] وغیرهم همه اتفاق کرده اند
برانکه مجامعت هیچ وقتی موافقتر از موسم بهار
نیست ...

Explicit, fol. 24b, 11

ونوعی نمایند که در وقت برگردانیدن پاره وشکسته
نشود تمام شد این کتاب مختصر المسمی بتحفة السلطان ...

This anonymous treatise on sexual medicine, in several *faṣl* (see Incipit), is titled *Tohfato s-soltān* in the scribe's colophon (see Explicit).

Not in PL or Monzavī.

No. 190 : MS 54 II

Anonymous

[*Farhang-e advīä*] [فرهنگ ادویه]

MS 54, 125 fols., 215 x 120 mm; binder's collection of seven works.
[*Farhang-e advīä*] on fols. 78–103.

For the description of the MS see **No. 164 : MS 54 I.**

Incipit, fol. 78a

بسمله. این نسخه است مفردات حکمت ملخص
اختیارات بدیعی وبعضی کتب دیگر...

Explicit, fol. 103b

دیگر پوست بیخ کبر مسهل خلط خام بود تمام شد فرهنگ ادویة [کذا]

This anonymous *materia medica* is titled *Farhang-e advīä* in the colophon (see above). It is divided into 26 *bāb* according to the indication of the drugs *a capite ad calcem.* In the preface it is said to have been excerpted from *Ekhtīārāt-e Badīʿī* and other books.[1]

1. See PL II 315, no. 584 (43), and **No. 20 : MS 36.**

No. 191 : MS 9 III

Anonymous

[*Khavāṣṣ-e ashyāʾ*] [خواصّ اشیاء]

MS 9 (ex Coll. Min.), 85 fols., 235 x 125 mm; scribe's collection of three Persian texts.
[*Khavāṣṣ-e ashyāʾ*] on fols. 48–63.

For the description of the MS see **No. 11 : MS 9 II.**

Incipit, fol. 48a

نان کماج * گرم و خشکست * مردم کارکن را نیکست *
مردم منعم را نسازد * بروغن بادام یا بروغن دنبه *

Explicit, fol. 63b, -1

... بسرکه خوش گرداند و هرچند ترش باشد بنمك
و بوی ابزارهای [؟] خوش گرداند]

End of *bāb* 28, fol. 63b, -5

عرق نعناع * میل بخشکی و سردی دارد * قوت معده
و صفرا دفع کند * درد پهلو و سرفه را بدست * با آش
نخود آب خورند

Beginning of unnumbered *bāb* on fol. 63b, -4

باب در آداب دیك پختن
آنکه در یك زور دو غذای مختلف نخورند ...

This is an anonymous, untitled treatise of 28 numbered *bāb* on the medicinal properties of foods, drinks, plants, animals, perfumes, ointments, etc., in tabular form; *bāb* 28 is followed by an unnumbered *bāb* of continuous text on the ways of preparing cocks, *dar ādāb-e dīk-pokhtan* (see above). In the first 28 *bāb*, there are, following the usual disposition of such works, five columns, giving: 1) the name (*nām* or *esm*), 2) nature (*ṭabīᶜat*), 3) virtue (*manfaᶜat*), 4) harmful properties (*mażarrat*), and 5) antidotes for such harmful properties (*dafᶜ-e mażarrat*). Beginning and end of the text are missing in this MS, and there are lacunae. Some fols. are misbound; their correct order is as follows: lacuna (one fol.?), 48–53, 55, 54, 58, 56, lacuna (from within *bāb* 13 to within *bāb* 15), 57, 59–61, lacuna (from within *bāb* 21 to within *bāb* 25), 62–63, lacuna (breaks off within *bāb* after *bāb* 28; see above). As far as preserved in the MS, the titles of the 28 *bāb* read as follows:

1. (beginning lost) — [در نانها]
2. (begins on fol. 48a, -2) — در آبها
3. (begins on fol. 49b, 2) — در دانها

4. (begins on fol. 50a, -2) — در گوشتها
5. (begins on fol. 51a, -4) — در گوشت مرغان
6. (begins on fol. 52a, 3) — در ماهیها وانواع آن
7. (begins on fol. 52b, 3) — در اعضای حیوان
8. (begins on fol. 53a, -1) — در آشها
9. (begins on fol. 55b, 3) — در کامخها
10. (begins on fol. 54a, 4) — در شیر و ماست
11. (begins on fol. 54b, -3) — در بیضها
12. (begins on fol. 58a, 5) — در سبزیها
13. (begins on fol. 56a, -3) — در توابل ودیگر انوارها
14. (lost)
15. (beginning lost) — [در میوهای خشك ؟]
16. (begins on fol. 57a, -1) — در شیرینها
17. (begins on fol. 59a, 3) — در حلواها
18. (begins on fol. 59b, 6) — در شربتها
19. (begins on fol. 60a, 5) — در شرابها
20. (begins on fol. 60b, -1) — در شرابهاء مست کننده
21. (begins on fol. 61b, 2) — در روغنها
22-24. (lost)
25. (beginning lost) — [در پوستینها]
26. (begins on fol. 62a, -4) — در هواها [[وریحانها]]
27. (begins on fol. 62b, -4) — در ریحانها
28. (begins on fol. 63a, -2; breaks off on fol. 63b) — در عرقها

No. 192 : MS 25 XI

Anonymous

[*Taqvīm-e advīä*] [تقویم ادویه]

MS 25 (ex Coll. Min.), 120 fols., 195 x 98 mm; scribe's collection of eleven works: ten from Yūsofī's *Majmūᶜä* and one anonymous text.
[*Taqvīm-e advīä*] on fols. 107b-115b.

For the description of the MS see **No. 47 : MS 25.**

Incipit

این مقاله بر هفت تقویم است تقویم اوّل در اغذیه
نان بدن را تقویت ... محدث سده است ... سکنجبین
عسلی ...

Explicit

شاهسفرم محلل فضول دماغست و فرموشی زایل گرداند
صاحب زکام را زکام زیاده کند نیلوفر با بنفشه این سخنان
که بترجمان لسان قلم بیان کرده جامع این رساله اختیاریست
که از تالیفات اعاظم حکما و افاخم اطبا نموده مامول
از ارباب ...

This treatise on the medicinal properties of victuals and aromatic plants is divided into seven *taqvīm*:

1. (begins on fol. 107b) foodstuffs (*aghẕīä*)
2. (begins on fol. 109b) beverages (*ashrebä*)
3. (begins on fol. 111a) fruits (*favākeh*)
4. (begins on fol. 112a) sweetmeats (*ḥalāvāt*)
5. (begins on fol. 113a) sorrel-like greens (*ḥomūżāt*)
6. (begins on fol. 114a) vegetables (*boqūl*)
7. (begins on fol. 114b) aromatic plants (*advīä-ye ṭayyebato r-rāyeḥä*)

These seven *taqvīm* consist of tables in four columns: a) name, b) virtue (*manfaᶜat*), c) negative effect (*mażarrat*), d) antidote (*dafᶜ-e mażarrat*).

No. 193 : MS 60 V

Anonymous

[*Taqvīm-e advīä*] [تقویم ادویه]

MS 60 (ex Coll. Min.), 74 fols., 240 x 150 mm; binder's collection in five sections. [*Taqvīm-e advīä*] on fols. 65–73.

For the description of the MS see **No. 177 : MS 60 II.**

Incipit, fol. 65a

بسر ارد [آیا یعنی بسر آرد ؟] بادها وانگرد مصلح او
بره وسرکه خورد نان ارزن طبیعت
گرم وخشك منفعت اسهال را تنگ است مضرت
گرمی وقولنج اورد مصلح ...

Explicit, fol. 73b, 1

هوای سر وسیر [؟] طبع گرم وتر است نفع گرم مزاج را سازد
مضرت سر ومزاج را نشاید مصلح غذای گرم خورند تمت
تمام شد

This incomplete treatise on the medicinal properties of foodstuffs, etc., is divided into 22 *bāb*. There is a lacuna between fols. 64 and 65, and the text starts within *bāb* 1, on *nānhā*. There follow: 2) *ābhā*, 3) *dānähā*, 4) *gūshthā* (end missing), 5) missing, 6) beginning missing, one paragraph headed *khāyä*, 7) *ashyā-ye gheẕāʾ*, 8) *torshīhā*, 9) *labanīyāt*, 10) *baiżhā*, 11) *sabzīhā*, 12) *meyvähā-ye tar*, 13) *meyvähā-ye khoshk*, 14) *shīrīnhā*, 15) *ḥalvāhā*, 16) *shorbathā*, 17) *sharābhā*, 18) *rowghanhā*, 19) *ʿeṭrhā*, 20) *morabba-yāt-e govāresh*, 21) *pūstīnhā*, 22) *havā-ye raiḥānhā*. The text is arranged under five rubrics: a) name, b) nature (*ṭabʿ*), c) virtue (*nafʿ*), d) harmful effect (*mażarrat*), e) antidote (*moṣleḥ*). It appears probable that this MS was copied from tables with these five columns.

No. 194 : MS 66 I

Anonymous

[*Taqvīm-e advīä*] [تقویم ادویه]

MS 66 (ex Coll. Min.), 130 fols., 310 x 215 mm; owner's collection of four medical works. (See also **Nos. 72, 165,** and **166**.) [*Taqvīm-e advīä*] on fols. 1-130.

Bound in black leather over thick, stiff cardboard; simple blind-tooled borders, three-medallion design inlaid with dark green leather, stamped in tan floral scrolls; inner covers pasted with Italian paper, dyed pink; watermarks: 1) in front, shield with crowned lion rampant sinister, and name BENTO PICARDO; 2) in back, six-pointed star and name E FIGLJ. One flyleaf each in front and back of Italian papers; watermarks: 1) in front, FABIANI 12; 2) in back, shield with crenellated tower, and in three lines C B, F, E M VEDOVA, resp. Binding slightly worn, especially corners. Written on Italian (exclusively?) papers of different provenance, medium thin, burnished, white; watermarks: 1) shield party per fesse, chief crowned half eagle displayed, base horse allant; 2) G M; 3) GIOR MAGNANI; 4) AL MASSO; 5) different coats of arms, obscure; first and last leaves soiled; after fol. 130 three leaves torn out; somewhat stained and worn.

12 x 8 fields in tables, 195 x 117 mm; blind-ruled; fields separated by thin crimson lines (except on fols. 27 and 35-37, where the page is not divided into fields), borders of two crimson and one blue lines; outer margins bordered on three sides by two thin crimson lines, 275 x 185 mm; black, crimson, blue; nos. I-II (fols. 1-130 and margins of fols. 2-63), small, elegant *shekastä-āmīz*, rubrics in no. I in large, distinguished *naskh*; no. III (margins of fols. 76-81a), medium-small, fine *shekastä-āmīz*; no. IV (margins of fols. 75, 81b-115), medium-sized, fine *naskh*. Diagonal lines, sometimes alternating between fields. Catchwords in I.

Nos. I-II copied, and no. I dated Saturday, 7 Jomādā II 1263/*Sunday*, 23 May 1847, by Maḥmūd Khorāsānī for ʿAbbāsʿalī Jarrāḥbāshī-ye Shīrāzī, the first owner of the MS; no. III also transcribed for him, by Aḥmad Semnānī on 4 Rabīʿ I 1264/9 February 1848; no. IV copied, and dated 4 Moḥarram 1265/30 November 1848, by Mīrzā Moḥammad b. Mollā ʿAlī Akbar Kāteb.

Marginal notes throughout.

On back inner cover *tamlīk* for ʿAbbāsʿalī Jarrāḥbāshī-ye Shīrāzī, written, and dated 10 Jomādā II 1266/23 April 1850, by Reżāqolī Jūzjānī.

Incipit, fol. 1b

بسمله. ادویه قوی مقوی مرحّر ابشن [؟] هاضم ش
۲ م مرحّر ش ۲ م جوزبوا مقوی هاضمه...

Explicit, fol. 130b

روغن هسته زردالو جهة ذحیر [کذا] فو جهة
معص قرنفل جهة معص این جلد کتاب
ازمال افقر عباد عباس الطبیب الجراح الشراری
در یوم...

In this anonymous, untitled work, the simple and compound drugs are listed according to their indication. A tabular work with the title *Ṭebb-e mojadval,* written in the thirteenth/nineteenth century, is listed in Monzavī (I 564b, no. 5276), but these may just be two examples of a common form of medical *vade mecum.*

No. 195 : MS 80

Anonymous

Mokhtaṣar-e mofīd مختصر مفید

MS 80 (ex Coll. Min.), 29 fols., 218 x 140 mm; **MSS 62, 80–83** are obviously parts of a scribe's collection of medical treatises that was only recently taken apart and bound separately.

Fols. 1a and 29b blank; for further description of the MS see **No. 150 : MS 62.**

Recipe, written by scribe, on fol. 27a. On fols. 27b–29a an excerpt from a larger work, also in the scribe's hand; *faṣl* 73:

در صاف کردن وکشتن دهاتها وابدهاتها وجواهر
ومانند آن بدانکه زر ونقره ومس ...

End, fol. 29a, 9

وهم بدین طریق بنتها [؟] تا چارده تپ بدهند
نقره کشته گردد

Incipit, fol. 1b

بسمله. الحمد لله حق حمده والصلوة علی نبیه محمد
واله اجمعین اما بدانکه این مختصری است
مفید که حکماء از برای نوشیروان عادل از کتاب
طب وخواص الاشیا بیرون آورده اند که اگر
روزی اورا بیماری واقع شود وحکماء حاضر
نباشند باین کتاب علاج کرده شود ...

Explicit, fol. 27a, 9

اگر زن سرمه یا سرکه بردارد آبستن نشود واگر
کودک دارد بیفتد والله اعلم بالصواب
تمت ...

This anonymous treatise on the medicinal properties of mineral, vegetable, and animal substances is described in the preface as a *Mokhtaṣar-e mofīd* (see Incipit); it was allegedly compiled for Anūshervān to serve as a medical *vade mecum* when no physician was at hand. It is divided into sixteen *bāb*:

1. در منافع انسان
2. در منافع بهایم
3. در منافع طیور
4. در منافع الاثمار
5. در منافع الاشجار المثمرة
6. در منافع سبزغام
7. در منافع پالیز وغیره
8. در منافع اخضریات
9. در غلات ومنافع او
10. در منافع حبوبات
11. در منافع سلیس [؟]
12. در منافع صموغ
13. در منافع جواهر
14. در منافع احجار گدازنده
15. در منافع احجار ستوده
16. در منافع احجار معدنی

Another MS of the same title, and ostensibly composed for Khosrow Anūshervān, is preserved at Tashkent; according to its preface, it consists of nineteen chapters, but actually it contains eighteen.[1]

1. Tashkent I, no. 537.

PL II 195, no. 348 (1).

No. 196 : MS 81

Anonymous

[*Javāhernāmä*] [جواهرنامه]

MS 81 (ex Coll. Min.), 15 fols., 220 x 140 mm; **MSS 62, 80–83** are obviously parts of a scribe's collection of medical treatises that was only recently taken apart and bound separately.

Fol. 15b blank; for further description of the MS see **No. 150 : MS 62.** Anonymous copy, dated 1240/1824.

Incipit, fol. 1b

بسمله. ارسطاطالیس حکیم گفت هرکه خاتم عقیق
در انگشت دارد از درد سینه وجگر ایمن باشد و پوشیدن
او اقامت سنت پیغمبران است بدانکه پیغمبر صلی الله
علیه وسلم خاتم عقیق را در دست داشتی...

Explicit, fol. 15a, -4

ودرچشم روشنی بیفزاید وجلا دهد ومبالغه کرده اند که
هرکه ان را با خود دارد از کید دشمن ایمن گردد والله اعلم
تمت...

This short, untitled tract on the medicinal and sympathetic properties of gemstones, coral, pearls, bezoar, and ambergris quotes from the Pseudo-Aristotelian book on stones. The mention of Gojarāt and other places in Hendūstān appears to suggest its place of composition. The text is divided into the following paragraphs:

1. (fol. 1b, 2) ʿ*aqīq* (cornelian)
2. (fol. 2a, 4) *marvārīd* (pearl)
3. (fol. 3a, 10) *yashm* (jasper)
4. (fol. 4a, 1) *fīrūzä* (turquoise)
5. (fol. 5a, 3) *zomorrod* (emerald)
6. (fol. 6a, 5) *bossad* (coral)
7. (fol. 6a, -4) *almās* (diamond)
8. (fol. 8a, 5) *yāqūt* (hyacinth)
9. (fol. 9b, 2) *laʿl* (ruby)
10. (fol. 10a, 6) *pādzahr-e ḥayavānī* (bezoar)
11. (fol. 11a, -2) ʿ*anbar-e ashhab* (ambergris)
12. (fol. 12b, 5) *lājvard* (lapis lazuli)
13. (fol. 14b, 7) *marjān* (small pearl?)

Not in PL or Monzavī.

No. 197 : MS 73 IV

ʿAṭāʾollāh b. Moḥammad Ḥosainī

Anīso l-majāles انیس المجالس

MS 73 (ex Coll. Min.), 131 fols., 205 x 145 mm; binder's collection of five works in two sections. *Anīso l-majāles* on fols. 98b–99a.

For the description of the MS see **No. 168 : MS 73 I.**

Incipit, fol. 98b

بسمله. شکر وسپاس خالق را که بقدرت کامله ابداع
جواهر عقلیّه مجرّده نموده وبتوسّط [کذا] آنها اختراع
اجرام مختلفه فرموده وبنجوم ثابته وسیّاره زیب وزینت
داده واز تاثیر افلاك در عالم کون وفساد وعناصر اربعه
وامتزاج آن انواع موالید بحسب استعداد برانگیخته
واز تعادل استقلال درکمیّات وکیفیّات مزاج انسانی را
که اعدل امزجه واشرف مخلوقاتست مرکب ساخته...

Explicit, fol. 99a, 1

معرفت پناه مشار الیه نوشته اینست رحمة الله علیه
تمت هذه الرسالة الموسوم [کذا] بانیس المجالس فی شهر...

In this MS, only the beginning of the preface and the end of the scribe's conclusion of *Anīso l-majāles* (see Explicit) are preserved; there is a long lacuna between fols. 98 and 99. This copy is a fragment of ʿAṭāʾollāh b. Moḥammad Ḥosainī's treatise on tobacco, tea, and coffee in a *moqaddemä* and three *bāb* which are subdivided into *faṣl.*[1] This MS provides a new *terminus ad quem* for the time of composition: it was copied in 1094/1682,[2] as against the MS in the Sepahsālār library dated 1142/1729.[3]

1. See Monzavī I 398 top, s.v. *Anīso l-majāles.*
2. See **No. 168 : MS 73 I.**
3. Sepahsālār, no. 7538 I (see also note 1 above for reference).

Not in PL; Monzavī I 398 top, no. 3698; Miklukho-Maklaĭ, p. 63, no. 254.

No. 198 : MS 58 III

Mīrzā Esmāʿīl Ṭabīb valad-e Mīrzā Sharīf

Dastūro l-ʿamal-e čūb-e čīnī دستور العمل چوب چینی

MS 58 (ex Coll. Min.), 147 fols., 213 x 153 mm; scribe's collection.
Dastūro l-ʿamal-e čūb-e čīnī on fols. 101–102.

For the description of the MS see **No. 135 : MS 58 I.**

Incipit, fol. 101a, 9

دستور العمل چوب چینی که مرحوم میرزا اسمعیل
طبیب ولد میرزا شریف مناسب احوال بنده نوشته
آنکه هر روز مقدار سه ۳ مثقال چوب چینی را خورده
نموده ...

Explicit, fol. 102a, -5

سفوف بجهت منع بخار نزلات که بجهت آزار
چشم مرزا محمد طبیب زاده بود تخم خشخاش
برداده [؟] نبات مغز هل تخم کشنیز ۵م
۱م ۲م ۳م
برداده [؟] کوبیده در پنج روز خورده شود.

The author's name appears only in the heading (cf. **No. 199 : MS 58 II**); the scribe states that the first recipe was formulated for himself.

Not in PL or Monzavī.

No. 199 : MS 58 II

Masīḥā Ṭabīb

Dastūr-e khwordan-e shīr-e olāgh دستور خوردن شیر الاغ

MS 58 (ex Coll. Min.), 147 fols., 213 x 153 mm; scribe's collection.
Dastūr-e khwordan-e shīr-e olāgh on fols. 100–101.

For the description of the MS see **No. 135 : MS 58 I.**

Incipit, fol. 100a

دستور خوردن شیر الاغ که مرحوم مسیحا طبیب بجهت آزار
حرقه البول چون که چهل روز از زایدن گذشته باشد ...

Explicit, fol. 101a, 7

گاهی پارچه نان باکباب بره یا فالوده یا فرنی میتوانند
خورد واما اگر دو مرتبه مطبوخ خفیف خورده شود
بهتر است.

The author's name appears only in the title to this short tract. It appears that he had died but recently when this MS was transcribed: the scribe refers to him as *marḥūm* (see Incipit).

Not in PL or Monzavī.

No. 200 : MS 54 IV

Anonymous

[*Farhang-e advīā*] [فرهنگ ادویه]

MS 54, 125 fols., 215 x 120 mm; binder's collection of seven works.
[*Farhang-e advīā*] on fols. 111–112.

For the description of the MS see **No. 164 : MS 54 I.**

Incipit, fol. 111a, -6

بسمله. فصل الالف انگبین شهد اجمود اجواین خراسانی

Explicit, fol. 112b

نمر درخت نیم نانخواه اجواین ناردین اسپند

This anonymous, untitled glossary of drug names in Arabic, Persian, and "Hendī" is divided into very short *faṣl* in alphabetical order. The text breaks off on fol. 112b, -1. Another MS of the same text, dated 1319/1901, is preserved in Punjab Univ.[1] The UCLA copy can serve to narrow down the period of composition: ca. 1150/1740 can be taken as a *terminus ad quem*.

1. Shīrānī II 384, no. 2084.

No. 201 : MS 54 III

Anonymous

[*Alfāẓ-e advīā*] [الفاظ ادویه]

MS 54, 125 fols., 215 x 120 mm; binder's collection of seven works.
[*Alfāẓ-e advīā*] on fols. 103b–111a.

For the description of the MS see **No. 164 : MS 54 I.**

Incipit, fol. 103b, 13

بسمله. باب الالف اره[؟] واسقیل و اسیقل عربی بصل
فارسی پیاز دشتی هندی کاندا گویند...

Explicit, fol. 111a, -8

...کوکهر و یتویق[؟] نمدی را گویند که از پشم میش
بود تمام شد الفاظ ادویه

This anonymous glossary of drug names in Arabic, Persian, and "Hendī" is titled *Alfāẓ-e advīā* in the colophon (see above). It is divided into *bāb* according to the Arabic alphabet.

No. 202 : MS 102

Anonymous

[*Farhang-e eṣṭelāḥāt*] [فرهنگ اصطلاحات]

MS 102, 29 fols., 385 x 235 mm

No real binding, MS loosely stitched together, in back a kind of cover, pasted together of three sheets of white Russian paper, covered with scribbles. Written on European (?) paper, medium thick, of rough surface, pinkish-grey; edges badly torn.

Black and red ink; Arabic entries in large, good *naskh*; Persian translations in much smaller *shekastä-āmīz*, by the same scribe. Fols. 11b–12a, 15b, 16a, 18a blank.

Anonymous, undated copy (end missing?); thirteenth/nineteenth century.

Reader's note on fol. 17b.

This Arabic-Persian glossary of medical terms is divided into three untitled sections. In the first, the names of particular and general diseases are listed in the usual order *a capite ad calcem*, ailments of joints and skin, and fevers (fols. 1a–15a). In the second section, terms of theoretical medicine, *ṭebb-e ʿelmī*, are explained, including the faculties (*qovā*) of the body, its spirits (*arvāḥ*), urinoscopy, and the pulse (fols. 16b–22a). The third and last part lists simple and compound drugs. No author or title is mentioned in this MS.

No. 203 : MS 73 III

Anonymous

[*Tafsīr iṣṭilāḥāt yūnānīya*] [تفسير اصطلاحات يونانيه]

MS 73 (ex Coll. Min.), 131 fols., 205 x 145 mm; binder's collection of five works in two sections.
[*Tafsīr iṣṭilāḥāt yūnānīya*] on fol. 97a.

For the description of the MS see **No. 168 : MS 73 I.**

Incipit, fol. 97a, 1

هو هذا تفسير كلمات يونانية وغيرها مستعملة في الطبّ
ماليقراطون هو ماء العسل افومالي هوان يؤخذ
الشهد فيغسل بالماء ويحفظ بذلك الماء من
غير طبخ اوذرومالي ...

Explicit, fol. 97a, -4

اوكسامالى هو خلّ قد خلط مع ماء الملح روزومالى
هو شراب يتخذ من عصارة الورد مع العسل
والله اعلم بعينه تم

In this short paragraph on "Greek and other terms" (see Incipit) the following names of honey- and grape drinks are explained: *mālīqarāṭūn* (μελίκρατον), *afūmālī* (ἀπόμελι), *ūdurūmālī* (ὑδρόμελι), *al-muʿassal*, *sharāb al-ʿasal*, *aṭ-ṭilāʾ*, *ūkusūmālī* (ὀξύμελι), *ūkusāmālī* (idem), *rūzūmālī* (ῥοδόμελι).

No. 204 : MS 120 II

Anonymous

[*Resālä dar bāb-e owzān va-makāʾīl*] [رساله درباب اوزان ومكائيل]

MS 120 (ex Coll. Min.), 187 fols., 222 x 120 mm; binder's collection of four works, nos. I–III copied by the same scribe. [*Resālä dar bāb-e owzān va-makāʾīl*] on fols. 35b–39a.

For the description of the MS see **No. 120 : MS 120 I.**

Incipit, fol. 35b

بسمله. اين رساله ايست درباب اوزان ومكائيل مصطلحه
درميان اطبا حبه يكجو ميانه است طسوج كه بفارسى طسو
گويند مقدار دوجو ميانه است قيراط چهارجو ميانه است
خرنوب شامى يك قيراط است كنكجى كه دربلاد هند نزد
زرگران وبعض ديگر مستعمل است بسه جو ميانه نزديك است ..

Explicit, fol. 39a, -2

اگر فرضا عدد شربات سى باشد ووزن مركب ده
شربت ان مركب ثلث درم خواهد بود زيرا كه نسبت
ثلث درم بده درم چون نسبت واحد است بعدد
شربات كه سى است وعلى هذا لقياس تمت [كذا]

This MS of a treatise on pharmaceutical weights and measures does not contain the name of the author or a title; the heading given above has been taken from the Incipit. The author discusses the various weights and measures, starting with the smallest and going on to bigger and bigger units. At the end he appends a short *zail* (fol. 39a, -6) on the dose of compound medicines in proportion to the dose of each of their ingredients. The sources of this treatise are works from three fields: medicine, Shīʿite *fiqh*, and Arabic lexicography. The author quotes from Avicenna's *Qānūn,*[1] ṣāḥeb-e *Zakhīrä,*[2] al-Qalānisī's *Qarābādhīn,*[3] and *Javāmeʿo l-advīä* by Zanjānī;[4] in canon law his sources are the well known Shīʿite scholars Jamāl ad-Dīn Ḥasan b. Yūsuf *al-ʿAllāma al-Ḥillī* with his *Irshād al-adhhān ilā aḥkām al-īmān,*[5] Jamāl ad-Dīn Muḥammad b. Makkī al-ʿĀmilī *ash-Shahīd al-Awwal* with his work *ad-Durūs ash-sharʿīya fī fiqh al-Imāmīya,*[6] and, in general, *foqahā-ye Emāmīyä.*[7] In Arabic lexicography he adduces Jauharī's *Ṣiḥāḥ*[8] and Fīrūzābādī's *Qāmūs.*[9] The last-named author is at the same time the latest of these explicitly named sources. The period of composition cannot, thus, be narrowly fixed, but a date after A.D. 1600 appears likely since the author is familiar with weights used in India among goldsmiths (fol. 35b, 4).

1. On the metrological appendix see Ullmann, pp. 319–20.
2. In all probability Esmāʿīl Jorjānī's *Zakhīrä-ye Khwārezmshāhī*; see **MSS 1–5.**
3. See Ullmann, p. 320.
4. In *Dharīʿa* (V 247, no. 1190) a book of this title is mentioned as having been composed by Ẓahīroddīn ʿEmādo l-Eslām al-Fāresī for Alp Arghūn, the ruler of Rayy; the author of *Dharīʿa* saw a copy of it that was in 981/1573 transcribed from, and collated with, a MS in al-Fāresī's own hand.
   It is by no means clear that the work mentioned in *Dharīʿa* is the same as that quoted by the author of the metrological treatise. The only other occurrence of a similar title is *Jawāmiʿ maʿānī l-khams maqālāt al-ūlā min K. Jālīnūs fī quwā l-adwiya al-mufrada . . .* by Ḥunain b. Isḥāq (Ullmann, p. 117). The author Zanjānī could not be identified.
5. GAL II 164, Supp. II 206, no. 3; cf. EI² III 390a, s.v. al-Ḥillī [Jafri]; he died in 726/1325.
6. GAL Supp. II 131; he was put to death for his Shīʿite convictions in 782/1380.
7. When mentioning them, the author adds the eulogy *raḥimahumu llāh,* in testimony of his Shīʿite faith (fol. 38b, 2).
8. Jauharī died ca. 400/1010; see EI² II 495b [Kopf].
9. Fīrūzābādī died in 817/1415; see EI² II 926a [Fleisch].

No. 205 : MS 86 III

Anonymous

[*Qarābāẕīn*] [قرابا ذين]

MS 86, 140 fols., 260 x 150 mm; scribe's collection in five sections.
[*Qarābāẕīn*] on fols. 70–105.

For the description of the MS see **No. 187 : MS 86 II.**

Incipit, fol. 70b

فايده اوّل دربيان سبب احتياج بدواى مركّب وكيفيت
تركيب ادويه مركبه بدان ايدك الله تعالى كه اكثر
اطّبا [كذا] متّفق اند دركتب ايشان مذكوراست كه
معالج اكثر درامراض دواى مفرد كافى دانند . . .

Explicit, fol. 105a, -5

حامی کبیر شش مثقال [کذا] حامی صغیره [کذا]
دو مثقال [کذا] خرما چهار مثقال [کذا] و رمپیه
وقیه مپسطون [کذا] صغیر ۲ درم قواس [کذا] یک
وقیه نیم یا طل [کذا] شش اقیه

This anonymous, untitled treatise on alchemical procedures and the preparation of compound medicines is divided into eight *fāyedä,* and these are subdivided into *ṭarīq,* sometimes wrongly styled *fāyedä.* The last section contains a brief discussion of pharmaceutical weights and measures.

No. 206 : MS 100

Anonymous

[*Qarābāẕīn*] [قرابا ذین]

MS 100 (ex Coll. Min.), 77 fols., 100 x 175 mm (*jong*)

Bound in flexible plain black leather; inner covers bare; worn, warped. Written on Russian paper, medium thick, burnished, white. On lacunae see below.

12–13 lines, ca. 50 x 80 mm; black with green rubrics, mostly left out; medium-large, ordinary *shekastä-āmīz.* Catchwords.

Anonymous, undated copy; thirteenth/nineteenth century.

This anonymous dispensatory includes at least 24 *bāb,* as far as can be gathered from this copy:

[3.] (beginning missing) *maʿjūnāt*
[4.] (begins on fol. 13b, 8) *eṭrīfalāt*
[5.] (begins on fol. 15a, 6) *īārajāt*
[6.] (begins on fol. 16a, 8) *aqrāṣ*
[7.] (begins on fol. 24b, -4) *ḥobūb va-moshelä va-ghair-e ān*
[8.] (begins on fol. 30a, 7) *safūfāt*
[9.] (begins on fol. 35b, -4) *ashrebä*
[10.] (begins with rubric on fol. 40a) *shorbat*
[11.] (begins on fol. 45a, 3) *sekanjobīn*
[12.] (begins on fol. 47b, 5) *morabbayāt*
[13.] (begins on fol. 50a, 7) *laʿūqāt*
[14.] (begins on fol. 52a, 4) *maṭbukhāt*
[15.] (begins on fol. 54a, 3) *naqūʿāt*
16. (begins as *bāb* 16 on fol. 55a, 1) *māʾo l-oṣūl*
[17.] (begins on fol. 56a, 5) *naṭūlāt*
[18.] (begins on fol. 58a, 7) *ṣaʿūṭāt*

[19.] (begins on fol. 59b, 7) *qaṭūrāt*
20. (begins as *bāb* 20 on fol. 61a, 1) *shīāfāt-e ʿain* (lacuna between fols. 69 and 70)
[21.?] (beginning missing) [*marham*] or [*ṭelā*]
[22.?] (begins on fol. 70a, -1) *sanūnāt*
[23.?] (begins on fol. 72a, 6) *ghargharāt*
[24.?] (begins on fol. 73a, 6) *żemādāt*; the text breaks off within this *bāb* on fol. 77b.

No. 207 : MS 24 VII

Anonymous

[*Advīä-ye morakkabä*] [ادويهٔ مركّبه]

MS 24 (ex Coll. Min.), 156 fols., 182 x 128 mm; binder's collection of eight works.
[*Advīä-ye morakkabä*] on fols. 111b–120a.

For the description of the MS see **No. 61 : MS 24 I.**

Incipit, fol. 111b, 1

بسمله. الحمد لله الذى خلق لكل داءٍ دواءً [كذا] والهمنا
منافع المفردات والمركبات ... [۱۱۱ب، ٤] وبعد بنابر التماس
من يجب استعانه كلمهٔ چند در بيان بعضى مركبات
مرتب ميرود ...

Explicit, fol. 120a, 2

شياف اخضر جرب وسبل را كه كهنه باشد وغلظة پلك
وناخنه كه بان حرارت نبود زنجار سه درم اسفيداج الرصاص
اشق صمغ عربى نشاسته از هريك يكدرم اشق را در اب
سذاب حل كرده بدان بسرشند وشياف سازند والله
اعلم بالصواب تم

This anonymous, untitled treatise on compound drugs is divided into five *bāb*: 1) decoctions (*sharāyeṭ-e maṭbūkhāt*), 2) electuaries (*maʿājīn*), 3) tablets and pills (*ḥobūb va-aqrāṣ*), 4) enemas and suppositories (*ḥoqan va-fatīlä*), 5) unguents, salves, and ophthalmic drugs (*adhān va-marāhem va-dārūhā-ye čashm*).

No. 208 : MS 28 V

Excerpts

[*Noskhejāt*] [نسخه جات]

MS 28 (ex Coll. Min.), 72 fols., 170 x 110 mm; scribe's collection of four works by Yūsofī and excerpts from various sources. [*Noskhejāt*] on fols. 68–72a.

For the description of the MS see **No. 64 : MS 28 I.**

There is a lacuna in the MS between fols. 67 and 68. The text on fol. 68a begins:

چرب کنند که بسیار نافع است نسخه سکنجبین افتیمونی
معمول میرزا محمد امین ...

On fol. 71a, 1 a quotation from ʿEmādoddīn Maḥmūd Shīrāzī on *āteshak* begins:

بدانکه اتشك در کتب اطبا مسطور نیست و یوسفی
حکیم درین باب خط کرده که نار فارسی وجمره را
از اقسام اتشك شمرده ...

Between fols. 71 and 72 there is another lacuna, and on fol. 72 there follow recipes for *marham-e āteshak.*

No. 209 : MS 29 IX

Roknoddīn

[*Noskhejāt*] [نسخه جات]

MS 29 (ex Coll. Min.), 119 fols., 200 x 135 mm; scribe's collection of ten works. [*Noskhejāt*] on fols. 109–111.

For the description of the MS see **No. 79 : MS 29 I.**

Incipit, fol. 109a, 5

شیخ رکن الدین میفرماید که هرکس این ایه را برنان
نویسد دربرده دهد تا بخورد ...

Explicit, fol. 111b, -5

واگر کسی گذشت خوکرا بیاویزند شب سریك را [؟]
دفع کند والله یعلم

This collection of recipes of medicines for various diseases, titled *favāyed-e okhrī* by the scribe (fol. 109a), was compiled by the otherwise unknown physician Roknoddīn (see Incipit above). They rely largely on magical procedures.

No. 210 : MS 68 III

Moḥammad Kāẓem Ṭabīb-e Khwānsārī Nehāvandī

[*Noskhejāt*] [نسخه جات]

MS 68 (ex Coll. Min.), 132 fols., 205 x 145 mm; binder's collection of seven works in two sections. [*Noskhejāt*] on fols. 53–74.

For the description of the MS see **No. 184 : MS 68 I.**

Incipit, fol. 53b

بسمله. الحمد لله ربّ العالمین والعاقبة للمتقین والصلواة
[کذا] والسلام علی خیر خلقه محمد وآله الطیبین الطاهرین
وهو یشفی بلطفه الکریم ولا حول ولا قوة الا بالله
بدانکه ایدك الله تعالی که دستور فاضل استاد افلاطون
دورانی ...

Explicit, fol. 74a, 9

هرگاه خواسته باشند قدری روغن بادام که بقدر بیست
مثقال باشد علاوه نمایند

This untitled collection of recipes for compound drugs was gathered by an unnamed student of Mīrzā Moḥammad Kāẓem Khūnsārī *aṣlan* Nehāvandī *maskinan* (fol. 53b, 5), who was the author of the recipes communicated here.

Not in PL or Monzavī.

No. 211 : MS 101

Anonymous

[*Noskhejāt*] [نسخه‌جات]

MS 101 (ex Coll. Min.), 20 fols., 88 x 155 mm (*jong*)

Bound in flexible burgundy-colored leather; simple blind-tooled borders; inner covers bare; one flyleaf each in front and back of thin Russian cardboard, printed on one side; binding in mint condition. Binding not original. Written on Eastern paper, medium thick, slightly coarse, greyish.

Varying number of lines on varying surface; different styles of handwriting by different scribes, from *naskh* to *shekastä*.

Anonymous, undated copy; thirteenth/nineteenth century.

This scrapbook contains an anonymous collection of recipes.

No. 212 : MS 58 IV

Materia medica and pharmacopoeia: extracts

MS 58 (ex Coll. Min.), 147 fols., 213 x 153 mm; scribe's collection.
Extracts on fols. 102–117.

For the description of the MS see **No. 135 : MS 58 I.**

Headings of paragraphs:

1. (fol. 102b) باب المراهیم مرهم سفید گوشت را برویاند
2. (fol. 103b) کتاب جواهرنامه

3. (fol. 105a) عقد زيبق
4. (fols. 106b–114a, 8) extracts from the first *maqālä* of *Ekhtīārāt-e Badīʿī* by Ḥājjī Zaino l-ʿAṭṭār (cf. **No. 20 : MS 36**, etc.)
5. (fol. 114a, 9) باب طريق ساختن شربتهای فواكه
6. (fol. 114a, -2) باب طريق ساختن ربوب فواكه
7. (fol. 114b, 2) باب طريق ساختن گل قند آفتابی
8. (fol. 114b, 5) روغن تخمجات وتنكيس وبادام ومثل او
9. (fol. 114b, 11) روغن رياحين
10. (fol. 114b, -2) تقطيرات وتيزابات
11. (fol. 115a, 3) گل حكمت
12. (fol. 115a, 4) تصعيد
13. (fol. 115a, -4) طريق ذبل [كذا]
14. (fol. 115b, 1) باب دربيان تعفين
15. (fol. 115b, -2) آتش مخفی
16. (fol. 116a, 6) ساحتن شربت ادويّه [كذا]
17. (fol. 117b, 1) طريق ساختن اطريفل صغير
18. (fol. 117b, 4) طريق ساختن ايارج فيقرا
19. (fol. 117b, 7) مطلا كردن

No. 213 : MS 58 VIII

Collection of extracts

MS 58 (ex Coll. Min.), 147 fols., 213 x 153 mm; scribe's collection.
Collection of extracts on fols. 134–147.

For the description of the MS see **No. 135 : MS 58 I.**

Headings of paragraphs:

1. (fol. 134a)

در بیان بعضی از رساین حکمای هند
باصطلاح هنود رساین بعضی کیمیای بدنست وآن
مخصوص است بادویهٔ [کذا] وتراکیبی که باعث حفظ
صحّت و طول عمر وتقویهٔ قوی واعضای رئیسه باشد...
[۱۳۴ب ۹،] دیگر رساین تری پلا است وآن عبارت
از هلیلجات است...

2. (fol. 136a; fol. 135b is blank) فصل دربیان عقاقیرهاست باب الالف...

This breaks off on fol. 138a within the letter *kāf*: کمادریوس بلوط الارض

3. (fols. 138b–147a) paragraphs on *jozām, khanāzīr, faṣd, ḥejāmat, maʿajīn,* taken from larger works.

No. 214 : MS 91

Ḥājjī ʿAlī ʿAskar Jarrāḥ and Āqā ʿAbdollāh Ṭabīb

[*Mojarrabāt*] [مجرّبات]

MS 91 (ex Coll. Min.), 101 fols., 85 x 145 mm (*jong*)

Bound in flexible plain black leather; inner covers bare; binding too narrow and too short for MS; worn and torn; MS almost totally out of binding, stitching mostly loose, many leaves unattached. Written on Russian and European papers: 1) fols. 1–75: Russian, medium thick, burnished, cream-colored; 2) fols. 76–101: European, medium thin, burnished, white; watermark: palmetto and G.P.

13–14 lines, 55 x 105 mm, on blind-ruled frame and lines; black with black overlinings; medium-small fair *shekastä*. Catchwords.

Anonymous, undated copy; a *terminus ad quem* is provided by a note on fol. 75b, dated 1246/1830.

Fols. 1a, 76–101, and margins filled with recipes in various hands; among them quotations from *K. minhāj,*[1] *Sharḥ al-Asbāb wa-l-ʿalāmāt,*[2] *Kefāyä-ye Manṣūrī,*[3] *Resālä-ye āteshak,*[4] *Toḥfato l-moʾmenīn,*[5] *Qarābāzīn-e kabīr,*[6] *Ṭebb-e Akbarī,*[7] *K. makhzan,*[8] *K. majmūʿo l-advīä,*[9] *K. Loṭfʿalī Khān*;[10] the following physicians are mentioned: Moḥammad Bāqer,[11] Moḥammad Ḥasan Ṭabīb, Mīrzā ʿAbdo l-Karīm Ṭabīb, Ākhond Mollā ʿAbdo l-Ghanī, Mīr Hāshem,[12] Ḥakīm Hāshem *al-mokhāṭab be-*Ḥakīm Moʿtamado d-dowlä va-l-Moʿtamado l-molūk[13] (*sic*!).

On fol. 1b, etc., an owner's stamp: Muḥammad Ḥusain, dated 1254/1838.

Incipit, fol. 1b

بسمله. از مجربات صاحبی خدایگانی مرحوم حاجی
علی عسکر جراح وسرکار خدایگانی آقا عبد الله طبیب

که بسیار خودشان بتجربه رسانیده اند و مفید است
نسخه شیاف سوزک بطریق فتیله منقول از مرحوم
مزبور حاجی ...

Explicit, fol. 75a, 7

اجزاء مذکوررا ممزوج ساخته ضماد ساخته ضماد نمایند
که بسیار مجرب است

This compilation of recipes on the authority of Ḥājjī ᶜAlī ᶜAskar Jarrāḥ and Āqā ᶜAbdollāh Ṭabīb (see Incipit) was done by an unnamed student of ᶜAlī ᶜAskar.

1. This could mean ibn Jazla's *K. Minhāj al-bayān fī-mā yastaᶜmiluhū l-insān,* or *Minhāj ad-dukkān* by al-Kūhīn al-ᶜAṭṭār (Ullmann, pp. 274–75 and 309, resp.).
2. Probably by Nafīs b. ᶜIwaḍ al-Kirmānī; see Ullmann, p. 170.
3. See **MSS 12–16a.**
4. Perhaps ᶜEmādoddīn Maḥmūd Shīrāzī's treatise on the subject; see **No. 99 : MS 46 II.**
5. See **MSS 115–121.**
6. Possibly ar-Rāzī's *al-Aqrābādhīn al-kabīr* is meant here; see Ullmann, p. 303. It appears more likely, however, that a book of a more recent period of composition is quoted here; a *Qarābāzīn-e kabīr* by Ḥakīm Moḥammad Ḥosain Khān is listed in Charminar, p. 239, no. 97. Possibly this author is identical with Moḥammad Ḥosain b. Moḥammad Hādī ᶜAqīlī ᶜAlavī; see note 8 below.
7. See **No. 131 : MS 122.**
8. Perhaps *Makhzano l-advīä va-tazkerä-ye ūlī n-nohā* by Moḥammad Ḥosain b. Moḥammad Hādī ᶜAqīlī ᶜAlavī; see **No. 140 : MS 89.** A *Makhzano l-advīä* was written by Nāẓemo l-aṭebbāʾ Sayyed Mūsā b. ᶜAqīl; see PL II 323, no. 113.
9. Not identified.
10. Not identified.
11. It is not clear which physician of this name is meant; ᶜEmādoddīn Maḥmūd Shīrāzī had a son Moḥammad Bāqer; see **No. 99 : MS 46 II**; PL II 251 and 264, nos. 428 and 452, resp.
12. These four not identified.
13. This is Moḥammad Hāshem b. Moḥammad Hādī Moᶜtamado l-molūk Sayyed ᶜAlavī Khān; see PL II 273, no. 475; **No. 142 : MS 124 II.**

No. 215 : MS 26 V

Pseudo-Loqman

Maᶜjūn-e nāfeᶜ-e Loqman معجون نافع لقمن

MS 26 (ex Coll. Min.), 103 fols., 178 x 120 mm; binder's collection of eleven works.
Maᶜjūn-e nāfeᶜ-e Loqman on fols. 56b, 1 to 57b.

For the description of the MS see **No. 62 : MS 26 I.**

Incipit, fol. 56b, 1

معجون نافع لقمن. صفت معجون ایست که معده را قوی
کند بلغم را برد ودرد معده ...

Explicit, fol. 57b

این همه را کوفته و بخته با سه وزن داروهاء مذکور شکر
با عسل ضم کرده معجون سازند و هر روز سه درم بخورند

The scribe attributed this recipe to the legendary pre-Islamic Arab sage Loqman.

No. 216 : MS 68 II

Anonymous

[*Moshammaʿāt*] [مشمّعات]

MS 68 (ex Coll. Min.), 132 fols., 205 x 145 mm; binder's collection of seven works in two sections. [*Moshammaʿāt*] on fols. 47–52.

For the description of the MS see **No. 184 : MS 68 I.**

Incipit, fol. 47a

در ذکر مشمعات اول مشمع مرداسنگ صفت آن
بگیرند مرداسنگ

Explicit, fol. 52b, -5

ازجهة رفع حموضت معده و حشاء حامض
وحرقة البول وکثرت سیلان ماده بسیار مفید
ونافع میباشد تاریخ ...

Fols. 47–52 contain a short collection of recipes, in the heading called *dar zekr-e moshammaʿāt* (see Incipit).

No. 217 : MS Ar. 96 VIII

Anonymous

[*Advīä*] [ادویه]

MS Ar. 96 (ex Coll. Min.), 159 fols., 212 x 150 mm; binder's collection of eight Arabic and Persian texts. [*Advīä*] on five loose leaves lying at the back of the MS.

For the description of the MS see **No. 144 : MS Ar. 96 I.**

Incipit, fol. 1a

می توان داد وبجهت [درهامش: بحسب] مزاج
مریض وبقرار قوّة آن ومقابل جلب طرطیر باید
واقل اوکنند وطریقه دیگر...

Explicit, fol. 5b, -1

وباید که نیم گرم باشد بگرمی شیر تازه دوشیده شکم
بکلّی پاك وخالی باشد]

These leaves are a fragment of an unidentified pharmacopoeia, composed in the nineteenth century, as is evidenced by European terms, e.g., طرطیر and ایپ ککوانا (fol. 1a, 1 and fol. 5b, 8, resp.).

No. 218 : MS 70

Pseudo-ᶜAlī b. Mūsā ar-Riḍā

Resālä-ye ẕahabīyä رسالهٔ ذهبیّة

MS 70 (ex Coll. Min.), 18 fols., 143 x 80 mm

Bound in dark brown leather over stiff cardboard; blind-tooled patterned borders and three-medallion design with blind-stamped floral scrolls; inner covers pasted with light blueish-grey paper; four flyleaves each in front and back of beige onionskin paper; binding virtually in mint condition. Binding not original. Written on Eastern paper, medium thin, slightly transparent, burnished, greyish; lacunae (see below) filled with similar paper; handwriting often obliterated by ink smears; whole MS restored.

10 lines, 90 x 45 mm, on blind-ruled frame and lines; borders of black, gold, two black, blue lines; two black hairlines close to edges; on fol. 1b *sarlowḥ*, left white except for frame; *basmala* written in white cloud on gold; black with crimson rubrics; medium-small, fine *nastaʿlīq*. Catchwords. Fols. 8–10, 15, and later substitutions, blank; fol. 18b has border, but no text.

Copied, and dated 1289/1872, by Ḥosain al-Mūsavī for *Ḥakīmbashī-ye dowlat-e ʿalīyä-ye Īrān* Āqā Mīrzā Mūsā Khān as a primer for Mūsā Khān's son Mīrzā Masīḥ Khān.

Incipit, fol. 1b

بسمله. بر ضمایر آگاه دلهای ارباب هوش پوشیده
نیست که نزهت طلبان ریاض معانی را شکفته
چمنی باین طراوت مشام آرا و تمام فیض گلشنی باین
شادمان نزهت نبوده...

Explicit, fol. 17a, -2

پس باید که بدین منوال طریقه صحت نگاه داری
و نفس خودرا در فرض هستداری [؟]

In this copy of *Resālä-ye zahabīyä* (see scribe's subscription, fol. 17b, 5), there are lacunae between fols. 7 and 11, and 14 and 16, later filled in with blanks, fols. 8–10, 15, resp.

The text of *Resālä-ye zahabīyä* that is represented in **MSS 70** and **71** is obviously identical with a version listed in Monzavī I 501a, nos. 4646–48 (copies no older than thirteenth/nineteenth century).

Cf. PL II 196, no. 350; Monzavī I 498b, nos. 4625–48; see also above in text.

No. 219 : MS 71

Pseudo-ʿAlī b. Mūsā ar-Riḍā

Resālä-ye zahabīyä

رسالهٔ ذهبیّه

MS 71 (ex Coll. Min.), 16 fols., 138 x 90 mm

Binding the same as in **MS 70**, except that the leather is dyed yellow; binding not original. Written on Russian (?) paper, medium thin, burnished, white; somewhat worn.

10 lines, 85 x 40 mm, on blind-ruled frame and lines; black with crimson rubrics; medium-small, fine *nastaʿlīq*. Catchwords. Fols. 1a, 16b blank.

Anonymous, undated copy; second half of thirteenth century/ca. 1835–80.

Incipit, fol. 1b, and Explicit, fol. 16b, -2, as in **No. 218 : MS 70.**

No. 220 : MS 96

Anonymous

Untitled treatise on alchemy, magic, and therapeutics

MS 96 (ex Coll. Min.), 177 fols., 186 x 132 mm

Bound in plain burgundy-colored leather over slightly flexible cardboard; inner covers pasted with white and grey paper in front and back resp.; two flyleaves in front, four in back, partly of Russian paper; binding worn and torn, spine repaired. Binding not original. Written on Eastern paper, thin to medium thin, transparent, burnished, cream-colored; some spots and stains; edges torn, repaired in greenish-grey Russian paper. On lacunae see below.

13 lines, 140 x 70 mm, on blind-ruled frame and lines; black with red rubrics; some designs for amulets in red; medium-sized good *nastaʿlīq*. Catchwords.

Collations by scribe.

Anonymous, undated copy (end missing); ca. 1100/1700.

Marginal notes by readers.

Incipit, fol. 1a

درج کرده شد از نصایح وسنن مرضیه تا طالبان زود
بمطلوب رسند وصواب ثمرات وخیرات این مجموعه
عجیب وغریب پادشاه عهد زمان ابراهیم
شاه سلطان مندرج باد آمین رب العالمین

The treatise represented by this MS is divided into 48 *bāb*, some of which are further divided into *faṣl*; in the beginning, one or two fols. are missing, containing the preface, and in the end, part of the last *bāb*, no. 48, is lost. No title or author's name is preserved in this copy. At the end of the preface it is said that this treatise is dedicated to Ebrāhīm Shāh Solṭān (see Incipit); he could not be identified.

There is a complete table of all 48 *bāb* on fols. 1a, 4 to 3b, -2:

1. در معني كلا مهاخر ا يتعالى عز وجل ونقش خاتم
سليمان عليه السلام وصفت ساختن آيينه زرين
وانچه خاصه بمعني فتح وظفر يافتن برخصمان ونگاهداشتن
خودرا ازاعدا

2. در معني دلايل فتح وظفر ونصرت برخصمان وبرلشكرهاء
انبوه وضبط كردن حصار بعلم امير المومنين علي رضي الله
عنه ودر معني انواع روحانيات ودريافتن كمين ومكر
دشمنان وساختن داروازكه درگوش اسب كند

3. (in nine *faṣl*)
در معني استخراج حكمت ارسطاطاليس حكيم كه بجهت
سلطان سكندر ذو القرنين رومي ساخته بود ودانستن
غالب ومغلوب

4. (in four *faṣl*)
در معني سلاحها پوشيدني كه درغايت سبكي وتنگي
باشد وهيچ سلاحي بران كار نكند وآب دادن
سلاحها كه بغايت برندگي وتيزي باشد وآنچه
هلاك كننده باشد ومرحم [كذا] بپذيرد [؟]

5. (in two *faṣl*)
در معني شكستن وباطل كردن دروازهاي آهنين
بنوعي وشكستن آهن وبرون نقش زر ازروي
سكه واشرفي بماليدن دست از قوت دارو

6. (in two *faṣl*)
در معني زيادت شدن حفظ وهوشياري وقوت عاقله
ورايهاي صواب واند يشهاي موافق <و> دريافتن كارهاي

مشکل و یاد کردن چیزهای گذشته و دیرینه و دانستن آبها
که درکدام موضع نزدیك است یا دوراست بجهت
کاویدن چاه و حوض

7. (in four *faṣl*)

درمعنی آتش زدن و بستر[؟] درمردمان و برچهارپایان
وکاه دانهای حصارکافران ومفسدان وفرستادن پیکان
وجاسوسان

8. (in two *faṣl*)

درمعنی آنکه درنظرخلقان با هیبت وعظمت باشد
وزبان همه خلقان برو بسته گردد ومطیع ومسخر اوگردد

9. (in four *faṣl*)

درمعنی حیوانات رونده وپرنده ونباتات وجمادات
وحاضتهای[کذا] ایشان

10. (in three *faṣl*)

درمعنی کیمیای قصیر ومسخرکردن جن وانس
واختصار طلایه

11. (in six *faṣl*)

درمعنی علمهای[کذا] مروارید ومرجان ورنگ
کردن سنگ بلور وعقد ژاله وعمله کافور وعملهای[کذا]
دیگر

12. (in four *faṣl*)

درمعنی معرفت اوقات سعد ونحس اختیارات وحجامت
کردن وفصد کردن وجامه نو بریدن ونو پوشیدن

13.

درمعنی دفع برف وژاله وموش وملخ وجانوران شیرومار
وکژدم وجمله گزندهگان ودرندهگان گرد او وگرد خانه
او وکشت او نگردد

14. درمعنی پیدا کردن دزد که دزدی کرده باشد بانواع حکمت حکماست

15. درمعنی غایب شدن از نظر خلقان و دریافتن وفای حکماء هند این نوع کوکه وا حو خوانند

16. درمعنی طلسمات وعجایبات از هر نوع نموده میشود

17. درعلاج درد سر ونیم سر وزکام ونزله ودراز شدن موی ودفع مستی

18. درعلاج دیوانگی وماخولیا [کذا] وبیهوشی ودوران سر

19. درعلاج خون بینی

20. درعلاج چشم

21. درعلاج گوش

22. درعلاج دمل وپختگی جراحت

23. درعلاج درد دندان ومحکم شدن بیخ دندان

24. درعلاج دفع ناسور وبواسیر

25. درعلاج قضیب وخصیه

26. درعلاج باد صرع

27. درعلاج باد خوره

28.
در علاج رشته

29.
در علاج هژده نوع جذام و برص

30.
در علاج سوختگی آتش و داغ آن

31.
در علاج زخم تیر و تیغ وغیره

32.
در علاج دفع مار و کژدم

33.
در علاج دیو و پری و کفتار

34.
در گرفتن حمل و دانستن کیفیت آن

35.
در علاج نهادن حمل عورت که بدرد زه مانده باشد

36.
در علاج اسقاط حمل و منع حمل

37.
در علاج افزوني شیر عورت که در پستان کم شده باشد

38.
در علاج گرد آمدن و محکم شدن پستان که سست شده باشد

39.
در علاج زیادت شدن لذت در جماع و تنگ ساختن فرج

40.
در معنی غذاهاي که باه بیفزاید و مني را زیادت کنند

41.
در علاج الفاظ [کذا. یعنی لفاظ؟] وامساك مني وادویه لذت مرد و زن

42.
در ساختن معجونات و مفرحات

43.
در علاج ساختن کل

44. درمعنى خضاب

45. دربيان حلوها و شيرينها

46. درمعنى ساختن سركه كه مريض
ومخموررا نافع آيد

47. درمعنى اختيارات سى روزه از قول پيغمبر
صلى الله عليه واله وسلم

48. درخواص اشياء متفرقه

The MS breaks off within *bāb* 48 (begins on fol. 177a, -4) on fol. 177b.

No. 221 : MS Ar. 53 II

Anonymous

al-Qīāfato n-nafsānīyä fī tartīb-e nowʿo l-ensānīyä

القيافة النفسانيه فى ترتيب نوع الانسانيه

MS Ar. 53 (ex Coll. Min.), 138 fols., 165 x 100 mm; binder's collection of several Arabic and two Persian medical texts. (See also **No. 149 : MS Ar. 53 III**.)
al-Qīāfato n-nafsānīyä fī tartīb-e nowʿo l-ensānīyä on pp. 26–146.

Bound in brown leather over stiff thick cardboard; simple blind-tooled borders; inner covers pasted with white Russian paper. Binding somewhat worn, especially along edges and around corners. Written on white Russian paper, medium thin, burnished.

Two Persian texts, pp. 26–146, 151–263: 13–16 lines, ca. 130 x 65 mm, on blind-ruled frame and lines; black; large, careless hand, vacillating between *naskh* and *shekastä*. Catchwords. Pages 147, 149, 150, 264–275 blank. Modern stamped pagination.

Copied, and dated Ṭehrān, Saturday, 28 Zū l-ḥejjä 1293/*Sunday*, 14 January 1877, by abū l-Ḥasan al-Ḥosainī al-Aʿrajī aṭ-Ṭabīb *al-molaqqab be-*Aresṭū an-Najafī *maskinan wa-madfinan inshāʾa llāh.*

On p. 148 a sketch of the human skull seen from the back, with numbered parts.

Incipit, p. 26, 1

کتاب القیافه. بسمله.
حمد خداوندی تعالی وتقدس سزاست که
باکمال نهانی از عقول وافهام ومدارك اوهام در
هر موجودی طریق ازمعرفت خد نهاده...

Explicit, p. 146, 8

جهة شهرت ومعروف گوئی بتکمیل
دراین علم مشغول گردد تمت
الرسالة المسماة بالقیافة النفسانیة فی ترتیب
نوع الانسانیة...

This anonymous treatise on physiognomy is divided into a *moqaddemä,* three *bayān,* and a *khātemä* (p. 28, 1). It was composed in 1287/1870 (p. 27, 12). In the scribe's subscription, its title is given as *al-Qīāfato n-nafsānīyä fī tartīb-e now*ᶜ*o l-ensānīä* (p. 146, 10).

Not in PL or Monzavī.

No. 222 : MS 69

Fożūlī (?)

[*Qeṣṣä-ye rūḥ*] [قصّهٔ روح]

MS 69 (ex Coll. Min.), 11 fols., 175 x 110 mm

Unbound, loose leaves in a folder of onionskin paper, off-white; most leaves torn at fold, no stitching. Written on Russian paper, medium thick, burnished, cream-colored. For lacunae see below.

10–15 lines, 120 x 68 mm, on blind-ruled frame and lines; black with black overlinings; according to the number of lines, medium-small to medium-sized, distinguished *nasta*ᶜ*līq.* Catchwords.

Collations by reader.

Anonymous, undated copy (end missing); ca. 1300/1900.

Incipit, fol. 1b

بسمله. حمد بحد خدایرا سزاست که ریاض بدن را
بآب روان پرورده وحسن را مظهر عشق و عشق را
زیور حسن کرده ودرود بیعدد معتمدیرا
رواست که علم او عقل را پیرایه است
وعقل او علم را سرمایه معتکف زاویه عجز
وانکسار فضولی خاکسار از محرکان سلاسل
حکایت و مؤسسان مبانی روایت چنین
نقل دارد . .

Explicit, fol. 11b, -2

اسکندر آینهٔ درانجا ساخته وعاد طرح ارم
درانجا انداخته به سی ونه قرن ازو مأثور
بدین سبب نامش بسینه مشهور از انجا
بمنزل رسیدند شنیدند که دراین]

The author of this untitled romance of the human soul, *rūḥ*, is called Fożūlī in this MS (fol. 1b, 4), not *Afżal*, as in the India Office MS of *Qeṣṣä-ye rūḥ*.[1] According to Ethé, the allegory follows the model of Fattāḥī's *Ḥosn-va Del*.[2] The soul, born in the world of omnipotence, *ʿālam-e jabrūt*, and dwelling on the plain of divinity, *fażā-ye lāhūt*, one day conceives a desire to travel and puts his (her?) foot into the world of humanity, *ʿālam-e nāsūt*. ***Rūḥ*** sees a country, *dīār*, called body, ***badan***, consisting of seven provinces, ***keshvar*** (not climes in this MS[3]), which are its limbs or parts, *andāmhā*; these are ruled by four brothers: blood, ***khūn***, yellow bile, *ṣafrā*, black bile, *sowdā*, and phlegm, ***balgham***. Successively all components and faculties of the human body are introduced in a similar fashion. This MS breaks off after the breast, *sīnä*, is reached on the soul's travels (see Explicit).

Since both the MS described by Ethé and this one are of recent date, the time of composition cannot in any way be exactly determined.

1. Ethé I 1591, no. 2929.
2. Fattāḥī died in 852/1448; on him see EI² II 865a, s.v. Fattāḥī [Bausani].
3. See Ethé (note 1 above) for reference.

See note 1 above for references to other MSS.

Index of Titles

The following index lists all titles of sources mentioned in this catalogue. In Part I, titles originally written in Arabic characters are entered in the order of the Arabic alphabet, without regard to different transcriptions of Arabic, Persian, and Turkish. Part II includes titles in other languages, in the order of the Roman alphabet. Titles of works contained in UCLA manuscripts are preceded by a †.

I

II

Index of Proper Names

With the exception of modern editors of texts and cataloguers of manuscript collections, all names occurring in this catalogue are here included.

I. Names Originally in Arabic or Hebrew Script

Listed according to the Persian-Arabic alphabet, *ibn* (b.), *abū* (a.), and the Arabic article being disregarded; the latter most often represented by a hyphen in front of the following word, e.g., -Ḥosainī. Alphabetical order is determined by (1) proper names in the strict sense (*ism ʿalam*), (2) elements following them, and, only when necessary, (3) elements preceding them. Brief identifications have been added in parentheses.

II. Other Names, Including Those in Watermarks

Index of Incipits

The following index lists only works the proper Incipits of which are preserved in the respective UCLA manuscripts. Texts have been divided into two groups, the first beginning with the customary eulogies and the other containing no such formulas, without appearing to be acephalous. The order within each group is strictly alphabetical; *basmala* and scribes' invocations of divine help having been left out, texts of the first group begin with *ḥamdala* in Arabic or Persian. The orthography adopted here does not follow peculiarities of individual manuscripts.

I. Incipits with eulogies

No. 103 : MS 46 V

الحمد لك والصلوة على رسولك بعد از
توفيق فراغ اربيان معالجه بفصد...

[رسالهٔ حجامه]

No. 148 : MS 61 III

الحمد لله الحكيم العليم الذّى يشفى بلطفه
السقيم والصلوة والسلام على من أوتى
بالدين القويم وعلى آله وأولاده الذّين...

مجمع التجارب

No. 88 : MS 105 II, et seqq.

الحمد لله الحكيم العليم والصلوة على من
أوتى الحكمة والكتاب الكريم وهو يشفى...

[قرابادين شفائى]

No. 160 : MS 26 XI

الحمد لله الّذى أرسل بالهدى من قال
العلم علمان...

[حفظ الصحّه]

No. 42 : MS 21

الحمد لله الّذى خلق الإنسان وجعله
أشرف مواليد الأركان والصلوة...

زبدة قوانين العلاج

No. 166 : MS 66 III

الحمد لله الّذى خلق السموات والارض
وصلّى الله على خير خلقه محمّد وآله
أجمعين الطيّبين الطاهرين امّا بعد...

مختصرة العوامّ

No. 207 : MS 24 VII

الحمد لله الذی خلق لکلّ داء دواء وألهمنا
منافع المفردات والمرکّبات .. [ادویهٔ مرکّبه]

No. 140 : MS 89

الحمد لله الذی عرفنا بنفسه وهدانا اولی النهی
بحمده وجعلنا من امّة حبیبه .. مخزن الادویه وتذکرة

No. 107 : MS 83

الحمد لله الکریم الجلیل الذی یشفی
بکمال حکمته ولطفه السقیم والعلیل .. [رسالهٔ چوب چینی]

No. 100 : MS Ar. 41 II, et seqq.

الحمد لله المحمود فی کلّ فعاله والصلوة
علی سیّدنا محمّد محمود احمد وآله
چون مرض که معروف بآتشک ... رسالهٔ آتشک

Nos. 47, 84 : MSS 25 VII, 29 IV, et seq.

الحمد لله المنعم لحیوة النفوس وصحّة الاجسام
والصلوة والسلام علی واضع قانون الشرع .. ستّهٔ ضروریّه

No. 77 : MS 24 II, et seqq.

الحمد لله النافع الحکیم العلّام والصلوة
علی زبدة الانبیاء ... دلایل النبض

No. 195 : MS 80

الحمد لله حقّ حمده والصلوة علی نبیّه
محمّد وآله اجمعین امّا بدان که .. مختصر مفید

No. 2 : MS 1, et seqq.

الحمد لله ربّ العالمین حمد الشاکرین
والصلوة علی نبیّه المصطفی
وآله اجمعین چون بتقدیر... ذخیرهٔ خوارزمشاهی

No. 14 : MS 11 *(see p. 21)*

الحمد لله ربّ العالمین حمد الشاکرین والصلوة
والسلام علی النبیّ المصطفی محمّد وآله
الطاهرین باید ... یادگار

No. 164 : MS 54 I

الحمد لله ربّ العالمین والصلوة علی رسوله
محمّد وآله اجمعین بدان که حق سبحانه... عین الحیوة

No. 19 : MS 56 II

الحمد لله ربّ العالمين والصلوة والسلام
على خير خلقه محمّد وآله اجمعين اعلم... القانونچة في الطبّ

No. 87 : MS 22 II

الحمد لله ربّ العالمين والصلوة والسلام
على خير خلقه محمّد وآله اجمعين امّا بعد... [رساله در بيخ چينى]

No. 138 : MS 59 I, et seq.

الحمد لله ربّ العالمين والصلوة والسلام
على خير خلقه محمّد وآله اجمعين امّا بعد... مفتاح الشفاء

No. 16 : MS 61 II

الحمد لله ربّ العالمين والصلوة والسلام
على خير خلقه محمّد وآله اجمعين وبعد... نزهة الملوك

No. 184 : MS 68 I

الحمد لله ربّ العالمين والصلوة والسلام
على خير خلقه محمّد وآله الطاهرين امّا بعد... [كحّالى]

No. 152 : MS 103

الحمد لله ربّ العالمين ∴ والصلوة والسلام
على خير خلقه محمّد وآله الطاهرين قال الشيخ... بسايط النبض

No. 44 : MS 22 I

الحمد لله ربّ العالمين والصلوة والسلام
على رسوله وحبيبه محمّد وآله
الطيّبين الطاهرين بدان كه... رسالهٔ ينبوع

No. 133 : MS 124 I

الحمد لله ربّ العالمين والصلوة والسلام
على سيّد المرسلين وعلى آله الطاهرين
امّا بعد... ميزان الطب

No. 132 : MS 123

الحمد لله ربّ العالمين والصلوة والسلام
على سيّد المرسلين وعلى آله واصحابه
اجمعين امّا بعد... مفرّح القلوب

No. 113 : MS 46 VII, et seq.

الحمد لله ربّ العالمين والصلوة والسلام
على محمّد خاتم المرسلين وخير البشر
على بن ابى طالب امير المؤمنين... [رساله در چوب چينى وقهوه وچاى]

No. 15 : MS 84

تقويم الصحّة

الحمد لله ربّ العالمين والصلوة والسلام
على نبيّه محمّد وآله اجمعين امّا بعد ...

No. 9 : MS 8, et seqq.

خفّى علائى

الحمد لله ربّ العالمين والعاقبة للمتقين
والصلوة على محمّد وآله اجمعين چون ...

No. 1 : MS 74 I

نور العيون

الحمد لله ربّ العالمين والعاقبة للمتّقين
ولا عدوان الّا على الظالمين وصلّى
الله على خير خلقه محمّد وآله الطاهرين ...

No. 210 : MS 68 III

[نسخه جات]

الحمد لله ربّ العالمين والعاقبة للمتّقين
والصلوة والسلام على خير خلقه محمّد
وآله الطيّبين الطاهرين وهو يشفى ...

No. 186 : MS 78 I, et seq.

نزهة الملوك

الحمد لله ربّ العالمين والعاقبة للمتّقين
والصلوة والسلام على رسوله محمّد وآله
اجمعين بدان كه ...

No. 180 : MS 86 IV

زبدة التجارات

الحمد لله ربّ العالمين والعاقبة للمتّقين
والصلوة والسلام على رسوله محمّد
وآله واصحابه اجمعين امّا ...

No. 154 : MS 74 II

تذكرة الكحّالين

الحمد لله ربّ العالمين وصلوته على محمّد
وآله اجمعين گفتار نخستين يادكنيم
در چشم وشرح دهيم ...

No. 20 : MS 36, et seqq.

اختيارات بديعى

امداد حمد بيحد واعداد سپاس
بيقياس مبدعى را كه آثار ابداع او
برهر ورقى از اوراق ...

Nos. 47, 54 : MSS 25 VIII, 24 IV, et seqq.

فواير اخيار

بدان چونكه گفتى سپاس ودرود ...

Reference	Title	Incipit
No. 218 : MS 70, et seq.	رسالهٔ ذهبیّه	بر ضمایر آگاه دلهای ارباب هوش پوشیده نیست که نزهت طالبان ریاض معانی را شگفته چمنی ...
No. 129 : MS 55	صالح العلاج	بر ضمیر منیر ارباب دانش و خاطر الباب بینش پوشیده نماند که نعت جلال احدیّت ...
No. 146 : MS 65	کیمیاء الشفاء	بر مبتدیان ترکیب معاجین جواهر انشاء اهم و واجب و بر متصدّیان تخمیر خمیرهٔ زواهر معنی لازم ...
Nos. 47, 75 : MSS 25 II, 26 III, et seq.	قصیده در حفظ صحّت	بعد از حمد حکیم دانا و تحیّت زبده رسل و انبیاء ...
No. 80 : MS 24 III, et seqq.	دلایل البول	بعد از سپاس حکیم مطلق جلّ ذکره و بعد از درود رسول برحق ...
No. 125 : MS 50	رؤوس المسائل	بعد از طی مراتب حمد و ثنای حکیم علی الاطلاق جلّت آلاءه ...
No. 179 : MS 58 VII	[معالجات]	بنام نگارندهٔ تحت و فوق که شد منبت عقل جان مست ...
No. 130 : MS 125	قرابادین قادری	ثنائی که شایان جناب مستطاب حضرت الهی تعالی است بجزوی نباید ...
No. 46 : MS 23	خلاصة التجارب	حمد بلا احصی حکیمی را سزد که بکمال حکمت و وفور عنایت ...
No. 222 : MS 69	قصّهٔ روح	حمد بیحد خدای را سزا است که ریاض بدن را بآب روان پرورده و حسن را مظهر عشق و عشق را ...

No. 106 : MS 82

حمد بیحد وسپاس بیعد مر حکیمی را
که دقایق حکمت او بیپایان است ... تحفهٔ خانیه

No. 147 : MS 57 II

حمد بیحد وستایش لا تحصی ولا تعدّ
نثار بارگاه وایثار پیشگاه کبریای حکیمی است ... ترجمهٔ برؤ الساعه

No. 221 : MS Ar. 53 II

حمد خداوندی تعالی وتقدّس
سزا است که با کمال نهانی ترتیب نوع الانسانیّة
از عقول وافهام ومدارك اوهام ... القیافة النفسانیّة فی

No. 108 : MS 86 V

حمد خداوندی را کش بدر کبریا
هست برابر بهم حشمت شاه گدا ... مفردات صحیح

Nos. 47, 61 : MSS 25 VI, 24 I, et seqq.

حمد نامحدود حکیمی را که بقانون حکمت
وکامل الصناعة رحمت رافع انواع امراض ... جامع الفواید

No. 126 : MS 47

حمد وثنائی که روایح عطر آن مجالس
خلوت نشینان عالم ملکوت را معطّر دارد ... [رسالهٔ حفظ صحّت]

No. 86 : MS 57 III

حمد وثنای بیشمار خالقی را که آثار
متنوّعه او در مخلوقات ظاهر وپیدا است ... فواید سعدیّه

No. 111 : MS Ar. 110

حمد وسپاس حکیمی را سزاست که
بحکمت کامله کیفیت مزاج را از
التیام عناصر متضادّه مختلف الاثر ساخته ... طبّ الائمّة

No. 105 : MS 88

حمد وسپاس سزاوار حکیمی است
که ترکیب بدن انسان را ... [رساله در تریاق کبیر]

No. 128 : MS 51

حمد وستایش * وسپاس بیقیاس
خالی از آلایش * که سواطع روایح ... حدیقة الحیوة

No. 141 : MS 104	حمدی که از کیفیت نشوهٔ مفرّح راح ریحان مجمع البیان عباراتش که...	بدایع الفنون
No. 47 : MS 25 IX, et seqq.	زبان را چه در اوّل این کلام زحمد و تحیّت...	تدبیر مأکول و مشروب
No. 127 : MS 73 II	سبحان الله رنگ آمیزی بساط حمد و سپاس حکیمی را که خرقه معرفت را بر قامت صحیح مزاجان...	خرقه
No. 127 : MS 73 II	سبحانك اللهمّ یا ذا الملك القدیم و یا طبیب کلّ الیم و سقیم...	خرقه
No. 115 : MS 115, et seqq.	سبحانك اللهمّ یا قدّوس و یا طبیب النفوس أتمّ لنا أنوار معرفتك و ارزقنا...	تحفة المؤمنین
No. 144 : MS Ar. 96 I	سبحانك اللهمّ یا من یداوی الارواح بطبّ الحقیقة و یعالج القلوب بحکمة الطریقة...	مرکّبات جوهریّة
No. 135 : MS 58 I, et seqq.	سپاس افزون از خواهش بیماران بشفاء و ستایش متجاوز از شوق دردمندان بلقاء...	زاد المسافرین
No. 182 : MS 76	سپاس بیقیاس بصیری را که دیده بصیرت اولی الابصار در ادراك الوان مصنوعات...	کنز الکحّالین
No. 159 : MS 124 IV	سپاس بیکران و ستایش بیپایان مر حکیم مطلق را سزد که...	دستور الفصد
No. 14 : MS 11	سپاس و ستایش مر خدای را عزّ و جلّ که منزّه است از هر جسد که...	یادگار

No. 124 : MS 49

سپاسی چون انفاس عیسوی روح پروا
وجان فزا * سزای بارگاه کبریای خالق است... عین الحیوة

No. 143 : MS 63

ستایش بیقیاس تحفه بارگاه حکیمی که
کلیّات عالم اسباب از مفردات مشیّتش... تذکرة العلاج

No. 43 : MS 77 V

سزاوار ستایش وسپاس مبدعی است
که باقتضای ذاتی او که... دانشنامهٔ جهان

No. 31 : MS 45

شکر نامحدود وسپاس نامعدود
خالقی را که هر ذرّه از ذرّات... دستور الاطبّاء عن قواعد الحکماء

No. 38 : MS 17, et seq.

شکر وسپاس پادشاهی را سزد وحمد
وثنای بیقیاس خالقی را که در
خلقت انسان دقایق حکمتش... [تشریح بدن انسان]

No. 197 : MS 73 IV

شکر وسپاس خالقی را که بقدرت کامله
ابداع جواهر عقلیّهٔ مجرّده نموده
وبتوسّط آنها اختراع اجرام مختلفه فرموده... انیس المجالس

No. 32 : MS 12, et seqq.

شکر وسپاس مر خالقی را که در خلقت
انسان دقایق حکمت بیپایان است... کفایهٔ مجاهدیّه

No. 175 : MS 52

لآلی تسبیح لباسی که موجب تحلیه
وتحلّی سامعه تکرار اذکار ساکنان
عالم بالا ویواقیت تمجید وتقدیس... مرصاد الاطبّاء

No. 157 : MS Ar. 60 II

لطایف حمد وثنا حکیمی را سزد که
بهر تشریح ابدان انسان وترویح
اجسام ایشان انوار حکمتش... خلاصة التشریح

No. 174 : MS 53

منهاج ادویه شفا حمد مسبّب
الاسباب است... منهاج المبتدئین

No. 110 : MS 105 I

هوالله الاحد الله الصمد که پایهٔ حقیقت
بیچونیش از دایرهٔ دریافت
واحاطهٔ شناخت برتر است ...

الفاظ ادویه

No. 153 : MS 64

یا مسهّل الصعاب سهّل لنا سلوك
طریق الصواب ...

[تشریح الامعاء]

II. Incipits without eulogies

No. 194 : MS 66 I

ادویهٔ قوی مقوی مرحرّ ابشن [؟] ...

[تقویم ادویه]

No. 196 : MS 81

ارسطاطالیس حکیم گفت هرکه
خاتم عقیق در انگشت دارد ...

[جواهرنامه]

No. 214 : MS 91

از مجرّبات صاحبی خدایگانی مرحوم
حاجّی علی عسکر جرّاح ...

[مجرّبات]

No. 204 : MS 120 II

این رسالهٔ است در باب اوزان ومکائیل
مصطلحه درمیان اطبّاء حبّه یك جو ...

[رساله در باب اوزان ومکائیل]

No. 155 : MS 124 III

این رساله مرتّب گشته برده مقاله
مقاله اوّل در امور طبیعی ...

[رسالهٔ قانونچهٔ فارسی]

No. 189 : MS 72 I

این مختصری است درباره ملتقط از
کتب طبّی مشتمل برچند فصل ...

تحفة السلطان

No. 192 : MS 25 XI

این مقاله برهفت تقویم است
تقویم اوّل در اغذیه ...

[رساله درخواص اشیاء]

No. 190 : MS 54 II

این نسخه است مفردات حکمت ملخّص
اختیارات بدیعی وبعضی کتب دیگر ...

[فرهنگ ادویه]

Entry	Title	Incipit
No. 201 : MS 54 III	[الفاظ ادويه]	باب الالف اره[؟] واسقيل ...
No. 165 : MS 66 II	[معالجات]	باب در امراض اذن وجع اذن چند نوع ...
No. 172 : MS 93 IV	[مثنوى در طب]	بحكمت همه حالها بگذران نگهدار تواند دار [كذا] ...
No. 152 : MS 103	بسايط النبض	بسايط النبض طويل دلّ على كثرة الحرارة ...
No. 104 : MS 87 II	[رسالۀ يخ چينى]	پوشيده نماند كه اين يخ در اين تاريخ مردم برآن اطّلاع ...
No. 150 : MS 62	برؤ الساعه	چنين گويد حكيم كامل فيلسوف فاضل محمّد بن زكريّاء الرازى ...
No. 151 : MS 29 X	برؤ الساعه	چنين گويد محمّد بن زكريّاء رازى طبيب كه در وقتى از اوقات در مجلس ...
No. 149 : MS Ar. 53 III	بدايع الحكمة ناصرى	چون بروزگار دولت ابدمدّت اعليحضرت سلطان ...
No. 112 : MS 26 IV	[طلب قوّت باه]	حكيم حاذق كامل نظام دولت ودين كه با تو چرخ ستيزه نماى نستيزد ...
No. 142 : MS 124 II	خلاصة قوانين العلاج	در ذكر خلاصة قوانين العلاج امراض بدن صداع بمعنى درد سر ...
No. 216 : MS 68 II	[در مشمّعات]	در ذكر مشمّعات اوّل مشمّع مردارسنگ صفت آن ...
No. 185 : MS Ar. 96 VI	[كحّالى]	در علاج چشم نوع الاوّل كه از خون باشد ...

	Title	Incipit
No. 215 : MS 26 V	معجون نافع لقمس	معجون نافع لقمس صفت معجونی است که معده را قوی کند...
No. 47 : MS 25 III	قصیده در لغات هندی	نام هر چیزی بهندی بشنو از من...
No. 203 : MS 73 III	[تفسیر اصطلاحات یونانیّة]	هذا تفسير كلمات يونانيّة وغيرها مستعملة في الطبّ ماليقراطون...
No. 173 : MS 29 VIII	[قطعه در طعم بد]	هر آن کوی بدرد ز خواب برخست...

Chronological List of Datable Works

A.H.	Title of Work	No. : MS
480	*Nūro l-ʿoyūn*	1 : 74 I
504-06	*Zakhīrä-ye Khwārezmshāhī*	2 : 1, et seqq.
506	*Khoffī-ye ʿAlāʾī*	9 : 8, et seqq.
[between 521 and 535]	*al-Aghrāżo ṭ-ṭebbīyä va-l-mabāheṣo l-ʿalāʾīyä*	13 : 6
[before 535]	*Yādgār*	14 : 11
[ca. 685]	*Ghīāṣīyä*	17 : 20, et seq.
[before 690]	*Taqvīmo ṣ-ṣeḥḥä*	15 : 84, et seq.
[before 745]	*al-Qānūnja fī ṭ-ṭibb*	19 : 56 II
770	*Ekhtīārāt-e Badīʿī*	20 : 36, et seqq.
[between 786 and 789]	*Kefāyä-ye Mojāhedīyä*	32 : 12, et seqq.
[ca. 800]	[*Tashrīḥ-e badan-e ensān*]	38 : 17, et seq.
[between 812 and 817]	[*Qarābāzīn*]	40 : 24 VIII
839	*Dastūro l-aṭebbāʾ ʿan qavāʿedo l-ḥokamāʾ*	31 : 45
[between 807 and 850]	*Sharāyeṭ-e jarrāḥī*	41 : 61 I
871	*Zobdat-e qavānīno l-ʿelāj*	42 : 21
879	*Dāneshnāmä-ye jahān*	43 : 77 V
[before 900]	*Resālä-ye yanbūʿ*	44 : 22 I
906	*Tadbīr-e maʾkūl va-mashrūb*	47 : 25 IX, et seqq.
[before 907]	*Resālä-ye Sohailīyä*	45 : 98
907	*Kholāṣato t-tajāreb*	46 : 23
913	*Favāyed-e akhyār*	47, 54 : 25 VIII, 24 IV, et seqq.
[before 917]	*ʿElājo l-amrāż*	60 : 60 IV
917	*Jāmeʿo l-favāyed*	47, 61 : 25 VI, 24 I, et seqq.
[before 937]	*Qaṣīdä dar ḥefẓ-e ṣeḥḥat*	47, 75 : 25 II, 26 III, et seq.
942	*Dalāyelo n-nabż*	77 : 24 II, et seqq.
942	*Dalāyelo l-bowl*	80 : 24 III, et seqq.
944	*Settä-ye żarūrīyä*	47, 84 : 25 VII, 29 IV, et seq.
[before 946]	*Qaṣīdä dar loghāt-e Hendī*	47 : 25 III
[before 946]	*Qaṣīdä dar asmāʾ-e ajnās-e advīä*	47 : 25 IV
[944? or 954?]	[*Resālä dar bīkh-e čīnī*]	87 : 22 II
[959?]	*Favāyed-e saʿdīyä*	86 : 57 III
[before 963]	[*Qarābāzīn*]	88 : 105 II, et seqq.
[before 974]	[*Resālä dar teryāq-e kabīr*]	105 : 88
977	[*Resālä-ye āteshak*]	99 : 46 II, et seqq.
977	*Toḥfä-ye Khānīyä*	106 : 82
979	[*Resālä-ye čūb-e čīnī*]	107 : 83
[ca. 970-80]	[*Dar taḥqīq-e mofarreḥāt-e yāqūtī*]	102 : 46 III
[ca. 970-80]	[*Resālä-ye bīkh-e čīnī*]	104 : 87 II
[before 990]	[*Resālä-ye ḥejāmä*]	103 : 46 V
[before 1015]	*Mofradāt-e ṣaḥīḥ*	108 : 86 V
1038	*Alfāẓ-e advīä*	110 : 105 I
[before 1046]	*Dastūro l-Honūd*	109 : 105 III
[before ca. 1050]	*Ṭibb al-aʾimma*	111 : Ar. 110
[before 1059]	[*Ṭalab-e qovvat-e bāh*]	112 : 26 IV
[before 1075]	[*Resālä dar čūb-e čīnī va-qahvä va-čāy*]	113 : 46 VII, et seq.
1082	*Roʾūso l-masāʾel*	125 : 50
1087	[*Resālä-ye ḥefẓ-e ṣeḥḥat*]	126 : 47

A.H.	Title of Work	No. : MS
1089	*Tohfä-ye Solaimānī*	123 : 48
[1080? or 1090?]	*Tohfato l-mo'menīn*	115 : 115, et seqq.
1096	*'Aino l-hayāt*	124 : 49
[ca. 1100]	*Kherqä*	127 : 73 II
[ca. 1100]	*Hadīqato l-hayāt*	128 : 51
1112	*Tebbo l-Akbar*	131 : 122
[before 1115]	*Sāleho l-'elāj*	129 : 55
[before 1126]	*Mofarreho l-qolūb*	132 : 123
[before 1126]	*Mīzāno t-tebb*	133 : 124 I
1126–1130	*Qarābāzīn-e Qāderī*	130 : 125
1141	*Zādo l-mosāferīn*	134 : 56 I, et seqq.
[after 1141]	*Meftāho sh-shefā'*	138 : 59 I, et seq.
[after 1185]	*Makhzano l-advīä va-tazkerä-ye ūlī n-nohā*	140 : 89
1215	*Badāye'o l-fonūn*	141 : 104
1216	*Kholāsat-e qavānīno l-'elāj*	142 : 124 II
[before 1249]	*Tazkerato l-'elāj*	143 : 63
[before 1249]	*Morakkabāt-e jowharīyä*	144 : Ar. 96 I, et seq.
[before 1250]	[*Tarjamä-ye Bor'o s-sā'ä*]	147 : 57 II
1252	*Kīmīā'o sh-shefā*	146 : 65
[before 1285]	*Badāye'o l-hekmato n-Nāserī*	149 : Ar. 53 III
[second half of 13th century]	*Majma'o t-tajāreb*	148 : 61 III

Chronological List of Manuscript Dates

A.H.	No. : MS
[ca. 600]	9 : 8
[before 700]	13 : 6
[ca. 850]	8 : Ar. 73 V
Rajab 907	20 : 36
[before 5 Zū l-qaᶜdä 913]	21 : 37
28 Zū l-qaᶜdä 922	22 : 38
last third of Ṣafar 940	66 : 30
27 Shavvāl 956	5 : 4
Shaᶜbān 963	61 : 24 I
[ca. 965]	61 : 24 II-VI
Ramażān 981	62 : 26 X
992	105 : 88
11 Jomādā I 996	15 : 84
Shavvāl 999	62 : 26 I-VII, XI
[10th century]	1 : 74
[10th century]	61 : 24 VII-VIII
[ca. 1000]	44 : 22 I
[ca. 1000]	87 : 22 II
[ca. 1000]	157 : Ar. 60 II, IV
[ca. 1000]	181 : 75
2 Zū l-ḥejjä 1021	43 : 77
[before 1042]	100 : Ar. 41
6 Rabīᶜ I 1046	23 : 38a
29 Jomādā II 1053	67 : 31
28 Shaᶜbān 1058	6 : 5
16 Moḥarram 1062	46 : 23
1069	110 : 105 II
4 Rabīᶜ II 1074	89 : 106
15 Rajab 1078	4 : 3
Ṣafar 1081-Moḥarram 1082	99 : 46
11 Rajab 1082	125 : 50
24 Jomādā II 1084	161 : 18
[before 1088]	91 : 108
Shavvāl 1094	168 : 73 IV
19 Zū l-ḥejjä 1096	32 : 12
[11th century]	11 : 9
[11th century]	24 : 39
[11th century]	31 : 45
[11th century]	42 : 21
[11th century]	58 : 35
[11th century]	94 : 111
[ca. 1100]	3 : 2
[ca. 1100]	12 : 10
[ca. 1100]	36 : 16
[ca. 1100]	68 : 32

A.H.	No. : MS
[ca. 1100]	114 : 87
[ca. 1100]	124 : 49
[ca. 1100]	126 : 47
[ca. 1100]	163 : 95
[ca. 1100]	177 : 60
[ca. 1100]	182 : 76
[ca. 1100]	220 : 96
21 Rabīᶜ II 1103	177 : 60 II
30 Rajab 1105	116 : 116
1115	129 : 55
[before 1117]	35 : 15
Ṣafar 1117	27 : 42
28 Rajab 1122	175 : 52
[between 1094 and 1123]	168 : 73 I, III
9 Rabīᶜ II 1123	168 : 73 II
Ṣafar 1126	92 : 109
4 Shaᶜbān 1128	38 : 17
13 Jomādā I 1130	110 : 105 III
[before last third of Jomādā II 1130]	120 : 120 IV
17 Rajab 1130	110 : 105 I
1130	111 : Ar. 110
19 Moḥarram 1136	63 : 27 I
25 Moḥarram 1136	63 : 27 II-III
8 Jomādā II 1136	164 : 54 I
[ca. 1140]	164 : 54 II
[first half of 12th century]	123 : 48
[before 1165]	176 : 92
9 Jomādā I 1170	14 : 11
20 Moḥarram 1181	25 : 40
[before 1187]	28 : 43
[before 23 Shavvāl 1196]	131 : 122
[12th century]	18 : 20a
[12th century]	45 : 98
[12th century]	90 : 107
[12th century]	95 : 112
[12th century]	96 : 113
[12th century]	97 : 114
[12th century]	118 : 118
[12th century]	128 : 51
[12th century]	162 : 19
[12th century]	169 : 85
[ca. 1200]	37 : 16a
[ca. 1200]	64 : 28
[ca. 1200]	85 : Ar. 98 VIII-XIII
[ca. 1200]	117 : 117
[ca. 1200]	119 : 119
[ca. 1200]	132 : 123

A.H.	No. : MS
[ca. 1200]	171 : 99
[ca. 1200]	186 : 78
[ca. 1200]	187 : 86
15 Jomādā II 1203	130 : 125
3 Shaʿbān 1210	33 : 13
15 Rabīʿ I 1215	141 : 104
14 Rabīʿ II 1216	133 : 124 III
1 Jomādā I 1216	133 : 124 II
16 Jomādā II 1216	133 : 124 I
[1216]	133 : 124 IV
23 Jomādā II 1230	174 : 53
[before 2 Zū l-qaʿdä 1230]	26 : 41
Rabīʿ I-II 1233	79 : 29
1233	120 : 120 I-III
17 Rabīʿ I 1235	36 : Ar. 102 IV
8 Shaʿbān 1235	69 : 33
6 Jomādā II 1236	17 : 20
Jomādā I 1240	150 : 80
1240	150 : 62
1240	150 : 81-83
7 Ramażān 1242	47 : 25
1244	34 : 14
[before 1246]	214 : 91
20 Zū l-qaʿdä 1247–6 Moḥarram 1248	122 : 121
[first half of 13th century]	140 : 89
25 Rabīʿ I 1252	146 : 65
8 Jomādā II 1254	153 : 64
6 Zū l-ḥejjä 1257	144 : Ar. 96 IV
6 Jomādā I 1258	137 : 7 I
1259	137 : 7 II
Ramażān 1261	135 : 58
5 Shavvāl 1261	134 : 56
7 Jomādā II 1263	194 : 66 I
[1263]	194 : 66 II
4 Rabīʿ I 1264	194 : 66 III
4 Moḥarram 1265	194 : 66 IV
1 Zū l-qaʿdä 1265	138 : 59 I
1265	138 : 59 II
1273	115 : 115
7 Zū l-qaʿdä 1274	70 : 34
Jomādā II 1275	136 : 57 I-II
[Jomādā II 1275]	136 : 57 III
3 Jomādā I 1276	189 : 72 I
Moḥarram 1280	44 : 22 I
1 Moḥarram 1282	2 : 1
17 Ramażān 1287	184 : 68 I
1289	218 : 70
28 Zū l-ḥejjä 1293	221 : Ar. 53 II-III
6 Jomādā I 1297	184 : 68 II
[second half of 13th century]	41 : 61
[second half of 13th century]	139 : 59a
[second half of 13th century]	143 : 63
[second half of 13th century]	144 : Ar. 96 I-III, V-VIII
[second half of 13th century]	219 : 71
[13th century]	30 : 44
[13th century]	74 : 93
[13th century]	93 : 110
[13th century]	152 : 103
[13th century]	156 : 67
[13th century]	170 : 94
[13th century]	184 : 68 III-VII
[13th century]	202 : 102
[13th century]	211 : 101
[ca. 1300]	222 : 69

List of Manuscript Parts Not Catalogued

MS	No.	*See page*
9 I	11	16
11 II	14	20
24 VI	61	77
25 I, V, X	47	65
26 VIII–IX	62	78
27 IV	63	79
29 VII	79	90
38a II	23	36
46 I, IV, VI, VIII	99	104
54 V–VII	164	191
58 V	134	155
60 I	177	210
67 I–III	156	182
68 V–VII	184	221
72 II–IV	189	226
73 V	168	195
77 I–IV, VI	43	58
78 II	186	224
86 I	187	224
87 III	114	126
93 I, III, V, VI	74	86
117 except last part	117	133
Ar. 41 I	100	108
Ar. 53 except II–III	149	176
Ar. 60, I, III	157	183
Ar. 73 except V	8	14
Ar. 96 III–V	144	167
Ar. 98 I–VIII, XIII	85	94
Ar. 102 I–III	39	52
Ar. 110 except preface	111	122

Concordance 1
Entry number : Library number

1	74 I	46	23	91	108	136	57 I	181	75
2	1	47	25	92	109	137	7 I	182	76
3	2	48	24 V	93	110	138	59 I	183	78 III
4	3	49	26 II	94	111	139	59a	184	68 I
5	4	50	27 III	95	112	140	89	185	Ar. 96 VI
6	5	51	28 III	96	113	141	104	186	78 I
7	Ar. 60 IV	52	29 VI	97	114	142	124 II	187	86 II
8	Ar. 73 V	53	Ar. 98 XII	98	85 II	143	63	188	26 X
9	8	54	24 IV	99	46 II	144	Ar. 96 I	189	72 I
10	7 II	55	27 II	100	Ar. 41 II	145	Ar. 96 II	190	54 II
11	9 II	56	28 II	101	Ar. 96 VII	146	65	191	9 III
12	10	57	29 V	102	46 III	147	57 II	192	25 XI
13	6	58	35	103	46 V	148	61 III	193	60 V
14	11	59	Ar. 98 XI	104	87 II	149	Ar. 53 III	194	66 I
15	84	60	60 IV	105	88	150	62	195	80
16	61 II	61	24 I	106	82	151	29 X	196	81
17	20	62	26 I	107	83	152	103	197	73 IV
18	20a	63	27 I	108	86 V	153	64	198	58 III
19	56 II	64	28 I	109	105 III	154	74 II	199	58 II
20	36	65	29 III	110	105 I	155	124 III	200	54 IV
21	37	66	30 I	111	Ar. 110	156	67 IV	201	54 III
22	38	67	31	112	26 IV	157	Ar. 60 II	202	102
23	38a	68	32	113	46 VII	158	120 III	203	73 III
24	39	69	33	114	87 I	159	124 IV	204	120 II
25	40	70	34	115	115	160	26 XI	205	86 III
26	41	71	59 II	116	116	161	18	206	100
27	42	72	66 IV	117	117	162	19	207	24 VII
28	43	73	78 IV	118	118	163	95	208	28 V
29	30 II	74	93 II	119	119	164	54 I	209	29 IX
30	44	75	26 III	120	120 I	165	66 II	210	68 III
31	45	76	28 IV	121	120 IV	166	66 III	211	101
32	12	77	24 II	122	121	167	68 IV	212	58 IV
33	13	78	26 VI	123	48	168	73 I	213	58 VIII
34	14	79	29 I	124	49	169	85 I	214	91
35	15	80	24 III	125	50	170	94	215	26 V
36	16	81	26 VII	126	47	171	99	216	68 II
37	16a	82	29 II	127	73 II	172	93 IV	217	Ar. 96 VIII
38	17	83	Ar. 98 X	128	51	173	29 VIII	218	70
39	Ar. 102 IV	84	29 IV	129	55	174	53	219	71
40	24 VIII	85	Ar. 98 IX	130	125	175	52	220	96
41	61 I	86	57 III	131	122	176	92	221	Ar. 53 II
42	21	87	22 II	132	123	177	60 II	222	69
43	77 V	88	105 II	133	124 I	178	60 III		
44	22 I	89	106	134	56 I	179	58 VII		
45	98	90	107	135	58 I	180	86 IV		

Concordance 2
Library Number : Entry number

Library Number	Entry number
1	2
2	3
3	4
4	5
5	6
6	13
7 I	137
7 II	10
8	9
9 II	11
9 III	191
10	12
11	14
12	32
13	33
14	34
15	35
16	36
16a	37
17	38
18	161
19	162
20	17
20a	18
21	42
22 I	44
22 II	87
23	46
24 I	61
24 II	77
24 III	80
24 IV	54
24 V	48
24 VII	207
24 VIII	40
25	47
25 XI	192
26 I	62
26 II	49
26 III	75
26 IV	112
26 V	215
26 VI	78
26 VII	81
26 X	188
26 XI	160
27 I	63
27 II	55
27 III	50
28 I	64
28 II	56
28 III	51
28 IV	76
28 V	208
29 I	79
29 II	82
29 III	65
29 IV	84
29 V	57
29 VI	52
29 VIII	173
29 IX	209
29 X	151
30 I	66
30 II	29
31	67
32	68
33	69
34	70
35	58
36	20
37	21
38	22
38a	23
39	24
40	25
41	26
42	27
43	28
44	30
45	31
46 II	99
46 III	102
46 V	103
46 VII	113
47	126
48	123
49	124
50	125
51	128
52	175
53	174
54 I	164
54 II	190
54 III	201
54 IV	200
55	129
56 I	134
56 II	19
57 I	136
57 II	147
57 III	86
58 I	135
58 II	199
58 III	198
58 IV	212
58 VII	179
58 VIII	213
59 I	138
59 II	71
59a	139
60 II	177
60 III	178
60 IV	60
60 V	193
61 I	41
61 II	16
61 III	148
62	150
63	143
64	153
65	146
66 I	194
66 II	165
66 III	166
66 IV	72
67 IV	156
68 I	184
68 II	216
68 III	210
68 IV	167
69	222
70	218
71	219
72 I	189
73 I	168
73 II	127
73 III	203
73 IV	197
74 I	1
74 II	154
75	181
76	182
77 V	43
78 I	186
78 III	183
78 IV	73
80	195
81	196
82	106
83	107
84	15
85 I	169
85 II	98
86 II	187
86 III	205
86 IV	180
86 V	108
87 I	114
87 II	104
88	105
89	140
91	214
92	176
93 II	74
93 IV	172
94	170
95	163
96	220
98	45
99	171
100	206
101	211
102	202
103	152
104	141
105 I	110
105 II	88
105 III	109
106	89
107	90
108	91
109	92
110	93
111	94
112	95
113	96
114	97
115	115
116	116
117	117
118	118
119	119
120 I	120
120 II	204
120 III	158
120 IV	121
121	122
122	131
123	132
124 I	133
124 II	142
124 III	155
124 IV	159
125	130
Ar. 41 II	100
Ar. 53 II	221
Ar. 53 III	149
Ar. 60 II	157
Ar. 60 IV	7
Ar. 73 V	8
Ar. 96 I	144
Ar. 96 II	145
Ar. 96 VI	185
Ar. 96 VII	101
Ar. 96 VIII	217
Ar. 98 IX	85
Ar. 98 X	83
Ar. 98 XI	59
Ar. 98 XII	53
Ar. 102 IV	39
Ar. 110	111

Typesetting and Preparation of Camera-ready Copy by
Freedmen's Organization
Los Angeles, California

Publications of the UCLA Center for Medieval and Renaissance Studies

HUMANA CIVILITAS Series (Undena Publications)

1. **On Pre-Modern Technology and Science: Studies in Honor of Lynn White, jr.** Bert S. Hall and Delno C. West, editors. 1976, 233 pages.
2. **The King's Progress to Jerusalem: Some Interpretations of David during the Reformation Period and Their Patristic and Medieval Background,** by Edward A. Gosselin. 1976. 131 pages.
3. **The Politics of an Erasmian Lawyer, Vasco de Quiroga,** by Ross Dealy. 1976, 33 pages.
4. **Persian Medical Manuscripts at the University of California, Los Angeles: A Descriptive Catalogue,** by Lutz Richter-Bernburg. 1978, xxii + 297 pages.

CONTRIBUTIONS Series (University of California Press)

1. **Medieval Secular Literature.** William Matthews, editor. 1965, 89 pages.
2. **Galileo Reappraised.** Carlo L. Golino, editor. 1966, 110 pages.
3. **The Transformation of the Roman World—Gibbon's Problem after Two Centuries.** Lynn White, jr., editor. 1966, 321 pages, hard cover and paperback.
4. **Scientific Methods in Medieval Archaeology.** Rainer Berger, editor. 1970, 459 pages.
5. **Violence and Civil Disorder in Italian Cities, 1200–1500.** Lauro Martines, editor. 1972, 353 pages.
6. **The Darker Vision of the Renaissance.** Robert S. Kinsman, editor. 1974, 352 pages.
7. **The Copernican Achievement.** Robert S. Westman, editor. 1975, 380 pages.
8. **First Images of America: The Impact of the New World on the Old.** Fredi Chiappelli, editor; Michael J. B. Allen and Robert L. Benson, co-editors. 1976, 2 vols., 957 pages.
9. **Friedrich Diez Centennial Lectures** (Supplement to *Romance Philology*, vol. XXX, 2). Edward F. Tuttle, editor. 1976, 30 pages.

PUBLICATIONS Series (University of California Press)

1. **Dissent and Reform in the Early Middle Ages,** by Jeffrey Burton Russell. 1965, 325 pages.
2. **Leonardo's Legacy: An International Symposium.** C. D. O'Malley, editor. 1969, 255 pages.
3. **Guide to Serial Bibliographies in Medieval Studies,** by Richard H. Rouse. 1969, 150 pages.
4. **The Decline of Medieval Hellenism in Asia Minor and the Process of Islamization from the Eleventh through the Fifteenth Century,** by Speros Vryonis, Jr. 1971, 532 pages.
5. **Christian Political Theory and Church Politics in the Mid-Twelfth Century,** by Stanley Chodorow. 1972, 300 pages.
6. **The Song of Roland: Formulaic Style and Poetic Craft,** by Joseph J. Duggan. 1973, 226 pages.
7. **Studies in Medieval Philosophy, Science, and Logic: Collected Papers, 1933–1969,** by Ernest A. Moody. 1975, 453 pages.
8. **Slavery and Serfdom in the Middle Ages,** selected essays by Marc Bloch. 1975, 276 pages.
9. **Marsilio Ficino: The *Philebus* Commentary, A Critical Edition and Translation,** by Michael J. B. Allen. 1975, 560 pages.
10. **Marius: *On the Elements*, A Critical Edition and Translation,** by Richard C. Dales. 1976, 206 pages.
11. **An Italian Lordship: The Bishopric of Lucca in the Late Middle Ages,** by Duane J. Osheim. 1977, 211 pages.
12. **Pope Alexander III and the Council of Tours (1163),** by Robert Somerville. 1977, 110 pages.

INDEPENDENT Publications

1. **Leonardo da Vinci: Studies for a Nativity and the "Mona Lisa Cartoon" with drawings after Leonardo from the Elmer Belt Library of Vinciana,** by Carlo Pedretti. 1973. 49 pages.
2. **In Honor of the Eightieth Birthday of Dr. Elmer Belt, Physician, Scholar and One Who Loves Nature,** by William A. Emboden, Jr. 1973. 20 pages, out of print.
3. **Boccaccio: Secoli di vita** (Proceedings of the International Symposium on Boccaccio, 1975). Marga Cottino-Jones and Edward F. Tuttle, editors. 1977. 310 pages (Angelo Longo Editore).
4. **Medieval and Renaissance Manuscripts at the University of California, Los Angeles: Preliminary Descriptions,** by Mirella Ferrari. 1978. 376 pages.

IN PREPARATION

1. Essays in Medieval Religion and Technology, by Lynn White, jr.
2. Anglo-Saxon Poetry: Conference Proceedings (1977). Daniel Calder, editor.
3. The Dawn of Banking: Conference Proceedings (1977).

JOURNALS

Viator: Medieval and Renaissance Studies (annually since 1970; University of California Press) is a hard-cover journal which averages 350–450 pages; its primary, but not exclusive, focus is intercultural and interdisciplinary research. *Viator* does not include reviews or current news.

Comitatus (annually since 1970, sponsored by the Center since 1973; Undena Publications) contains articles in the field of Medieval and Renaissance studies by University of California graduate students.